# Community Care in Practice

## Services for the Continuing Care Client

Edited by

ANTHONY LAVENDER

*Department of Clinical Psychology*
*Maidstone*

and

FRANK HOLLOWAY

*Kings College Hospital*
*London*

**JOHN WILEY & SONS**

Chichester · New York · Brisbane · Toronto · Singapore

*Library of Congress Cataloging in Publication Data:*

Community care in practice: services for the continuing care client/
  edited by Anthony Lavender and Frank Holloway.
        p.      cm.—(The Wiley series in clinical psychology.)
    ISBN 0 471 91294 8 (cloth)      ISBN 0 471 92040 1 (paper)
    1. Community mental health services—Great Britain.      I. Lavender,
Anthony.      II. Holloway, Frank.      III. Series.
    [DNLM: 1. Community Mental Health Services—Great Britain.
2. Long Term Care—Great Britain.      WM 30 C7275]
RA790.7.G7C66 1988
362.2'0425—dc19
DNLM/DLC
for Library of Congress                                                              88-10749
                                                                                         CIP


*British Library Cataloguing in Publication Data:*

Community care in practice service for the
  continuing care client. —(The Wiley
  series in clinical psychology).
  1. Great Britain. Mentally disordered
  persons. Community care
  I. Lavender, Anthony      II. Holloway, Frank
  362.2'1

  ISBN 0 471 91294 8 (cloth)
  ISBN 0 471 92040 1 (paper)


Typeset by Acorn Bookwork, Salisbury, Wiltshire
Printed and bound in Great Britain by Anchor Brendon Ltd, Tiptree, Essex

# Contents

vi

# List of Contributors

PETER BATES — Social Worker, Nottingham Rehabilitation and Community Care Services, 114 Thorneywood Mount, Nottingham NG3 2PZ

TRAOLACH SEAN BRUGHA — Senior Lecturer in Psychiatry, University of Leicester, CSB Leicester Royal Infirmary, PO Box 65, Leicester LE2 7LX

PAUL CLIFFORD — Principal Clinical Psychologist, Programme Coordinator (Rehabilitation and Resettlement), National Unit for Psychiatric Research and Development, Lewisham Hospital, Lewisham High Street, London SE13 6LH

PHILIPPA GARETY — Lecturer in Psychology, Institute of Psychiatry, Decrespigny Park, Camberwell, London SE5 8AF

FRANK HOLLOWAY — Consultant Community Psychiatrist, Department of Psychological Medicine, Kings College Hospital, Camberwell, London SE5 8AF

JOHN HOWAT — Consultant Psychiatrist, Clinical Services Director, Nottingham Rehabilitation and Community Care Services, 114 Thorneywood Mount, Nottingham NG3 2PZ

SU KINGSLEY — Service Manager—Mental Health, St Ann's Hospital, St Ann's Road, London N15 2TH

ANTHONY LAVENDER — Principal Clinical Psychologist, Department of Clinical Psychology, Red House, Oakapple Lane, Maidstone ME16 9NW

BRIGID MACCARTHY — Scientific Officer, MRC Social Psychiatry Research Unit, Institute of Psychiatry, Decrespigny Park, Camberwell, London SE5 8AF

JOHN MAHONEY — Service Manager—Merton Services, Springfield Hospital, 61 Glenburnie Road, London W2 4HS

STEEN P. MANGEN — Lecturer in European Social Policy, The London School of Economics, Houghton Street, London WC2 2AE

JOE PIDGEON — Social Worker, Nottingham Rehabilitation and Community Care Services, 114 Thorneywood Mount, Nottingham NG3 2PZ

STEPHEN PILLING — Principal Psychologist, Islington Health Authority, Whittington Hospital, Highgate Hill, London N19

SHULAMIT RAMON — Lecturer in Social Work and Course Convenor, Social Work Studies, The London School of Economics, Houghton Street, London WC2 2AE

GEOFF SHEPHERD — Top Grade Clinical Psychologist, Psychology Department, Fulbourn Hospital, Cambridge CB1 5EF

GILLIAN SHEPPERSON — Social Work Team Leader, Community Support Team—Mental Health, 55 Vicar Lane, Chesterfield, Derbyshire

ANTHEA SPERLINGER — Top Grade Clinical Psychologist, Psychology Department, Goldie Leigh, Lodge Hill, Abbey Wood, London SE2 0AY

DAVID TOWELL — Fellow in Mental Health Policy and Development, Kings Fund College, 2 Palace Court, London W2 4HS

TONY WAINWRIGHT — Principal Clinical Psychologist, Camberwell Resettlement Team, St. Giles Hospital, St. Giles Road, Camberwell, London, SE5 7RN

# Series Editor's Preface

Though this book appears in the Wiley Series in Clinical Psychology, the issues that it deals with confront all mental health workers whatever their background. In recent years, increasing attempts have been made to provide mental health services as far as possible in the 'community' rather than in mental hospitals. The reasons for this movement are complex. In part, it was a reaction against the high financial cost but poor quality of many traditional hospital services. However, there has also been a good deal of optimism about the potential of good community based services.

It is now clear that it is no simple matter to organize good community services. At their worst, they can simply transplant to a new setting the unattractive features of hospital services. They are also not cheap. This has left responsible mental health professionals to grapple with the complex and difficult problem of creating good community services within the constraints of limited resources.

The creation of such services requires a broad range of professional skills and resources, and it is hard to imagine that any single person would have had the breadth of perspective to deal with it adequately. This book successfully integrates the variety of approaches that the topic requires. Indeed, it sets new standards in work on community care in its comprehensive scope and breadth of perspective.

After an introduction to the issues as they have arisen, both in Great Britain and elsewhere, the book is divided into three main sections. The first concerns policy issues and objectives, such as the constraints of financial resources and trained staff within which service planning has to work. Next, the various components of community provision are considered, such as day care, residential facilities, work and the family. Finally, case studies are presented of particular community care projects that have important general implications.

Community care is now being planned on a big scale, but too often it is attempted with little apparent understanding of the principles involved. This thoughtful and comprehensive book is timely and meets a real need.

FRASER WATTS
*Series Editor*

# Section A

# *Introduction*

Community Care in Practice
Edited by A. Lavender and F. Holloway
© 1988 John Wiley & Sons Ltd

# Chapter 1

# Introduction

## ANTHONY LAVENDER and FRANK HOLLOWAY

This book is concerned with the issues and practical struggles involved in establishing community-based services for people with severe and long-term mental health problems. In order to achieve this we have included a historical and international overview, an examination of the major issues relating to service planning, an analysis of the components of a community-based service and finally some critical accounts of services in the making. The aim is both to stimulate thought about the provision of these services and to help ensure that the new services are an improvement on those they are replacing. The contributors have been chosen not on the basis of a single ideology but rather to reflect the current thinking and practice involved in providing community-based care. The common link is that all have been concerned that the movement towards providing care in the community will result in an improvement in the quality of services offered to consumers.

The movement to establish community care is not new. During the past four decades hospital staff have been discharging people energetically from the large mental hospitals. However in the latter half of the 1970s and 1980s the movement to provide community-based services has received fresh impetus from the attempt of government and regional health authorities to close these hospitals. This impetus is due both to a genuine desire to improve the quality of the service and an equally genuine desire that the replacement services should be cheaper. Given these mixed motives the will to actually provide community care is fragile, especially when it begins to become clear that the new services are likely to be more expensive, and restrictions on public expenditure becomes a matter of government strategy. A similar point has already been eloquently made by Jones and Fowles (1984) in the prologue to *Ideas on Institutions*. If a collapse in this impetus is to be avoided it is a matter of urgency that we demonstrate that the new services offer a significant improvement in the quality of care for the long-term client.

3

Before proceeding further it is important to describe the people with long-term mental health problems. This term immediately raises the problem of labelling, and whether it or any other label is appropriate for this client group. The reader will probably be familiar with the linguistic contortions many well-intentioned staff find themselves performing, when trying to choose a label that does not devalue the clients. A sample of some of these labels is as follows: lunatics, inmates, mad, mental patients, chronics, burnt-out schizophrenics, chronic schizophrenics, chronically mentally ill, old long-stay, new long-sta ʒ, new long-term.

The issue is an important one because it is in essence concerned with the nature of the individual's primary difficulty. This primary difficulty is clearly important to face, and as far as possible to understand, in order that appropriate help can be provided. However, from the list above it will be evident that the label sometimes attached to this client group often both obscures the nature of the difficulty and has serious consequences in terms of devaluing that individual. The question then raised is what is an appropriate name; that is, one which will not devalue the people but will provide some indication of the problem and thereby enable funds to be identified to meet the needs of the group. It is perhaps useful to start such a search with an inquiry into the nature of the primary difficulty.

The primary difficulty usually involves an inner experience of a particularly disturbing nature. This can include: (1) a strong feeling that people with whom you come in contact are against you and are plotting, sometimes with elaborate means, to attack or keep you under surveillance; (2) a distressing experience, such as hearing arguing voices or seeing images that nobody else can see or hear; (3) a strong belief in an idea or an explanation about events in your life that others neither believe nor understand; (4) a feeling of great despair out of which it seems impossible to break; (5) a feeling of the greatest optimism and belief in yourself that seems to others completely unjustified by your circumstances and that seems to be often followed by deep despair; (6) a feeling of severe isolation from other human beings where any contact becomes a painful experience to be avoided. These are just some examples of the kinds of experiences from which people referred to in this book are likely to suffer for long periods during their lives. From a sufferer's point of view the experience is that of a disturbance of the emotions that affects both thinking and action.

These experiences have, within the medical tradition, been defined as symptoms, and certain patterns of these symptoms have been identified to which particular diagnostic labels have been attached. For example, the experiences described in (2), that is hearing two voices arguing when there is no tangible source, is likely to result in the person being diagnosed as suffering from schizophrenia. Thus an individual coming into contact with psychiatric services receives a particular label because they describe a particular pattern of experiences that has been labelled, in this example, schizophrenia.

There are, however, a number of problems with the use of diagnosis. Firstly, in everyday clinical practice the diagnostic labels can easily come to be applied sloppily. Secondly, the experiences to which the diagnostic labels are applied are so unique to each individual that the use of diagnosis can obscure important differences. Thirdly, the stigma attached to the diagnosis has serious consequences on individuals' lives both in terms of their own and others' expectations. (It is, however, worth pointing out that many of these people have suffered from the stigma associated with being odd or eccentric before coming into contact with psychiatric services.) This can result in people, particularly professionals, acting in a uniform way that disregards their individuality. Some would argue that the diagnostic process is useful in terms of the prescription of certain treatments, such as medication, that have general effects on a range of disturbing experiences and in prescribing a prognosis to a condition.

At present there are many theories about the origins of these primary disturbances involving genetic, chemical, psychological and social explanations. Although there is good evidence for all these having some explanatory value none can be said definitively to be the sole cause, in spite of the strength of people's personal beliefs in a particular theory. Disputes about the origins of these experiences are often a reflection of the power battles between different professional groups rather than arguments based on 'real' evidence. In the midst of all this are usually the clients or patients, trying to make sense of their own and the professionals' behaviour. Unfortunately simple answers cannot truthfully be given.

People suffering with the disturbing experiences previously described frequently have other and often related problems which interfere with their ability to live 'ordinary' lives in the community. Indeed it is often these related problems that determine whether people require the help of statutory services. These related problems may include inability to hold down a job, difficulty maintaining stable relationships or lack of the basic skills necessary for everyday living. Additionally the treatments that clients have received often lead to other problems, such as the 'side' effects of medication and/or the effects of spending years segregated from other members of the community in a psychiatric hospital. Thus individuals with these disturbing experiences often have a series of other interrelated problems for which they require help. It is perhaps worth adding that people without the disturbing experiences described, but with many of the related problems, are also often supported within the services described in this book.

Having examined the experiences of the people with whom this book is concerned, and how these experiences have resulted in the application of certain labels, we return full circle to the issue of whether there is a more appropriate label. Whatever is decided, it is clear that many of the people who have these experiences require help over long periods. For this reason the term 'continuing care clients' has been used, because this describes the care that is needed without attempting to provide a summary label that aspires to describe the individual's experience. There are problems with this term, especially its vagueness, but for the present this suits our purposes. This term has not been forced on the contributors; indeed they have been encouraged to use their own terms. This policy has been adopted so that the chapters reflect 'actual' practice. Readers should consider the issues raised here about the use of client labels as they progress through the book.

The purpose of this book is to examine how community services are being, and might be, created to meet the needs of this continuing care client group. The rationale for the organization of the book is self-evident. This introduction is simply intended to give a brief indication of the experiences and problems this group of people face, and which community-based services must address.

The book has been organized into four sections. The first, 'Introduction', includes a chapter by Shulamit Ramon in which she traces the history of community care in Britain, with particular reference to the political, financial and professional influences on this movement. Clearly an awareness of the history of community care, particularly the mistakes of the past, holds out the possibility that these mistakes can be avoided in the future. In addition to the historical perspective it is important to be aware of what has been tried in other countries, and in Chapter Three Steen Mangen provides an analysis of community care movements internationally, with special reference to Italy and the United States of America. This chapter is an attempt to avoid the tendency of people involved in the development of community-based services to become insular and fail to learn from the experiences of other nations.

The second section provides an analysis of the major issues in service development. Su Kingsley and David Towell in Chapter Four provide an introduction to the complex tasks and issues which need to be tackled within both the existing services engaged in the process of transition and the new community-based alternatives that are being developed. Of major importance to this process is the funding of the new services. In Chapter Five John Mahoney provides a description and critical analysis of the major sources of funding. The need to evaluate newly established services is often only contemplated after they have been established. This is clearly problematic and many valuable opportunities are missed. For this reason Geoff Shepherd's chapter on evaluation has been included at an early stage in the book. In this chapter he outlines the major methods and measures that are likely to prove useful in evaluating, and therefore developing, community services. The final chapter in the second section concerns staff training. Here Tony Lavender and Anthea Sperlinger examine the current needs for staff training, and explore how a training model can be built into existing and new services. It is evident that unless such training strategies are adopted the new services will quickly become as stale and institutionalized as many of the services they are replacing.

The third section explores the components of a community-based service. All people in the community require housing and Philippa Garety in Chapter Eight examines the options currently available for continuing care clients. Day care is to a large extent the core of a community-based service, and for this reason has been given extra space within the book. Thus in Chapter Nine Frank Holloway provides an analysis of current day care provision and a synthesis of the roles that these services need to adopt in a comprehensive community-based service. In Chapter Ten Stephen Pilling explores the concept of work and its relevance for people with long-term mental health problems. In addition he discusses critically a number of employment schemes, and makes some suggestions about future developments. The ability of staff to support the families and friends of clients is clearly vital to the success of community-based services. In the last chapter in this section Brigid MacCarthy critically discusses what is involved in providing that support.

The fourth section of the book is concerned with providing some working examples of community care in action. These examples are not chosen because they provide blueprints for others to follow, but because the analysis presented within each chapter is likely to have relevance for many involved in established and developing services. In Chapter Twelve Tony Wainwright, Frank Holloway and Traolach Brugha provide a description of the day care services within an inner-city area and evaluate that service from the perspectives of both Health Services Research and Normalization. Paul Clifford follows this with an analysis from a psychoanalytic perspective of the move of a hospital/ward-based group of staff and patients into a house in the community. The final chapter in the section, by John Howat and his colleagues, includes a description and analysis of the services being developed in Nottingham. Of particular importance in this process have been the attempts to help place continuing care clients with 'ordinary families', and for the services to gain some monitoring and control over the private sector.

Overall the purpose of the book is not to provide a series of blueprints for the provision of community-based services for continuing care clients. Rather it is to help those involved in developing, or in positions to influence the development of, continuing care services to think through the issues more thoroughly and to discover more creative and constructive solutions for consumers.

## REFERENCE

Jones, K., and Fowles, A. J. (1984). *Ideas on Institutions*, Routledge & Kegan Paul, London.

Community Care in Practice
Edited by A. Lavender and F. Holloway
© 1988 John Wiley & Sons Ltd

Chapter 2

# Community Care in Britain

## SHULAMIT RAMON

'Community Care' has been with us as a slogan and a guideline for policy for more than a quarter of a century. In this chapter an attempt will be made to trace and understand the meanings attributed to the term, and its significance in shaping British policy and practice with the continuing care client. In investigating these themes attention will be given to the views and activities of professionals, politicians, voluntary organizations, direct and indirect users of the psychiatric services and the media.

The continuing debate in the social sciences literature highlights how problematical 'community care' and 'community' are as concepts (Abrams, 1977). A community usually implies more than a physical neighbourhood; it focuses on collective membership limited by geographical proximity, the sharing of local social institutions and an interest in ensuring the well-being of the collective and its individual members. Community care is therefore concerned with the means by which the well-being of vulnerable groups in the locality is ensured. In the literature a distinction is drawn between care by the community and care in the community (Abrams, 1977). The first has always existed, though one of the explanations for the increase in formal care (i.e. care by the state, by a local authority) in the past century, and especially since the last world war, is the reduction in the care provided by the community. In order to understand the way services have developed one must look at the type of community care advocated in different periods and by different groups within each period, the nature of the social institutions established to provide care and the groups seen as requiring special social attention.

## BETWEEN THE WARS, 1918–39

At the end of the First World War psychiatric services consisted primarily of mental hospitals run by counties. The cost of treatment for poor people was covered by the county. The middle classes had to pay for themselves and at times to ask for coverage from charities. The rich usually went to the existing private hospitals, of which there were only 38 by 1930 (Parry Jones, 1972). Apart from the Mental Aftercare Association, a voluntary organization founded in the 1870s, there was little or no residential provision for patients discharged from the mental hospital. Outpatient psychiatric care was almost unknown.

Several developments took place in psychiatric practice between 1918 and 1939 which foreshadowed the major changes that later occurred to psychiatric community care (PCC). An era of optimism concerning organic psychiatry began with the discovery of Salvarsan, a treatment for the syphilitic infection which causes general paralysis of the insane. Insulin coma, psycho-surgery and convulsive therapy were all initiated between the wars. Each was heralded in turn as the solution to psychosis. Psychological understanding and interventions also made great strides into psychiatry. Psychological treatment of shell-shocked soldiers in the First World War, the introduction of child guidance clinics, the establishment of the first non-hospital service for adults (the Tavistock, in 1920) and the attribution of psychological motivation to factory workers' frustration on the job were the most important examples in this direction (Ramon, 1985a; Stone, 1985).

The 1930 Mental Treatment Act took account of these developments. Voluntary admission became possible for the first time in British psychiatric history, although the 1930 Act made such admissions a cumbersome process. Local authorities were requested to provide aftercare services for ex-patients, although this was not made compulsory.

## THE SECOND WORLD WAR AND THE 1950s

During the Second World War a public psychiatric service operated as part of the wartime general medical service. It was the first time that such a service was offered on a universal basis and as a matter of right. This feature of the service was enhanced with the introduction of the National Health Service (NHS) in 1948. Despite initial reluctance psychiatric services became an integral part of the NHS. As spending on the NHS as a whole rose there was an expansion of psychiatric services in terms of financial resources, manpower and buildings. However, spending on psychiatric patients always remained proportionally less than that devoted to patients in the rest of the NHS.

The first therapeutic communities were initiated during the war, in two settings run by teams of psychoanalytically oriented psychiatrists (Jones,

1952). The communities were for soldiers who suffered from severe neurosis and psychopathy. They allowed a freer dialogue between staff and residents, in which residents were encouraged to explore the dynamics of their interpersonal relationships. Residents were also given greater responsibility and autonomy. Therapeutic communities became a model for what can potentially be achieved with continuing care clients. Therapeutic community principles have been influential in the subsequent development of both residential and day services.

An open-door policy was initiated towards the end of the war. This meant that large numbers of psychiatric patients of all categories were discharged after much shorter periods of hospitalization. At the same time the rate of readmission rose sharply and the average length of stay decreased dramatically (Registrar General, 1959). The policy was instigated by hospital superintendents as a means of reducing the overcrowding in psychiatric hospitals. Their readiness to open the wards indicates that they had become convinced no harm would ensue as a result of this policy, either to the patients or the public. In effect the superintendents who initiated this move believed in the value and ability of leading a non-institutionalized life for the majority of the inpatients. The fact that this was conceived and implemented without a public outcry indicated that there had been a fundamental change in public attitude towards the non-violent mentally ill (i.e. the overwhelming majority).

Inside the hospitals more wards became open. In some places rehabilitation wards were established in which patients were prepared for the move outside, as well as being kept positively active. Little attention was paid to possible harmful effects of discharge, or to the type of supportive services required outside the hospital. Even less thought was given to the services needed to prevent admission in the first place.

Independently day care was initiated for the discharged patients, in the form of social clubs and later as day hospitals and industrial sheltered workshops. In some areas of Britain the pattern of services changed with the introduction of district psychiatric services. The facilities for out-patients were enlarged, although the hospital remained the core of the service.

The anti-psychotic drug chlorpromazine was introduced to Britain in 1954, and imipramine, an antidepressant, in 1957. The existence of effective psychotropic medication generated a new sense of optimism amongst psychiatrists. It has subsequently been claimed that the change in the psychiatric system during the 1950s was primarily due to the introduction of psychotropic drugs. However, chronologically it was not the case (*Lancet*, 1954; Scull, 1975), although it could be argued that these drugs influenced developments in the 1960s.

The psychologization of everyday life which started in the 1920s gathered momentum during the war. This trend reduced the gap in people's minds between the 'normal' and the 'abnormal'. Greater tolerance of people who exhibited psychiatric symptoms developed, because there was a conceptual framework for understanding the reasons for their behaviour and a belief that there were psychological methods of managing this behaviour (for example psychoanalysis and behaviour modification). Indeed this shift enabled the public to entertain the idea that such people do not necessarily need to be removed from ordinary life, or need to be removed only for short periods. A view also developed that everyone was potentially psychologically vulnerable and in need of professional support. During the war psychologists participated in the mass screening of recruits to the army. Social workers were involved in the evacuation of families and children, many of whom could not be classified as the 'usual social work client', i.e. the poor.

The psychologization of everyday life, and the higher social status accredited to psychologists and social workers coincided with increasing criticisms of psychiatric hospitals as environments which produced apathy, and physical and mental deterioration (Rees, 1957; Brown, 1959). These problems were, and still are, common among the long-term residents of any institution, not only the mental hospital. In British psychiatry a small but eminent group of psychiatrists, and most social workers, accepted that the inability to function socially was in part due to the effect of illness and in part to the effect of institutionalization. It was claimed that up to a quarter of the inpatient population could live outside (*Hansard*, vol. 574, p. 1055), a rather modest claim by today's standards. This anti-institutional stance gained credibility among politicians. They were attracted to the humanistic message of desegregation and to the belief that care in the community was going to be cheaper. The first calculations of cost of day hospital places demonstrated that they were considerably cheaper than a hospital bed (Farndale, 1964).

Politicians and all parties declared themselves to be in favour of community care, which came to mean the move out of the hospital of the majority of residents, including the long-term client. Very little thought went into the types of services required outside hospital, the role of the hospital in a future service or the transition process for both residents and staff. The politicians and those professionals interested in such a move were thinking about care in the community, and not about shifting the bulk of care to informal or voluntary carers. Most politicians interested in mental distress, always a tiny minority in both houses, came from the back benches of the Labour Party (Ramon, 1985a). An explanation for this recurring pattern is that the Conservative Party is not interested in the unsuccessful component of the population, unless such a group is engaged in criminal activity (Ramon, 1985a). It should, however, be stated that the Labour Party as a whole was not that interested in mental distress. There has never been either a special-interest group in the party on this issue or a clear policy in the party manifesto. The obvious reason for this lack of interest is that the mentally distressed were, and are, neither vote-catchers nor a strong pressure group.

The test of the strength of the politicians' commitment to community care came to the crunch when the Royal Commission on the Law related to Mental Illness (Cmnd 169) was appointed in 1954 after scandals concerning overcrowding in psychiatric hospitals. It recommended that the duties of local authorities for aftercare and housing for discharged patients should become mandatory. The recommendation was based on the experience from 1930 onwards, which clearly demonstrated the unevenness of local authority provision and the low priority given to services for the mentally distressed. While the government accepted most of the recommendations of the committee, including the radical proposal to set up mental health review tribunals, it refused to make local authorities' duties mandatory. On the surface it is not difficult to understand this refusal, as such legislation would cost central government money to implement. However in fact the Ministry of Health was convinced that community care would cost less than hospital-based care. Why then was its development not forthcoming? It has been hypothesized that the Ministry, led by the prevalent beliefs of the British psychiatric establishment, could not envisage a radically different service from the one offered at the time (Ramon, 1985a). It therefore preferred to encourage an incremental approach of local shifts of personnel from the mental hospital to district services, which would follow the same philosophy but be located outside the hospital. In short, the Ministry and the majority of psychiatrists and nurses did not view community care as really different from hospital-based care; they argued that they needed more of the same, an argument which is heard today. This approach to community care, typical of the British establishment, contrasts with conceptual and practice developments in the United States at the same time. There community mental health centres were legislated for in a special Bill and financed by the Federal Government from 1963.

The 1959 Mental Health Act had little to say about community care; in fact the term does not appear in the Act. Surprisingly it has become known as the Act which heralded the era of community care in psychiatry. Politicians and professionals congratulated themselves on the development of a more humane psychiatric system. However, the texts of the period leave little doubt that there was no critical reappraisal of what required change and how it might be achieved.

**The voluntary and private sectors**

The voluntary sector had been involved on a small scale in the aftercare of ex-patients since the nineteenth century. The different small mental health associations united into one national body in 1946, the National Association for Mental Health, which later became MIND. During the 1950s MIND became a pressure group for new mental health legislation and a group committed to community care. At the time it was barely involved in initiating new projects.

The number of private hospitals dwindled considerably between the wars. The introduction of the welfare state, and the NHS as a part of it, increased the reliance on publicly funded facilities. While private consultations continued to be on offer, no significant private sector existed in terms of hospitals, outpatient clinics or aftercare facilities. However, from the 1950s onwards some former mental hospital residents went to live in private accommodation, often in seaside resorts. As the arrangements were made privately, they were not known to any local public service, and the premises were usually not inspected (Bennett, 1983).

FROM 1959 TO 1979

The 1960s began with the declaration of the then Minister of Health, Enoch Powell, that the primary objective for the psychiatric services was a cut of 20,000 beds in the next 20 years. This was justified on the grounds of the progress made by psychiatry and the wish for desegregation. The White Paper 'Community Care' (Cmnd 169) followed in 1963. It generated very little enthusiasm or practical developments, because it remained at the level of unspecified generalities. The predicted cut in bed numbers was based on calculations of future trends of length of stay, rather than on the number of people admitted per year. By the end of the 1970s it could be observed that these calculations were correct, as 50 per cent of those admitted did not stay for more than a month (DHSS, 1982). The number of people coming in for the first time declined, while the number of readmissions increased. This implies that services were more successful at preventing first admissions than working with long-term clients who formed the majority of readmissions.

By the end of the 1970s care in the community had become a reality for many long-term clients even if they continued to use an inpatient unit for brief periods. The main forms that this service took included:

1. GP consultation and prescription of medication, including major tranquillizers;

2. outpatient clinic appointments;
3. home visits by community psychiatric nurses in some areas;
4. day care facilities—i.e. day hospital, day centre;
5. group homes and hostels;
6. a few therapeutic communities (e.g. the Richmond Fellowship);
7. brief periods of hospitalization.

The first social work attachment to a health centre, where support was offered to people with emotional problems, took place in 1966. An intensive crisis intervention service, based on home visiting, was offered in the Barnet area. It was initiated by social workers and psychiatrists (Ratna, 1978). Despite very promising results both of these innovations (especially the second) have remained a minority practice.

While the use of the GP for an initial psychiatric consultation was frequent before 1960, the reliance on psychotropic drugs has led to greater use of GPs for the maintenance of people with long-term psychiatric symptoms. There was no parallel increase in the amount of psychiatric training for GPs.

British research on the impact of long-term living in psychiatric hospitals concluded that it was necessary to change the regime in hospital in order to minimize the effect of the institution. Amongst British researchers there was disagreement about the relative importance of the effects of the institution and the biological impairments associated with mental illness. A greater application of behaviour modification techniques, initiated by psychologists, was allowed to take place in some hospital wards with long-term patients. The results were encouraging in demonstrating the rehabilitative potential of a group that had been largely given up by other psychological therapies (Trower et al., 1978).

During the 1960s psychiatrists believed that when the older generation of long-stay patients eventually died there would be only few new long-term clients. This assertion was rejected in the late 1970s when the evidence accumulated of a growing number of readmissions of people in the age range 25–35 years. Furthermore, there was enough evidence to indicate that their living pattern outside the hospital was quite similar to that of the institutional patient inside (McCowen and Wilder, 1975). This has led on the one hand to the reinforcement of the emphasis on the disease model, and on the other hand to the realization by some professionals that merely being outside the hospital would not prevent institutionalism. An institutional atmosphere could be equally re-created in day facilities and sheltered accommodation outside the hospital.

Research into the impact of the family environment on the long-term client revealed that the latter did better when living outside the family than staying within it. This observation led to an interest in the role of the emotional environment in the course of mental distress. However, surprisingly little interest was devoted to the problems experienced by the relatives. The findings of these interwoven strands of research became the basis of British mainstream psychiatry's thinking and service planning on community care (Wing, 1972).

Anti-psychiatry attempted to rock the boat when in the late 1960s it juxtaposed the relationships between society and the family with the deviancy approach to inpatients. The importance of anti-psychiatry was dual. Firstly, it rejected hospitalization, giving a central place to communal living and individual psychotherapy (Laing, 1971). The communal living was to be sustained by a mixture of people who suffer from acute mental distress, those who do not, and professional support. Secondly it triggered off considerable media attention, most of it positive, in the early 1970s. Equally it led to very hostile reactions from professionals and politicians. Its message was rightly understood to be not only about psychiatry, but about the place of nuclear families and the negative aspects of family relationships.

Social workers were particularly intrigued by the anti-psychiatry message. This related to changes within social work at the time. Social work had become less focused on psychological intervention with individuals and more interested in the social context. The growth of community work during the 1960s and 1970s exemplifies this trend (Mayo, 1975), though to assume that the majority of social workers were 'trendy Hippie Lefties' is quite incorrect. Moreover, social work views were broadly similar to those of successive Labour governments in the 1960s and 1970s. Given that Labour was elected to office in 1964, 1966 and 1974, it would seem that these views represented the mood of the country at the time. The then prevailing mood of social reform was weaker but similar to movements elsewhere in Europe. This, and the fact that their dominant position in the psychiatric services was not seriously threatened by the type of community care advocated by British politicians, including the Labour Party, are two reasons why psychiatrists did not resist the cut in bed numbers that occurred.

The growing interest in community care as a panacea for all vulnerable groups during that period also led to the creation of the personal social services departments (SSD), which were expected to provide such care. For the first time social workers were able to unite across different fields and the government was ready to allow social services to have more concentrated power. The new groups of employees in these departments also reflect the change in the concept of care in the community, which shifted in the 1970s to include home helps, residential workers, welfare rights officers and a new, fairly large, group of middle managers.

The separation of the health and social services, which existed throughout the history of modern Britain, received a seal of approval in 1970. For the psychiatric service it meant that social workers were from now on employed by a SSD and not by the health authority of the hospital in which they worked. Those not working directly in a hospital or child guidance clinics would combine mental health work with other types of social work. With the increase in child care work a decrease in mental health work carried out by generic teams became a fact of life (Fisher *et al.*, 1984). As a result very little psychiatric community care work was done by social services teams. Furthermore, because social workers in the hospitals tended to follow the pattern of work of the rest of the clinical team they too were barely involved in setting up community care services. However they continued to be more involved in planning the discharge of an individual client than were any other members of the clinical team, mainly because they were doing most of the liaison work with outside agencies.

While casework with individuals and families was not at odds with mainstream British psychiatry's view of community care, the community work stream in social work proposed a rather different direction. This was more concerned with the involvement of users of services in the planning and provision of services, in giving users more control over resources and in demystifying the monopoly of professional expertise in the process. However, community work did not involve setting up facilities for mentally distressed people.

### The voluntary and private sectors

The community work message, rather than its methods of work, was to an extent taken up by some of the voluntary organizations involved in mental health. Perhaps paradoxically the community participation ethos encouraged the growth of associations such as the National Schizophrenia Fellowship, a relatives group which accepted traditional psychiatric views and patronage. It offered relatives moral support and established sheltered workshops for discharged people who were diagnosed as suffering from schizophrenia. MIND embarked on the dual objectives of lobbying for more legal rights to patients and initiating pioneering projects. Private hospitals played no significant role in the British psychiatric system during the 1960s and 1970s. However, a growing number of patients were discharged into profit-making private residential facilities.

## POLICY DIRECTIONS IN THE 1970s

Three White Papers on mental distress appeared between 1975 and 1978. They highlight most of the major issues of psychiatric care at the time, although the solutions proposed bear the hallmark of the thinking of the DHSS, influenced primarily by the Royal College of Psychiatrists.

The Butler Committee on 'mentally abnormal offenders' (Cmnd 6244) was set up in response to the situation in which a few of the many long-term clients who lived outside the hospital were offending or perceived as potentially violent. This subgroup includes patients with a mixture of diagnoses including personality disorder, schizophrenia, manic-depressive disorder and severe neurosis. The committee wished to find for this group a setting which would offer psychiatric treatment and protect society by means of seclusion. It recognized the unsatisfactory state of affairs concerning the problematical diagnosis of psychopathy and the poor track record of psychiatric intervention with this clientele. It proposed the establishment of regional secure units solely for mentally ill offenders. The importance of the Committee and its recommendations to this text is that together they represent the limits of care in the community in Britain.

The document 'Better services for the mentally ill' (1975, Cmnd 6233) reiterated commitment to community care, but admitted that very little had been achieved since 1959, and that insufficient resources had been allocated to it. The White Paper, which has since become the blueprint for the official allocation of manpower and facilities, expected multidisciplinary teams to work together, and reinforced the district unit of services as the core of local psychiatric service. Implicitly community care meant local services. Psychiatric wards in the general hospital were seen as part of the locality, and were expected to replace the psychiatric hospital for people in an acute crisis. With the exception of offenders, other users of the psychiatric services were expected to be dealt with in outpatients or day care facilities. Although unsaid, the message was that there was no role for the psychiatric hospital, but that equally there was no need for a radical change in the repertoire of psychiatric interventions in the period of transition and after the disappearance of the mental hospital.

The review of the 1959 Mental Health Act (Cmnd 7320) took place in 1978 at a time when the Secretary of State was a former officer of MIND. A prolonged process of consultation took place prior to the publication of the paper, where the only group not represented directly were the service users. With a view to legislation, the review suggested several proposals related to the rights and conditions of the 5 per cent of the inpatient population who were detained compulsorily. Only BASW (the British Association of Social Workers) proposed to legislate community care orders, which would have been a combination of a probation order and guardianship. Such an order would have involved a specified contract between the client and a local authority social worker about such matters as attendance at day centres, outpatient clinics and place of residence. In effect, local authorities' duties concerning community care would have had to become mandatory. The DHSS saw the proposal as impractical, while MIND viewed it as limiting users' liberty.

The direct involvement of the DHSS in establishing psychiatric community care was limited to financing a few selected projects. Of these the Worcester development project and services in Camberwell are the best known (Tombs and Bennett, 1987; Wing 1982).

## TRENDS IN THE 1980s

The pace of change in thinking about community care and related activities has accelerated considerably since 1980. There are both political and professional reasons for this. The issues at the political level are the more significant. The government is committed to cutting down public sector expenditure and to privatizing services. In this view the ultimate objective of community care would be to hand over care to the informal carers, unpaid volunteers and private entrepreneurs. In line with this approach the DHSS is pursuing the closure of large psychiatric hospitals. Financially this is logical because of the high cost of keeping the old Victorian hospitals in good order, especially as the number of patients is decreasing and unit costs are rising. The DHSS therefore has found attractive the professional message that the majority of inpatients could live outside if the right supports were provided. Following the report by the House of Commons Social Services Select Committee (1985) the DHSS has committed itself to provide the necessary bridging resources. With Departmental blessing regional health authorities are allocating a one-off sum for each person who leaves a psychiatric hospital to the service which will take on responsibility for the ex-patient. While the size of this 'dowry' varies from £11,000 to £20,000 per person, it is a useful incentive for the health and social services to become really interested in the closure of the mental hospitals.

The collaboration between these two major services is riddled with difficulties and conflicts (Glennester and Korman, 1986; Audit Commission, 1986). The health services feel that social services are dragging their feet in planning and executing plans. The latter feel strongly that the health authorities prefer to establish their own services and not to transfer the money to the social services. Behind the difficulties in cooperation and the power struggles are different approaches to community care and different professional groups. In addition there is a reality in which social services departments' resources have been cut more drastically than those of the health service. The need to work together cannot be overstated, especially at the level of the continuing care clients who are caught in the transition from hospital to community.

In 1983 COHSE suggested that all services related to community care for the mentally distressed become part of the NHS, a proposal motivated partly by self-interest and partly in recognition of the need to unify the services under one roof. While an equal plea could be made for the move of workers to social services, the issue of fragmentation and slowness of execution of plans needs to be better resolved. Neither COHSE's proposal nor MIND's suggestion to establish a unified category of mental health worker has received serious attention either at the DHSS or in professional circles, although a recent report by the Audit Commission has revived the proposal of a unified mental health service (Audit Commission, 1986). Furthermore, the Commission raises the intriguing possibility of creating care authorities responsible specifically for the elderly, people with mental distress and developmental handicap. Such authorities will receive joint funding from the health and social services, but will be self-managed rather than jointly managed.

The DHSS is unclear how the closures should be carried out, or what should be the shape of the alternative services. This lack of clarity allows regions and districts to do their own thing. Differing strategies for closure emerge. For example the closure of one hospital took place by the transfer of all of its residents and nearly all of the staff to several other hospitals (Reid, 1986). In contrast the closure of another hospital has been carried out by moving all residents to hostels and group homes in the locality, while the staff have moved into local mental health centres (King, 1987).

Similarly, there are no national guidelines concerning the preparation of the staff to move out of the hospitals. Every authority has been left to its own devices, with exceptions such as the programmes offered by the King's Fund. Furthermore, the commitment of the government and health authority to hospital closures is questioned, for example, by the permission to open a new private psychiatric hospital in North London only a few miles away from the site of a large public hospital which is earmarked for closure.

A new and important group has emerged—the Health Service General Managers. They come predominantly from an administrative background, although some general managers have been practitioners. The requirement for general managers to focus on planning objectives and methods has given them a very different perspective on the development of services. In addition, the greater power given to managers in the NHS, coupled with a greater measure of flexibility, enables those managers who wish to develop community-based psychiatric services to be more effective than in the past.

## The voluntary and private sectors

Over recent years the voluntary sector has become more prominent in the whole area of community care. This higher profile is due to the government's readiness to encourage this sector and to increase public attention to the activities of certain voluntary organizations. The imminence of closure of the large hospitals has also led to the creation of a united front of those who oppose such closures, including relatives' associations.

For the first time since the 1920s there has been a considerable increase in private sector provision for the continuing care client. This has involved primarily accommodation, either in adult fostering or in 'landladies' schemes. In some cases those providing accommodation are ex-psychiatric nurses. This development is actively encouraged by the DHSS, which now pays directly to private landlords, through board and lodging charges, bypassing the local authority. In addition the number of new private psychiatric hospitals are being developed. All are financed and run by American corporations. So far, most of them cater for rich people with mild symptomatology. However, one private hospital in Cambridgeshire specializes in looking after those who are seen as requiring secure facilities.

The spread of the private sector is controversial. It puts at risk the jobs of employees within the public sector. Its activities are much more difficult to monitor than within the public service. However, it is clear that careful monitoring is required to ensure that the continuing care client is not merely hidden away. By directing resources to the private sector the government is now limiting the flexibility of local authority services. However, the private sector may offer a more flexible and efficient service because it is less bureaucratized. The American experience with private for-profit organizations justifies reservations about the expansion in this country of the private sector (Brown, 1985).

## New legislation

The Mental Health Amendments Act of 1983 follows closely the 1959 Act in relation to community care. It has not added any new responsibility to any given service concerning community care, apart from the requirement on the approved social worker to consider alternatives for hospitalization at the time of investigating a request for compulsory admission.

## The professionals' perspectives

The lack of clarity within the DHSS reflects the absence of an overall vision about community care among the majority of British professionals, in spite of the existence of a number of promising new projects and new ideas. This lack of vision may stem from the emphasis within professional training on individual symptomatology and the traditional British preference for pragmatism and resistance to change. However, we now possess much more empirical knowledge than in the past on several key issues related to psychiatric community care. This knowledge base comes only in part from the British psychiatric system itself. Most of it comes either from abroad (the US, Holland and Italy) or other welfare areas in Britain. It is up to the providers, planners and users of psychiatric services to work out how to interpret and use this evidence.

We now have knowledge of the harm done to people with long-term mental illnesses by hurried closures of mental hospitals, and by the lack of suitable support in the community (Brown, 1985). Research has shown that most continuing care clients are poor people, whose access to ordinary life opportunities is largely blocked by being poor (Kay and Legg, 1986). It is, however, clear that most continuing care clients cannot only survive outside the hospital but can, given the right support, improve the quality of their lives (Ramon, 1985b; Stein and Test, 1978). In some cases this improvement is dramatic. The needs of informal carers are now being increasingly recognized (Butterworth and Skidmore, 1981). Publications have defined the areas and types of support that long-term clients require (Watts and Bennett, 1983).

However, if the continuing care client is to stand a reasonable chance of leading a less segregated life than in the former mental hospital system the attitudes in neighbourhoods and the media must change (Ramon, 1985b). In developing community care an important issue is the preparation of staff who must move outside the hospital (Towell and Davies, 1984). We must also learn how to involve neighbourhoods in the mixture of formal, informal, public and private care for the continuing care client that will develop (Bulmer, 1986). There is no doubt that psychiatric community care is not financially a cheap option. It is primarily a labour-intensive service, although the personnel need not consist only of highly trained people (Frank, 1981).

Although much is now known about the community care services of the future it is not clear how best to manage small groups of younger people who are beginning to become long-stay or who, in the absence of long-stay hospital beds, have become what in America have been termed 'the young chronic drifters'. The future of services for the mentally ill offender is also unclear, and the current pattern of services for them appears unsatisfactory.

With increasing political pressure for change the latent attitudes of professionals to psychiatric community care have become manifest. Currently there is a polarization of views. On the one hand there is a belief that psychiatric hospitals are necessary. On the other hand people are convinced that such facilities are unnecessary and should be replaced by non-institutionalizing community services. People working in hospitals, especially those that are earmarked for closure in the near future, tend to believe in the need for long-term hospital care. However, this view is not

just motivated by self-interest. There is also a glorification of the psychiatric hospital as a caring and protective institution. It is asserted that the
psychiatric hospital is here to stay because a significant proportion of
people suffering from long-term mental illnesses cannot live outside such
institutions given the impact of their illness (Jones and Fowles, 1984). This
repudiation of the critique of the total institution seems to be based on a
national failure to meet the needs of the continuing care client outside the
hospital, and on some belief that total institutions are in essence valuable.

Can all continuing care clients manage outside the hospital? The answer
to this question depends to a large extent on one's belief about the
aetiology and prognosis of mental illness, and whether the current pattern
of community care is indeed all that could and should be on offer.

The view that hospitals are unnecessary, and should be replaced by
community services, is held by a minority of social workers and psychologists who reaffirm the critique of the institutions which was first articulated
in the 1950s. Their focus is on providing real opportunities for normalization and on empowering users (Wolfensberger, 1982; Milroy and Hennel-
ley, 1984). For them the appropriate role of the professional is that of the
enabler, who steps into a more directly supportive role only when required, and on a temporary basis. This group of professionals believe that
the meaning of community care is care by the community, where to a large
extent the community is one of users and their carers. Their approach
follows the growth of self-help groups in mental health and other areas,
which have shown very positive response from users. Lessons have been
learnt from women's and ethnic minorities groups on how to enable the
development of assertion and advocacy of those who lack power in society.

The majority of professional providers fall between those who romanti-
cally glorify the institution and those who see their role solely as an
enabler. They are less sure today than before that all continuing care clients
can live outside a protective environment, but do not assume that this
environment must be a hospital. They are very sceptical of the government's commitment to psychiatric community care and fear that the
closure of hospitals may be used as an exercise in reducing services.
However, the majority of those who have made the move to work outside
the hospital are enthusiastic about working in the community.

Finally, a further logical though radical development is the attempt to
involve users in groups that advise on policy. Such attempts are currently
encouraged by some health authorities, social services departments and
MIND (Davis, 1985). Other user groups have organized themselves without the support of formal organizations, for example Survivors Speak Out
and CAPO. These tend to be highly critical of the input of professionals. A
substantial number of the users active in these groups have come from the
continuing care clientele.

The psychiatric system and professionals working within it are going through a major period of transition, in which a number of 'sacred cows' concerning community care are being questioned. Positions of power are being threatened and new relationships between professionals and non-professionals, providers and users must emerge. Furthermore, as a society we will need to re-examine our traditional response to the continuing care client in the light of these changes. For a growing number of providers and users the development in psychiatric community care has become a challenge. This is perhaps the best indicator of the viability of the direction in which policies are now going, even if the present manifestations of community care policies are likely yet again to change in the future.

## REFERENCES

Abrams, P. (1977). Community care: some research problems and priorities, *Policy and Politics*, **6**, 125–51.

Audit Commission (1986). *Making Community Care a Reality*. HMSO, London.

Bennett, D. (1983). The historical development of rehabilitation services. In F. N. Watts and D. Bennett (eds) *The Theory and Practice of Psychiatric Rehabilitation*, Wiley & Sons, Chichester.

Brown, G. (1959). Social factors influencing length of hospital stay of schizophrenic patients, *British Medical Journal*, **2**, 1300–2.

Brown, P. (1985). *The Transfer of Care*, Routledge & Kegan Paul, London.

Bulmer, M. (1986). *Neighbours: The Work of Philip Abrams*, Cambridge University Press, Cambridge.

Butterworth, G. and Skidmore, D. (1981). *Caring for the Mentally Ill in the Community*, Croom Helm, London.

Davis, A. (1985). Coventry Crisis Intervention Team: the consumers' view. *Social Services Research*, **14**, 1.

Department of Health and Social Security (1982). *Personal and Health Statistics*, DHSS, London.

Farndale, W. (1964). *The Day Hospital Movement in Britain*, Pergamon Press, Oxford.

Fisher, M., Newton, C., and Sainsbury, E. (1984). *Mental Health Social Work Observed*, George Allen & Unwin, London.

Frank, R. (1981). Cost benefit analysis for Mental Health Services: a review of the literature, *Administration in Mental Health*, **8**, 161–76.

Glennester, H., and Korman, N. (1986). *Closing a Hospital: Darneth Park Project*, Bedford Square Publications, London.

House of Commons (1985). Second Report from the Social Services Committee Sessions 1984–1985. *Community Care: with special reference to adult mentally ill and mentally handicapped people*, HMSO, London.

Jones, M. (1952). *Social Psychiatry*, Tavistock, London.

Jones, K., and Fowles, A. J. (1984). *Ideas on Institutions*, Routledge & Kegan Paul, London.

Kay, A., and Legg, C. (1986). *Discharge to the Community: a review of housing and support for people leaving psychiatric care*, Housing Research Group, The City University.

King, D. (1987). Replacing the mental hospital with better services. In S. Ramon (ed.) *Psychiatry in Transition*, Zwan, London.

Laing, R. D. (1971). The Politics of the Family, Tavistock: London.

*Lancet* (1954). Editorial: Unlocked doors, *Lancet*, **2**, 953.

McCowan, P., and Wilder, H. (1975). Lifestyle of 100 Psychiatric Patients, Psychiatric Rehabilitation Association.

Mayo, M. (1975). Community development: a radical alternative? In R. Bailey and M. Brake (eds) *Radical Social Work*, Arnold, London.

Milroy, A., and Hennelly, R. (1984) *Exploiting Infinity*. MIND Annual Conference, MIND Publications, London.

Parry Jones, W. (1972). *The Trade in Lunacy*, Routledge & Kegan Paul, London.

Ramon, S. (1985a). *Psychiatry in Britain: meaning and policy*, Croom Helm, London.

Ramon, S. (1985b). The Italian Psychiatric Reform. In S. Mangen (ed.) *Mental Health Care in the European Community*, Croom Helm, London.

Ratna, L. (1978). *The Practice of Psychiatric Crisis Intervention*, Napsbury League of Friends, St Albans.

Rees, T. P. (1957). Back to moral treatment and community care, *Journal of Mental Science*, **103**, 303–13.

Registrar General (1959). *Statistical Review of England and Wales*. Supplement on Mental Health, HMSO, London.

Reid, H. (1986). Instead of Banstead, *Openmind*, **22**, 14.

Scull, A. (1975). *Decarceration*, Prentice Hall, London.

Stein, L. I., and Test, M. A. (1978). *Alternatives to Mental Hospital Treatment*, Plenum Press, New York.

Stone, M. (1985). Psychology and industry in the interim wars period, Ph.D. thesis, London School of Economics.

Tombs, D., and Bennett, C. (1987). The evaluation of the Worcester Project. In S. Mangen and S. Ramon (eds) *Community Mental Health Care in Europe: developments and constraints, international Journal of Social Psychiatry*, Monograph.

Towell, D., and Davies, A. (1984). Moving out from the large hospitals: involving the people (staff and patients) concerned. In *Care in the Community—Keep it Local*, MIND, London.

Trower, P., Bryant, B., and Argyle, M. (1978). *Social Skills and Mental Health*, Methuen, London.

Watts, F. N., and Bennett, D. (1983). *The Theory and Practice of Psychiatric Rehabilitation*, Wiley, Chichester.

Wing, J. K. (1972). Principles of evaluation. In J. K. Wing and A. M. Hailey (eds) *Evaluating a Community Psychiatric Service*, Oxford University Press, Oxford.

Wing, J. K. (1982). Long-term community care: experience in a London borough, *Psychological Medicine* Monograph, Supplement 2.

Wolfensberger, W. (1982). *Normalization: The Principles of Normalization in Human Services*, Toronto, National Institute for Medical Research.

Community Care in Practice
Edited by A. Lavender and F. Holloway
© 1988 John Wiley & Sons Ltd

Chapter 3

# Implementing Community Care: an international assessment

## S. P. MANGEN

In the past 25 years most Western countries have enacted reforms of mental health policy. This review provides a cross-national assessment of the success of these reforms in terms of their impact on services for long-term psychiatric clients. Although the discussion of policy issues is cast in a broad comparative framework, detailed case studies of the United States and Italy are provided, since both countries have experienced sharp declines in the size of the inpatient sector, each for different reasons. There have been numerous obstacles to the implementation of reform. Principal among them are: inertia due to a lack of commitment on the part of politicians, administrators and key sections of the mental health professions; structural factors such as the dysfunctional political division of responsibilities for health and social services; lack of organizational co-ordination at the local level; and a chronic under-financing of services exacerbated by complex and sometimes conflicting funding systems. The major conclusion is that, whatever the system of mental health care, it has been the long-term mentally ill who have been deprived of adequate resources and who continue to be in receipt of 'Cinderella' services.

### Mental health care systems

The varying institutional arrangements of welfare states among European countries and in America have a direct bearing on the nature of mental health systems. Although all these states share a heritage of a locally administered network of asylums emanating from the nineteenth century, there remains considerable international variation in legislative provisions, political and administrative responsibility for services, and the status of service providers (that is, whether services are supplied directly by the public sector, voluntary bodies or by private profit-making enterprises). There are differences, too, in the organization of the psychiatric profession, not least in the extent to which independent office practice coexists with the hospital-based services and is the dominant provider of outpatient treatment. Where this has occurred in conjunction with the development of private inpatient facilities it has led to a form of 'two-tier' psychiatry that in some countries is an important feature of the mental health system and critically distinguishes the careers of psychiatric clienteles. Finally, countries also differ in the extent to which psychoanalysis has developed as a formal alternative to the strong neuropsychiatric tradition.

In most countries reviewed here it was not until the 1960s that changes in the mental hospital system were first initiated, at least in terms of psychiatric hospital bed capacities. Whilst England and Wales and the United States record early and substantial reductions in this sector, in France, the Federal Republic of Germany, Spain and Portugal an absolute decline was not reported until the 1970s. In some countries—most notably France—these reductions were partly offset by substantial bed additions in general hospital psychiatric units. Studies of other institutional provisions strongly suggest that, to a significant degree, the decline in the inpatient sector has come about by the transfer of elderly and other long-term patients to high-support nursing and residential homes. This practice is evident in France and Germany and is best documented in the case of the United States. Transfers of this kind do not appear to have been a major feature of the Italian experience, although some patients have moved to old people's homes. However, as will be discussed later, some highly contested evaluations of services in Italy argue that the decline in inpatient numbers has been achieved merely by a change of nomenclature, some patients having become 'ospiti' (guests) with little real change of status. Unfortunately, the paucity of official statistics on other psychiatric services frustrates attempts to compare the speed at which specific policies on community-based care are being implemented internationally.

## The emergence of mental health reform as an issue

The post-war expansion of the welfare state has facilitated growth and diversity among the health and welfare professions, as new specialisms have been added to existing professional territories and have stimulated moves to practise outside and sometimes independent of the hospital base. Castel (1981) has interpreted these developments as representing the 'aggiornomento' of psychiatry, providing it with fresh opportunities to annexe new terrains and specialities catering, if not for the whole popula-tion, at least for those large groups of clients regarded as being most 'at risk'. These events are hardly likely to be conflict-free. Innovations in providing community-based care, for example, may threaten established roles to which many professionals attach high value. Furthermore, care systems are becoming increasingly pluralist, with gradual expansion of the number and range of providing agencies that must be taken into account in negotiating reform policies. To these must be added various old-established and newly emerging pressure groups, including patients' and relatives' organizations, which are attempting to exert influence in some countries. In addition some health trade unions have been mobilizing to oppose changes which they see as leading to a deterioration in conditions of employment, or to the threat of job losses in cases of hospital closures. It is for reasons like these that the issue of psychiatric reform has become politicized.

But the politicization of the issue goes deeper. In professional and academic circles two major critiques have dominated the debate in the past quarter century about the need for change inside the psychiatric system. On the one hand, proposed solutions have stressed a 'technical' approach relying on various forms of sectorization of outpatient and inpatient services, whilst others have espoused a more radical anti-institutional model of care which has brought into question the whole social and political purpose of psychiatry. This discourse has been in evidence nearly everywhere, but has perhaps been most polarized in France from the late 1950s and in Italy from the mid-1960s (Balduzzi and Balduzzi, 1981).

Political and administrative developments occurring in allied fields have also been critical in shaping reform issues. Since the late 1960s increasing importance has been attached to libertarian concerns. There has been a growing salience of issues surrounding the status of various social and ethnic minorities. Radical social critiques about the coercive functions of the welfare state have been published at a time of disillusionment with its performance, best evidenced perhaps in its inability to eradicate long-term unemployment with the consequent emergence of 'new poverty'. Increasingly, the legitimate concern of planners with the resource implications of policies is being overtaken by narrower preoccupations with effecting budgetary cuts where it is easiest to do so, in order to resolve the many funding 'crises' of the welfare state. Administrative reorganization and decentralization have either been proposed or adopted in part to counter the general disillusionment with centralized, bureaucratized and inflexible large-scale systems of welfare delivery. There has been concern, too, that the increasing professionalization and specialization of care has marginalized the consumer in the decision-making processes and has also raised questions about the adequacy of systems of accountability.

In all these debates the cost implications of reform have dominated official thinking, even if 'community care' has been initially espoused for its apparent clinical soundness and popular appeal. More recently, however, the potential merits of this model of care as a cheaper option have given way to the recognition that full implementation of the policy could call for substantial additional financial outlays. Current strategies therefore argue for 'value-for-money' options. However, in comparative terms, the economics of community care provide an insufficient explanation of the reform impetus. Sedgwick (1981) in a detailed discussion argues that health costs were spiralling long before certain countries took action to supplement the expensive hospital base of their mental health system with a range of outpatient services. The Federal Republic of Germany is a case in point. In others, reforms were implemented during the heyday of the post-war welfare states, long before the current fiscal crisis concentrated official minds firmly on cost containment and the shedding of public sector responsibilities. Several countries—France and Britain are examples—are now having to cope with the effects their policies have had in producing a long-term decline in the inpatient population which has created serious problems of overcapacity in decaying and increasingly redundant hospitals. On the other hand, there is evidence that potentially costly institutional solutions have not been entirely discarded in these times of pressure on the public purse, as is demonstrated by the current Italian proposals to re-establish medium-stay inpatient facilities, which are discussed later.

The prominence of each element in the emergence of psychiatric reform as an issue varies among the countries discussed here, but some convergent trends can be detected. There has been growing recognition of—if limited attempts to remedy—the dysfunctional effects of organizational divisions of responsibility between health and welfare agencies and the inadequacies of social security programmes as they affect long-term clients. Attempts at reorganization of the mental health system have involved a geographical sectorization of services including internal sectorization of mental hospitals, which has been frequently accompanied by capital programmes to improve physical conditions. The problem of hospital overcapacity has been occupying planners in some countries and is being resolved through selective closure programmes, often involving further transfers of responsibilities for the care of some patient groups to other welfare sectors. The creation of alternative inpatient facilities in the form of psychiatric units in general hospitals, although implemented in all the countries discussed, has generally progressed slowly and in most cases relatively few are sufficiently resourced to fulfil catchment area responsibilities.

The growing reliance on voluntary and private profit-making provision has in some countries reinforced the constitutional 'subsidiarity' tradition of public services and has been accompanied almost everywhere by some withdrawal of direct public sector involvement. More recent psychiatric legislation stressing the equality of status between the mentally and physically ill has acknowledged the rights of patients to treatment and has sometimes conferred the right of patients' consent to treatment. The benison of self-help has been rediscovered and, whilst this policy has been especially nurtured by centre right political parties in several countries, there are suspicions that it might be exploited in an attempt to conceal a depletion of assistance being offered by formal services. Whilst the essential role of informal carers is now more widely recognized, there are unresolved questions about the often intolerable burden on the family, which in turn raises the question of unpaid female labour and its compatibility with coexisting policies promoting women's equality.

## THE CASE STUDIES

As these brief profiles of developments demonstrate, the history of psychiatry is replete with examples of how influential innovators—whether clinicians, officials, politicians or journalists—have been able to exploit wider political events to create favourable opportunities for mental health reform. The case studies identify key figures in the USA and Italy. In this context, mention should be made of their counterparts elsewhere. These include the French psychiatrists, Bonnafé and Tosquelles, celebrated for their work on 'institutional psychotherapy', who were instrumental in gaining ministerial support in 1960 for the formal initiation of the 'psychiatrie de secteur'. In Germany a Christian Democrat MP, Walter Picard, exploited the favourable political circumstances surrounding the establishment in 1969 of a Brandt-led government committed to an expansionary social programme to campaign for mental health reform, a strategy that eventually resulted in the appointment of a major commission of inquiry. The subsequent report has been the basis of German mental health planning in the 1970s and 1980s.

However, even when the stimulus provided by individuals and pressure groups has been strong, and has attracted sufficient political support to enact reform, implementation has frequently been a slow process. The case studies are evidence of the fact that the speed of innovation in these (and other) countries has been determined by the interaction of a wide range of constraints. Principal among these are organizational dysfunctions, inadequacies of funding, inertia among professionals, the low profile of mental health as a public issue and serious deficiencies in information-gathering which frustrate effective planning.

Coordination between deinstitutionalization strategies and efforts to create locally-based 'community' services has been a universal problem because of the contradictory nature of reform policies, especially regarding funding arrangements. Each mental health system under review contains perverse incentives to perpetuate inefficient utilization of resources, preventing cost-effective transfers of financial responsibilities between different care sectors. Administrative structures, for example, often serve to protect vested interests, since it is rare that benefits derived from innovations which accrue in one (locally-based) sector automatically compensate losses—notably the loss of employment—in other sectors. This kind of constraint is reinforced by resistance to change among some professionals who, for the most part, have experienced an exclusively hospital-based training.

Too many resources which could be deployed to provide locally-based services are trapped in providing institutional care. Although the redistribution of funding is argued in the interests of cost containment—and several countries have attempted reforms—the fundamental problem everywhere arises from the lack of an across-the-board means of financing new services which would permit the easy transfer of monies. Instead, funding systems are compartmentalized and in certain countries, such as Germany, are reliant on a heavy legalism and are competitive so that each funder is motivated to limit liabilities. In the absence of comprehensive reform, several countries have been attempting to resolve the funding of the operational costs of community services such as day centres, workshops and hostels. Difficulties have arisen because many of these provisions are discretionary rather than statutory and have to rely on patients' entitlements to means-tested social assistance or invalidity pensions. To a large extent, then, the establishment of new services is determined by ease of reimbursement through welfare benefits. This unsatisfactory state of affairs poses major problems of financial insecurity for the smaller, more recently established services in the private non-profit sector.

These case studies provide ample evidence that lengthy delays in general implementation have resulted in marked regional inequalities in the provision of new services, especially those for the long-term user. This situation is unlikely to be improved in the short run, given the widespread retrenchment in social expenditure. Indeed, it is likely that effective planning capacities have been declining in the 1980s, since several of the national policies were formulated in times of a buoyant economy only to be implemented in a period of recession. Furthermore, decentralization of public agencies and the increasing resort to various forms of privatization significantly extend the number of interested parties who need to be included in negotiations if planning is to be effective.

## COMMUNITY CARE POLICIES IN THE UNITED STATES OF AMERICA

In 1955 there were 558,922 resident inpatients in the 350 American state mental hospitals; by 1982 there were only 125,200. This sharp rate of decline, amounting to over 75 per cent of capacity, did not begin to abate until the late 1970s. The fiscal implications of maintaining large decaying and discredited hospitals had prompted deinstitutionalization on a scale unparalleled anywhere in the world. Two states stand out as pioneers, although as we shall see their policies could hardly be regarded as exemplary: New York and Governor Reagan's California, the latter having experienced an eighty percent reduction in the state hospital patient population (Martindale and Martindale, 1985). During the 1960s deinstitutionalization policies were aided by federal funding programmes targeted at mental health and by the introduction of Medicaid, Medicare and Supplemental Security Disability Income (SSDI) which provided a source of new money to pay for alternative care settings. As we shall see, not all these facilities have proved to be desirable, and welfare monies have permitted an unfortunate new 'trade in lunacy'.

These developments, however, did not lead to a coordinated programme of discharge to a variegated locally based network of 'community' facilities; rather, much of the decline in inpatient numbers is attributable to 'transinstitutionalization', principally of elderly patients to other large health and welfare establishments. By the mid-1970s, for example, there were 85,000 former mental hospital patients in nursing homes (Fagin, 1985). There has also been a high discharge rate of other long-stay groups to cheap hotel and board-and-lodging accommodation, a lot of it of dubious quality, resulting in scandals of criminal exploitation and violence against patients. Much of the remainder is accounted for by the national problem of homelessness among the discharged mentally ill, due in part to the reluctance of some state hospitals to admit severely disturbed or potentially violent patients.

Deinstitutionalization policies were being adopted by the individual states in the 1950s at the time when federal initiatives to develop a more positive conceptualization of alternatives to the mental hospitals had been taking shape. The 1947 National Mental Health Act, which established the National Institute of Mental Health as an agency to stimulate innovations in care, owes much to the endeavours of Albert Deutsch, a journalist who was an ardent campaigner in the early post-war years and whose influential articles were subsequently republished as *The Shame of the States*. A further impetus to maintain the reform effort emanated from the mounting empirical critiques of mental hospitals by such authors as Stanton and Schwarz (1954) and Goffman (1961). Publication of the report of the Joint Commission on Mental Health in 1961 presented the newly elected President Kennedy with one of his first platforms for social reform, and his supporters were able effectively to counter the massive lobbying against the reform organized by the American Medical Association which feared insidious socialization of the health system (Martindale and Martindale, 1985). The report, which Kennedy in the first-ever presidential address on mental health affirmed as a 'bold' new approach, laid the groundwork for a federal community care programme in service areas profoundly neglected by the public bodies hitherto responsible: the states and local authorities. The main recommendation was that community mental health centres (CMHCs) should be established at a ratio of one per 50,000 population to provide a full range of general psychiatric care.

Federal legislation followed two years later in the form of the 1963 Community Mental Health Centres Construction Act which released 200 million federal dollars in the form of matching grants to run for a four-year period to cover up to 75 per cent of capital costs of each project, after which continued funding was to be solely a state and local authority responsibility. Proposals for the funding of staff, which were initially dropped in the face of stiff opposition from the American Medical Association, were enacted two years later, when uptake of the programme had proved slow due to the reluctance of some states to match federal monies to build the centres when they were not to be assisted with staffing costs. Subsequent legislative amendments carried the funding programme through to the mid-1970s.

One of the principal concerns of the Act was to provide for the seriously mentally ill, who hitherto had been the kind of patients trapped in the state hospitals for want of any alternative. The new CMHCs were to prevent unnecessary admissions by providing five key services: inpatient facilities, outpatient treatment, day care and night clinics, 24-hour crisis intervention, and a consultancy and education programme. The centres became the first structure in which the multidisciplinary team approach was seriously adopted, although in practice medically qualified staff have tended to occupy the most senior positions. However, with the expansion of the CMHC network, there has been some withdrawal of involvement by psychiatrists who regard the centres as fulfilling a social welfare rather than a clinical role. Staff rates among nurses, clinical psychologists and social workers have grown rapidly. Many psychiatrists were, in any case, employed part-time and combined CMHC work with private practice.

## Implementing the programme

Between 1965 and 1974 expenditure on the Community Mental Health Centre programme amounted to 1000 million dollars (Armour, 1981). Originally, it was envisaged that there would be over 2000 centres, but this was subsequently scaled down to 1500. By 1974, however, there were only

400 centres. Nonetheless, the programme was to produce a dramatic diffusion in the psychiatric care system which occurred during a period of a 'psychologization' of everyday life with an explosion of alternative therapies in the 'psychoboom' of the late 1960s and 1970s (Castel *et al.*, 1982).

The ten years from the mid-1960s were also a period during which libertarian issues in mental health were effectively raised. The New York Civil Liberties Union initiated a national campaign of litigation, facilitated by the introduction of legal aid schemes. Theirs was a two-flanked attack: to contest the legality of compulsory detentions and to demand improved standards of services. However, critics of this strategy have pointed out that court judgments in favour of service improvements did not call forward additional resources, and were ineffective in ensuring enactment. By and large, litigation merely forced shifts in state funds from one service area to another. However, the rise of legalism had the effect of encouraging an ongoing decline of state involvement with mental illness services. Local non-profit-making agencies increasingly took centre stage, many of the CMHCs being in the voluntary sector. According to Curtis (1986) the privately delivered but publicly funded system is now larger in some states than the public sector.

One of the chief drawbacks of the CMHC programme arises from the fact that it did not provide a means of creating a unified system for planning and funding the whole range of psychiatric services. Instead, it involved a tripartite collaborative funding between Washington, the states and the local authorities, whilst the state mental hospitals continued to be funded almost entirely from state tax sources. Critically, there has been a poor coordination of activities between centres and the state mental hospitals, some of whose functions they were to replace. The National Institute of Mental Health, the institution charged with overseeing the programme, issued only broad guidelines and the lack of any strong accountability meant that there was scope for considerable reinterpretation on the ground. No real evaluative planning criteria were developed to assess the progress of the programme. Nor did the anticipated consumer participation play a prominent role.

The programme was in essence a pump-priming exercise, albeit of massive proportions. But reluctant state and local authorities, which would both have to contribute funds, could not be forced to take part. It has also proved inadequate in guaranteeing permanent local funding for new community services. By the mid-1970s the programme still accounted for only 5 per cent of the total national mental health budget.

## Critique and prospects

The community mental health centres were the centrepiece of federal initiatives, but by the end of the 1970s many catchment areas were without a centre. The 1978 Commission appointed by President Carter, whilst expressing its commitment to the ideal of the centres, accepted much of the general criticism of the programme, especially the neglect of the long-term mentally ill. The ill-fated 1980 Mental Health Systems Act was in part aimed at alleviating the lack of coordination and improving services for chronic patients. However, events were overtaken by the 1980 Presidential election. The Reagan administration carried forward the spirit of 'new federalism' by replacing many of the federal categorical grants with non-earmarked block grants. Federal funding of programmes was simul-taneously reduced by 25 per cent, a cutback that has permeated the whole of the mental health system. All that remained was the federal Community Support Programme which has funded 20 pilot mental health projects for long-term clients. State funds remain the largest direct source of financing chronic care, and in many states over 80 per cent of this expenditure is allocated to the state hospitals (Talbott and Sharfstein, 1986). Medicare and SSI benefits have enabled the states to shift part of their burden of financing chronic care onto federal sources.

With the withdrawal of large-scale federal funding, community services are tending to provide interventions that are the most easily reimbursed, since most local authorities have not stepped in to make good the deficits. There are reports that some CMHCs are bordering on bankruptcy (Scull, 1986); others are surviving on Medicaid/Medicare payments and have gradually shifted their efforts to providing inpatient care which generates greater revenues than day and outpatient treatment. Thus, many centres may have become less community-orientated and this raises the question of whether they are openly competing with the state hospitals for in-patients (Dowell and Ciarlo, 1983).

One positive effect which can be attributed in part to the CMHC programme has been the enormous growth in outpatient psychiatry which accounted for almost three-quarters of treatment episodes by the mid-1970s. Dowell and Ciarlo (1983) cite research indicating that the pro-gramme's impact on resident inpatient rates has been relatively modest, although its contribution to reducing admission rates has been stronger. In practice, most centres have not fulfilled the alternative role to the mental hospital that was part of the original intention. However, the more enter-prising CMHCs have instigated outreach programmes that have been reasonably successful in attracting poor clients, although most of the elderly mentally ill continue to elude them. For the most part, the work of the centres reflects the predilections of their staff; there have been criti-cisms that clinically they have tended to play safe by undertaking routine work with a select clientele and have often declined to take 'difficult' patients presenting to emergency clinics. Thus, the patient profile is typified by the young, middle-income patient suffering from mild to moderate symptoms. Paradoxically, the budgetary cuts that have been imposed in the 1980s might go some way to redressing this imbalance, as centres increasingly seek out welfare patients offering guaranteed sources of reimbursement. However, it is apparent that most CMHCs continue to provide little in the way of a service to ex-inpatients: Scull (1986) refers to recent NIMH data suggesting that nationally only 4 per cent of the centres' intake comprised patients discharged from the state hospital system.

Meanwhile, the massive deinstitutionalization programme of the states has continued, despite a report of the American Psychiatric Association in 1984 which termed it a 'major societal tragedy'. During the 1970s over 75 hospitals were closed in the face of opposition provoked by fears for the local economy. The policy was in practice rarely positively conceived but, rather, was a rapid means for shedding responsibilities for long-term patients. The practice of 'transinstitutionalization', whereby many clients end up in large nursing homes, some of highly dubious quality, has partially offset the decline in the state hospital population and has done nothing to reduce their marginalized status. Moreover, other ex-patients fare no better but are in prison, cheap hotels or are destitute. Although some state hospitals continue to accept patients the locally based services reject, many are increasingly reluctant to admit the severely disturbed, for whom there is often no alternative but the prison cell. According to NIMH data, only 7 per cent of long-term patients are now left in the state hospitals. On the other hand, there was a more than 100 per cent increase in patient numbers in nursing homes in the early 1970s, a transfer made possible by the introduction of federal and state welfare programmes. In the 1960s and 1970s, in fact, private nursing homes were something of a boom industry as welfare payments rolled in, but the retrenchment of the 1980s has seen some large undertakings go bankrupt.

Currently, it is estimated that over one million ex-inpatients live in private households, sometimes sharing with their relatives; 750,000 reside in nursing homes; and between 750,000 and 1,500,000 live in other settings, many being in prison or on the streets (Talbott and Sharfstein, 1986). Indeed, there have been several exposés of the scandal of homelessness among the mentally ill. In 1984 *Newsweek* magazine calculated that between a third and a half of all homeless were former inpatients. The situation is well known to be worst in the largest cities, a study in New York City estimating that the proportion of the homeless who are 'mentally disabled' could be as high as 60 per cent (Curtis, 1986). In recent years the City has been employing mobile clinical teams to work among the homeless. However, this policy is not without its opponents, the New York Civil Liberties Union being among those, who argue that it provides a smokescreen diverting attention away from the fact that inadequate resources continue to be allocated to creating vital housing and care facilities.

THE ITALIAN EXPERIENCE

In Italy legislative reform came about largely through pressure from an alliance forged between left-of-centre politicians, trade unions and the movement, 'Psichiatria Democratica', whose chief ideologue was Franco Basaglia. Support was organized in parliament by the small but effective Radical Party, the need for reform being argued within the context of wider demands for the establishment of a comprehensive national health service. However, proposals for mental health reform were first seriously mooted in the early 1960s when parliamentary interest was shown in the newly introduced French policy of sectorization. Although the Communist Party introduced a bill on sectorization in 1965, all that was achieved was a relatively modest amendment of the 1904 basic legislation to permit voluntary admissions to public mental hospitals and sanction the crea-tion of outpatient 'mental hygiene' clinics. The 'events' of 1968 probably had more effect in Italy than anywhere else in Europe (Simons, 1980) and subsequently led to demands among the trade unions and the left for widespread social reforms. The enactment of regionalisation policies in 1970 provided real political opportunity for mental health reform in some parts of the country, since it sanctioned a substantial degree of decentra-lization of policy-making, with the transfer of health responsibilities from the old provinces to the 20 regions, and created a unified structure for local health planning and organization. Central government has retained few policy-making powers; variation in both the character and quality of health and welfare facilities is therefore inevitable. There have been criticisms that the lack of national coordination compromises the principle of geographi-cal equity. A national health plan which should have been prepared immediately after the establishment of the national health service in 1978 is still awaited.

Some authorities judge that ten regions had begun seriously to imple-ment community care policies before the passing of the basic legislation, Law 180, in 1978 (Balduzzi and Balduzzi, 1981). Four psychiatric hospitals had been closed prior to the legislation. After regional devolution some of the traditionally 'red' regions in central Italy formulated their own plans for psychiatric reform. But reform initiatives also extended to a few northern regions dominated by the Christian Democrats, such as the Veneto. Some of the earliest and best-documented local experiences are those of Gorizia initiated by Franco Basaglia in 1963, Perugia and Trieste (Ramon, 1985).

**La Libertà e Terapeutica**

The Italian reform was strongly influenced by Psichiatria Democratica (PD), a movement formed in 1974 to unite committed progressives, largely though not exclusively among professionals. PD was to change the balance of power within Italian psychiatry. Clinically, it espouses eclecticism; there is no one formal therapeutic model. The role of psychotropic medication is tolerated, even accepted, but electro-shock treatment is rejected. Anti-psychiatry is also regarded as theoretically unsound, since for PD the private is always political (Ramon, 1985).

PD's most celebrated campaigner has been the late Franco Basaglia, who in the early 1970s emerged as the leading reform personality and theorist. In the Gorizia team's best-known book, *L'Istituzione Negata*, Basaglia argued that the innate contradictions of the asylum are fundamentally irreconcilable: namely, how to care for and liberate in an environment of marginalization and custodialism (Basaglia, 1968). For him the mental hospital was an arena for political struggle. Madness can only be con-quered as a social problem, for what psychiatry terms sickness society calls dangerous. Madness can only be overcome by dismantling the rigid hierarchical set of relationships that the asylum represents. Success in achieving this depends on the wider involvement of progressive workers' and students' movements (Basaglia, 1980). Within a year of his move from Gorizia to Trieste the local mental hospital had been all but emptied according to a carefully orchestrated programme: patients organized their own newspapers; patient cooperatives were formed; festivals organized for the local populace, including hospital closure celebrations; and a close alliance forged with local politicians and trade unions. The walls of the mental hospital were torn down and the remaining patients were con-ferred with the status of 'ospiti'.

## The passing of the Act

Because of immediate political pressures, Law 180 was drafted and passed quickly without prior evaluations or parliamentary inquiries. In their petition for reform Psichiatria Democratica had succeeded in collecting the necessary half-million signatures which, according to the Italian Constitu-tion, would have set in train a national referendum on the question of the reform of the 1904 legislation. Referenda on social issues, notably divorce, had caused political embarrassment in the past, particularly for the Chris-tian Democrats. There was an understandable desire on the politicians' part to avoid any repetition and, in any case, mental health policies were principally a concern of the regions, so implementation would largely not be Rome's affair. Thus, the Law eschews the imposition of a rigid blueprint which would unnecessarily constrain the regions. Excluded from the scope of the legislation were the six forensic hospitals, private hospitals and other residential institutions, and services principally intended for substance abusers.

Law 180 was a compromise between what PD reformers would have proposed and a strategy that would carry the professional mainstream along. It did not represent a complete vindication of the anti-institutional stance: compulsory admission was to continue as an option; the mental hospitals were retained, at least in the short run; and a prominent role was allocated to psychiatric 'diagnosis and cure' (D&C) units in general hospitals. However, the legislation promoted the full integration of psychiatry into the rest of medicine, and formalized public sector commitment to provision of alternatives to the mental hospital. All this was to be achieved, not by a crude programme of deinstitutionalization, as Italian critics interpreted the experience in the United States, but by a careful rehabilitation strategy worked out locally.

There was an explicit policy not to have too long a transitional period for the closure to admissions to the mental hospitals. This was to prevent a prolonged implementation period. First admissions to public hospitals were stopped but readmissions were allowed until December 1980, although in the event this was prolonged until December 1981. Building permissions for new hospitals could no longer be sanctioned and those in the pipeline were rescinded. Fundamental was the freeing of psychiatry from juridical control, authorization of compulsory admissions being transferred from the magistracy to the local mayor. Periods of commitment were reduced and procedures were tightened to make such admissions exceptional rather than routine (Giancanelli, 1981). Compulsory admissions to private hospitals were discontinued in 1978. The great strength of the Law was the shift in focus away from a person's individual psychopathology to the right to treatment and to the services available to cope with mental disorder. The hospital's hegemony was to be broken. Instead, a decentralized system of formal and informal care was envisaged offering preventive, treatment and aftercare facilities from a non-mental hospital base. Community mental health centres were to be the key element in the new network and were to provide a full range of in-house and domiciliary services, collaborating closely with local welfare, housing and education services (Ramon, 1985).

The few planning norms contained in the legislation refer to acute inpatient beds. A maximum of fifteen beds per 200,000 population was permitted, which were to be located in the community mental health centres to be established, or in D&C units in general hospitals which, in place of the old mental hospitals, were to be the location for emergency admissions. In addition, the legislation provided that no more than fifteen beds in private psychiatric hospitals could be licensed to obtain reimbursement from the national health service for new admissions and, moreover, these hospitals are not permitted to confine themselves to psychiatric inpatient work.

## Assessments of the Italian reform

The debate on the Italian reform centres around the question of whether the problems that have occurred are due to poor or non-implementation, or whether the reform itself is based on unsound and untested principles. The late 1970s were scarcely a propitious time to embark on major and potentially expensive innovations and, critically, the state did not allocate additional funds to promote the policy. Nonetheless, proponents of the reform argued that the Law had to be enacted quickly to maintain momentum: waiting for a gradual development of alternative facilities, they considered, might lead to ossification of the reform process, with the mental hospital retaining its central role, as it does in other psychiatric systems. Others argue that the reform legislation was strong on abolition of the old but short on conceptualization of the new, and that it destroyed incremental but more soundly-based initiatives that were already under way in various parts of the country. They point out that the acid test of the reform lies in its poor performance in the larger cities, and that centres of excellence have tended to be small and medium-sized free-standing towns, often with a relatively plentiful supply of housing for discharged patients, and where coordination among local health districts has not been a major problem.

Assessments of specific aspects of the 'Italian' experience must allow not only for marked regional variation in implementation, but also for the comparative lack of routine official statistics. As in a number of other European countries, inpatient bed numbers in Italy were declining before enactment of the law in 1978. In fact, the trend began in the late 1960s and gathered pace from the mid-1970s. It is therefore difficult to assess reliably how much of the decline is attributable to the reform legislation. Currently there are about 35,000 beds, about half of the number existing in 1978. However, the trend of decline varies substantially across the country and between the public and private sector, the latter having experienced a smaller contraction. This disparity also applies to numbers of bed-days. Since enactment there has been only a 1 per cent decline in the proportion of total bed capacity taken up by psychiatry (38 per cent) in the south compared with a 9 per cent reduction in northern and central regions (Morosini et al., 1985). Moreover, by Anglo-Saxon standards the proportion of compulsory admissions has on average remained high, and in recent years has begun to climb again (Basaglia, 1987): in the south they amount to 45 per cent of the total (Morosini et al., 1985), but in contrast in Trieste only seven commitments were made in 1983 (Ramon, 1985).

Many of the patients remaining in the mental hospitals have been given the status of 'ospiti'. Although legal advantages accrue from this policy, there have been claims that, in reality, the change has meant little for some patients who reside on long-term wards that are frequently kept locked (Jones and Poletti, 1986). Of the 52,000 resident patients in 1978, 38,000 were still there in 1981 (Perris and Kemali, 1985). Currently, the mental hopitals are in a vacuum, their longevity largely being assured until the last cohort of patients dies, since alternative facilities for the old long-stay are generally lacking and there is no policy of massive disposal of elderly patients to nursing homes, although some are transferring to old people's homes. Public sector cutbacks have contributed to a further deterioration of the physical state of many hospitals, although in some there has been considerable outlay in converting premises into group homes and in creating rehabilitation units.

Reform implementation has been dismally slow in some regions where, apart from inpatient beds, there is an almost total lack of alternative provisions. Tansella and colleagues (1987) discovered, for example, that apart from CMHCs there are only 32 day care facilities in the country (1:1.8 million). There is also a chronic shortage of both staffed hostels (1:660,000) and unstaffed hostels (1:150,000). Although the value of these structures is contested by some professionals, who perceive a danger of new forms of institutionalism, there have been entirely valid criticisms that in practice the reform in most areas has relied too much on the willingness of relatives to make good the deficits in formal care resources. As such 'community' care becomes a spuriously cheaper option. Several relatives' organizations have emerged at the national level, though their views differ on the direction they wish new policies to take.

Given the relative lack of alternative services, it is perhaps not surprising that admissions to D&C units are becoming more routine than was originally envisaged, even though less than 60 per cent of the planned units have been built (Lovell, 1986). Many within the PD had argued that psychiatric beds should be decanted throughout the general hospital rather than 'ghettoized' in a separate unit. Separate provision has, however, been the norm, and in some cases the units occupy remote positions on hospital sites, with the consequent danger that they may reproduce the isolation of the old asylums. In some hospitals there is an insistence that the units are kept locked, and that patients who leave the premises must be accompanied by nursing personnel. Some units occupy cramped and unsatisfactory accommodation with few clinical facilities and little provision for rehabilitation.

The impact of the reform on private inpatient and residential facilities has received considerable attention. The private hospital occupies a somewhat ambivalent position within the politics of the Italian NHS. Some central and southern regions are heavily dependent on private psychiatric beds. Private facilities of all kinds, many of them run by religious orders, have long enjoyed a hegemony of provision, and these regions historically have been poorly equipped with public services. The emerging conclusion is that there may be a potentially limitless role for these institutions as substitutes for the back wards of mental hospitals, especially in the hospitalization of the older patient with a long psychiatric career. The clinics are admitting many patients who were formerly long-stay residents in public hospitals. It has been found that their patients remain for longer periods with shorter intervening spells between discharge and readmission. Patient turnover is therefore low (Perris and Kemali, 1985). Moreover, continuity of care is a considerable problem because the private hospitals do not have sector responsibilies and accept patients from a wide geographical area.

It is not possible to disentangle the statistics on the prison population to assess the effects on the reform there; nor is it possible to ascertain whether the increase in bed-days in forensic hospitals is due to an increase in the numbers of patients being referred, or to increases in the length of stay, or both (Tansella et al., 1987).

Lovell (1986) argues that there is no evidence of mass 'dumping' of patients, although there have been incidences of 'wild discharges' in some areas, and newspapers have published numerous articles on the plight of the 'abandonati'. A study of three areas in which psychiatric case registers operate indicates that 'new long-stay' are not accumulating in hospitals, although large numbers continue to require long-term care in the community (Tansella et al., 1987).

Doctors in private office practice have survived the establishment of the national health service. Doctors are contracted to treat public patients in addition to their work with private patients. Research on social class and diagnostic profiles indicates the existence of a form of 'two-tier' psychiatry, private practice being more involved with higher-income groups and with patients suffering from neuroses and public sector inpatient and outpatient services being more closely associated with the treatment of patients with psychosis and, more generally, those with low incomes (Bollini et al., 1984).

## Prospects

There is little doubt that the achievements of the reform may now be under threat, and PD is marshalling support to defend it. A serious handicap arose from the economic climate prevailing in the early stages of implementation which coincided with the period when the recession was entering its deepest phase. In 1980, not long after the institution of the national health service, the Italian government imposed a moratorium on new posts and the health service generally was subjected to stricter cost-containment measures. In 1982 health care expenditure was reduced by one-fifth. Non-replacement of staff and reliance on short-term contracts have hit community services more than the hospitals, which continue to receive the lion's share of the mental health budget. Several regions which were among the most enthusiastic reformers have blown cold, and there is a growing body of centre and right-wing opinion pressing for legislative amendments. Proposals to establish medium-stay institutions, often by conversion of mental hospital premises, have been discussed since the early 1980s and legislation has been in draft form since 1982. At present, the Italian parliament is studying the various proposals to create institutions for different client groups judged in need of long-term residential care. It is envisaged that these institutions would consist of 200-bed units, 80 beds being reserved for the mentally ill. Additional monies would become available to implement these plans if accepted. There have also been proposals to amend the procedures for compulsory admission, extending the limit for detention from 7 to 15 or even 30 days.

In the meantime, regions such as Lombardy are going their own way, and have created rehabilitation centres with staffed residential facilities in some of their old mental hospitals. Other regions, sensing that legislative amendment was likely, have been exceptionally late in introducing their own regional plans for full enactments of the reform. Legislation in Naples, for example, was not promulgated until 1983 and implementation so far has been less than enthusiastic (Scala and Gritti, 1985). Lovell (1986) suggests that in 1984 almost half of the regions had failed to designate the full range of services for which the local health districts were to be responsible.

## CONCLUSION

Each national plan for mental health reform has had to respond to a specific mental health system. However, in all countries reforms have been conceptualized within the framework of some form of sectorization to provide a service network giving pride of place, at least in theory, to locally based services. The new policies have emphasized the multidisciplinary approach to therapy, and have specified that a comprehensive range of preventive, treatment and aftercare facilities should be created to fulfil one of the wider goals of preventing unnecessary hospital admissions. Yet in most states a nebulous future was prescribed for the mental hospitals, at least in the middle run, and, although some countries are now engaged in extensive hospital closure programmes that are cost-led, only in Italy was policy formulated with a clear view to abolishing the mental hospital network.

A crucial constraint in reform implementation has been the lack of an adequate means of across-the-board financing of the kinds of services the long-term client is likely to require. The process of creating new facilities has been slow, and incremental advances have meant that provisions are typically piecemeal, with marked geographical variation in availability. To a large extent the establishment of vital locally based services is determined by ease of reimbursement, either through some form of social assistance, earmarked government budgets, general taxation or sickness and invalidity insurance. Some countries have attempted reform whilst maintaining the 'liberal' character of their health system: France and Quebec, for example, have instituted the 'global budget' system of financing hospital and outpatient care, although the system in France is to be reformed again because of opposition from the social insurance schemes to honouring part of their new liabilities. Others, notably the German-speaking countries, have retained the traditional system of reimbursing treatment via the item-of-service system, perpetuating the innate dangers of rewarding overprovision of outpatient and inpatient services. Only in Italy has a new mental health system been accompanied by a comprehensive reform of the health service, albeit with the retention of private office practice. Some countries have examined ways of reducing reliance on social assistance reimbursement for the costs of long-term care by extending the insurance principle. The Netherlands and Luxembourg have introduced 'heavy-risk' insurance to finance chronic care of various kinds and, for a time, the German federal government considered this possibility.

The various compromise solutions have particularly retarded the development of community services for the high-contact user. Some systems maintain illogical distinctions between 'treatment' and 'care' in assessing liabilities for the costs of care (for example, France) and in others there is a meticulous policing of a reimbursement system that seeks to distinguish 'medical', 'social' and 'occupational' rehabilitation (for example, West Germany). It is not only the users who suffer from these disjunctions but also some providers. Many of the agencies providing rehabilitative and residential facilities for this clientele are small and recently established, and can be heavily dependent on public sector subsidies, in addition to social assistance reimbursement for the costs of care (for a review of the situation in Germany, see Mangen, 1985). At the same time, the central role of office psychiatrists in Continental systems—in Germany, for example, they were afforded near-monopoly rights to provide outpatient treatment—has meant that a form of 'two-tier' psychiatry has been created whereby poor patients and those suffering from psychoses use public 'community' services, and the middle- to high-income patient consults the office practitioner, treatment being partly if not wholly reimbursed through health insurance.

Calls for strategic planning of mental health services have come precisely at a time when actual planning capacities have been declining. Plans formulated in periods of relative economic prosperity have faced implementation in the post-oil crisis recession. Moreover, increasing reliance on private non-profit and profit-making agencies, together with the decentralization of policy-making, have contributed to the plural character of the psychiatric system by multiplying the number of agencies which, to be effective, must be incorporated into the planning process.

Essentially, the long-term client is the victim of the contradictions contained in policies on community care, the vocabulary in which psychiatric reform was articulated. Once uncritically promoted as the ideal model of care, this panacea is increasingly being called into question, and the benefits of old institutional solutions are now being re-examined in some circles in a more positive light. In the meantime, the search for cheap solutions has seen the adoption of policies of 'transinstitutionalization' in many countries, that has given rise to a regrettable new 'trade in lunacy', creating new social spaces in which the logic of the asylum has been reproduced.

Cross-nationally, there is now little consensus about a blueprint for community care, either in terms of the range of services to be established, the degree to which the system should be directed by professionals or acknowledge and incorporate a central role for informal care, or, more critically, about its wider social functions.

## REFERENCES

Armour, P. K. (1981). *The Cycles of Social Reform: Mental health policy making in the United States, England and Sweden*, Washington University Press of America.

Balduzzi, E., and Balduzzi, C. (1981). La Loi Psychiatrique du 13 Mai 1978: Introduction au Probleme, *L'Information Psychiatrique*, **57**, 567–80.

Basaglia, F. (ed.) (1968). *L'Istituzione Negate: Rapporto da un Ospedale Psichiatrico*, Einaudi Editore, Turin.

Basaglia, F. (1980). Problems of law and psychiatry: the Italian experience, *International Journal of Law and Psychiatry*, **3**, 17–37.

Basaglia, F. (1987). Preface. In Scheper-Hughes, N., and Lovell. A. (eds) *Psychiatry Inside Out: selected writings of Franco Basaglia*, Columbia University Press, New York.

Bollini, P., Muscettola, G., Piazza, A., Puca, M., and Tognoni, G. (1984). Mental health care in southern Italy: a case control evaluation of the quality of care. Istituto Mario Negri, Milan (mimeo).

Castel, R. (1981). *La Gestion des Risques: de L'Anti-Psychiatrie a L'Apres Psychiatrie*, Editions de Minuit, Paris.

Castel, F., Castel, R., and Lovell, A. (1982). *The Psychiatric Society*, Columbia University Press, New York.

Curtis, W. R. (1986). The deinstitutionalisation story, *The Public Interest*, **85**, 34–49.

Deutsch, A. (1948). The Shame of the States. New York, Harcourt Brace Jovanovich Inc.

Dowell, D. A., and Ciarlo, J. A. (1983). Overview of the community mental health centres programme from an evaluation perspective, *Community Mental Health Journal*, **19**, 95–125.

Fagin, L. (1985). Deinstitutionalisation in the USA, *Bulletin of the Royal College of Psychiatrists*, **9**, 112–18.

Giancanelli, F. (1981). La Metamorphose Possible: Réflexions sur la Reforme de la Psychiatrie en Italie. *L'Information Psychiatrique*, **57**, 607–13.

Goffman, E. (1961). *Asylums: essays on the social situation of mental patients and other inmates*, Penguin, Harmondsworth.

Jones, K., and Poletti, A. (1986). The 'Italian Experience' reconsidered, *British Journal of Psychiatry*, **148**, 144–50.

Lovell, A. (1986). The paradoxes of reform: re-evaluating Italy's mental health law of 1978, *Hospital and Community Psychiatry*, **37**, 802–8.

Mangen, S. P. (1985). Germany: the enquete and its aftermath. In Mangen, S. P. (ed.) *Mental Health Care in the European Community*, Croom Helm, London.

Martindale, D., and Martindale, E. (1985). *Mental Disability in America since World War Two* Philosophical Library, New York.

Morosini, P. L., Repetto, F., De Salvia, D., and Cecere, F. (1985). Psychiatric hospitalisation in Italy before and after 1978, *Acta Psychiatrica Scandinavica*, (Suppl. 316), **71**, 27–44.

Perris, C., and Kemali, D. (1985). Focus on the Italian psychiatric reform: an introduction, *Acta Psychiatrica Scandinavica* (Suppl. 316), **71**, 9–14.

Ramon, S. (1985). The Italian psychiatric reform. In Mangen, S. (ed.) *Mental Health Care in the European Community*, Croom Helm, London.

Scala, A., and Gritti, P. (1985). The impact of psychiatric reform on inpatient services in a metropolitan area of southern Italy: the Naples case, *Acta Psychiatrica Scandinavica*, (Suppl. 316), **71**, 151–7.

Scull, A. (1986). Mental patients and the community: a critical note, *International Journal of Law and Psychiatry*, **9**, 383–92.

Sedgwick, P. (1981). *Psychopolitics*, Pluto Press, London.

Simons, T. (1980). Psychiatrie im Übergang: von der Verwaltung der sozialen Ausgrenzung zum sozialen Dienst. In Simons, T. (ed.) *Absage an die Anstalt: Programm und Realität der demokratischen Psychiatrie in Italien*, Campus Verlag, Frankfurt.

Stanton, A. H., and Schwarz, M. S. (1954). *The Mental Hospital: a study of institutional participation in psychiatric illness and treatment*, Basic Books, New York.

Talbott, J. A., and Sharfstein, S. S. (1986). A proposal for future funding of chronic and episodic mental illness, *Hospital and Community Psychiatry*, **37**, 1126–30.

Tansella, M., De Salvia, D., and Williams, P. (1987). The Italian psychiatric reform: some quantitative evidence. *Social Psychiatry*, **22**, 37–48.

# Section B

# *Planning Community Services*

Community Care in Practice
Edited by A. Lavender and F. Holloway
© 1988 John Wiley & Sons Ltd

Chapter 4

# Planning for High-quality Local Services

## SU KINGSLEY and DAVID TOWELL

Any examination of the changes in psychiatric services in different parts of Britain over the past decade or more would show considerable variations in both the pace and nature of local development. At best, as other chapters in this book report, there has been some growth in high-quality services, often quite small in scale, which reflects the energy and ability of local innovators. However the current context (Towell and McAusland, 1984) is one in which incremental growth is being overtaken by pressures for more rapid and large-scale changes, particularly associated with the decentralization of NHS institutional provision.

These pressures present a period of opportunity; and a period of risks. As both the House of Commons Social Services Committee (1985) and the Audit Commission (1986) have argued forcibly, the national strategic framework and financial policies within which change is occurring are far from adequate. There is also considerable evidence that weaknesses in traditional approaches to planning and implementation at local level may mean that opportunities for real improvements in services will be wasted (Etherington and Bosanquet, 1985).

Where improvements are evident they often appear to be due to the efforts of one or two key individuals—this has created difficulties in generalizing and sustaining changes. These 'innovations' frequently remain only that, and do not fulfil their potential of changing services on a larger scale. However, in those cases where broader shifts are being achieved (for example in Exeter Health Authority) it is apparent that the local context for change provided fertile ground for local change leaders to work in. This suggests the importance of working and persevering at change, rather than reliance on charismatic individuals; and requires recognition of the long-term nature of change which needs nurturing, rather than occurring overnight.

It follows, then, that the development of high-quality services requires

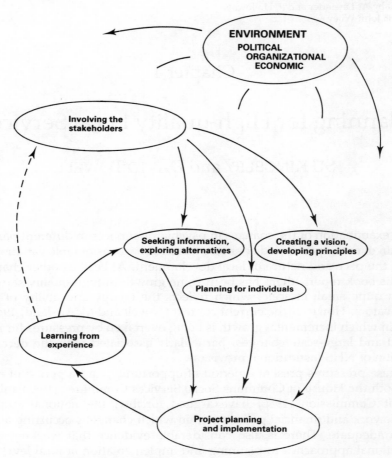

Figure 4.1   Elements in an organic model of service development.

attention not only to the design of these services but equally to the design of the *process* of service development itself.

The approach to planning, described in this chapter, seeks to integrate the process and content of service design to create an organic model of service development. Its major themes and their interrelationships are illustrated in Figure 4.1. The figure seeks to represent planning as a number of overlapping activities which require regular review and revision. The planning task is one of repeated cycles, rather than a linear series of steps. The model includes six main elements:

1. commitment to involving a broad range of stakeholders in the future pattern of psychiatric services in contributing their expertise and experience to the process of service development;
2. stress on the importance of planning for individuals and therefore developing methods for directly involving service users in this participative approach;
3. recognition that the development of high-quality services must start from clarity about the values and principles which define quality, and be guided by a shared vision of what would constitute a desirable future;
4. investment in a variety of information-seeking activities designed to map potential demand, increase awareness of how services impact on individual users and explore alternative ways of meeting needs which will be consistent with these principles;
5. recognition that plans need to be revised and reformulated as lessons are drawn from the experience of implementation;
6. careful attention to the way all these activities can be incorporated into the formal decision-making structures of the larger public agencies (particularly the NHS and local authorities) responsible for providing local psychiatric services.

This process is intended to be dynamic. The challenge of planning for new patterns of services is to go beyond existing and known forms of provision. This will require a robust framework for dealing with and adapting to changing circumstances, while always maintaining a clear end in view.

The model has emerged from work with managers and professional staff (NHS, local authorities and voluntary agencies), from over a third of the local services in England and Wales. In elaborating these ideas emphasis will be placed on the development of services to meet the needs of adults with severe psychiatric disabilities. This description gives particular attention to the features of the model which are not common in much current practice, beginning from the importance of seeing planning as everybody's business.


INVOLVING THE STAKEHOLDERS

Health service development has traditionally been led by professional interests, although this has been extended since the 1974 reorganization to include key service managers who have a broader focus on the overall provision of services, (see Butts et al., 1981; Glennerster et al., 1983; Tallis, 1981). Designing major changes in the pattern of service delivery needs to involve a much wider group of interests—including both providers and recipients. A series of questions may be helpful in identifying representatives of these broader interests. Who has a legitimate concern with the future pattern of psychiatric services? As the situation changes, who will be able to influence decisions? Who stands to gain? Who stands to lose? In a group considering community mental health centres, a response to these questions produced a list of seventeen agencies which included the Samaritans, local housing officers, a counselling agency, service users, various groups of professional service workers, mental health voluntary organizations, health authority members, relatives and carers groups, and local branches of national specialist agencies.

Other groups considering different aspects of psychiatric services are likely to produce lists with a similarly wide range of interested parties. Traditionally many of these agencies have been excluded from important decisions concerning service development, although their contributions are potentially very valuable. They represent a wealth of interest and energy which creative planning can harness. In particular, people who are current and past service users, relatives and carers, and front-line staff all have perspectives on the ways in which services are delivered, but have not generally been involved or consulted in the development of new services.

In planning community-based services, where much of the eventual success of the service will depend on the support of a network of groups and agencies with no single body in overall control, building shared commitment at an early stage is an essential process.

## Mobilizing multi-agency groups

The starting point for creating wider service-development networks can vary. Where major developments are concerned, however, it is important that at the centre of these networks there is a core of senior managers (like the joint planning groups suggested in the Nodder (DHSS, 1980), and MIND (1983) proposals) able to integrate planning with the formal decision-making structures of the NHS and local authorities. Such collaboration is, of course, likely to be promoted where authorities have made commitments to a joint approach; reflected, for example, in agreeing to pool financial resources in a programme budget (Glennerster et al., 1983) for mental health services.

However, participative planning requires much wider involvement. In North Lincolnshire Health Authority, for example, a group of 23 people from all levels of the service, and including service users, relatives and informal carers, were brought together to generate designs for a future service (Collin, 1985). The wide membership of the group meant that it encompassed a much broader range of backgrounds and experience than is common in planning groups—and this meant that much greater attention had to be paid to how the group worked together, to ensure that everyone had an equal opportunity to take part.

Another example of joint action between different agencies comes from the 'Coalition for Community Care', a voluntary group, initiated by three CHCs and their local MIND associations in West London. The aim of the coalition is to focus attention on the need for joint strategies for mental health service development, in an area where joint working has been severely handicapped by overlapping geographical boundaries and unclear responsibilities. The 'Coalition' now has members from the local statutory providers as well as concerned individuals, users and ex-users of mental health services, and other voluntary groups. It has become an important neutral meeting ground where perceptions and ideas can be shared between groups with diverse backgrounds and interests.

The large size of these groups is of course a challenge in itself. Working in a group of 30–40 people requires new techniques, and is a very different experience from the small committee structures more common in traditional service planning. Meetings need careful organizing, and this is likely to involve small group work and well-managed large group sessions, to ensure opportunities for everyone to participate. Larger groups are also likely to bring in people who are unaccustomed to committee procedures and who may need specific encouragement in order to participate fully. There are already a number of examples which illustrate how large planning groups can be enabled to work effectively. In North Lincolnshire an external facilitator was brought in to design a process through which the group could work together. The large group used an exercise which enabled them to agree on some common guidelines for service development. They then split into smaller task groups of four to six people, to work on detailed proposals for developing particular aspects of the service. These proposals were brought back to the larger group for approval before being put to the then District Management Team. Coalition for Community Care and forums in Lambeth, Islington and Lewisham have all been helped by paid workers who, in addition to doing administrative work for the group, also arrange a programme of meetings, sometimes with outside speakers or leaders, providing opportunities for the group to think through major issues.

Alternatively, a group which starts from a small core may draw in local expertise through setting up a series of subgroups around specific topics, each of which then creates a new nucleus attracting other people. This cascade or pyramid system has been used successfully in places where districts have identified localities as a basis for service planning and delivery.

## Community participation

Bringing local community representatives into service planning is a much more challenging task than bringing together different professional agencies. We have little real experience in Britain of community participation to fall back on, and that which we do have often looks like empty tokenism. (For example, the lone consumer whose voice is swamped and whose confidence is undermined in a committee of experienced professionals.) Yet there are good reasons for extending participation to the community, as illustrated by Exeter's experience of 'locality planning' (Court, 1984; King and Court, 1984). By contributing their knowledge and expertise, local people can improve the quality of service planning and help to make maximum use of available resources. Participation in planning can ease implementation, through defusing opposition at an early stage and re-routing concern into productive activities. Local participation is an important channel through which planning groups can receive initial feedback. Finally, since community care must also be about desegregation it demands an active involvement from the community, not simply passive acquiescence.

It is important to start here by thinking small. Traditionally the smallest unit for planning in the NHS has been the health district—with a population of between 200,000 and 500,000 and an area ranging from a crowded few square miles in an inner-city area, to rural districts which stretch 50 miles in one direction and 40 in the other. The current trend towards decentralization in social services and housing departments has demonstrated that the areas with which local residents identify are much smaller than this, usually including only 5000–10,000 people (Barclay, 1982). Further, as interest has grown in coordinating the efforts of statutory services with voluntary agencies and informal carers it has become evident that this is more feasible within a small locality. So in planning the future pattern of mental health services there is much to be said for seeking ways to develop planning based on neighbourhoods and small localities, rather than planning which attempts to suit the needs of a whole health district in a blanket way. At the same time, experience in social services decentralization has already shown that a framework of specialized services remains important, providing support to local services, and actively liaising between local and district services. People with continuing care needs are likely to be especially vulnerable to isolation, and consequently may be overlooked by services not charged specifically with ensuring that their needs are met.

Experience in Exeter and elsewhere suggests ten preconditions if community participation is to be productive:

1. local people should be viewed as a resource, with innovative ideas for meeting needs, not simply a source of additional demands;
2. the local community's concern to develop an appropriate local service

should be respected—it is in the community that mental health problems arise and most people, even with severe psychiatric disabilities,
are already living outside hospitals;

3. participation should offer an opportunity for local people to influence
   plans and priorities, not merely a public relations exercise in disguise;
4. local views and questions need to be taken seriously—naivety may be
   a result of lack of information, but can also point to fundamental issues
   which sophisticated approaches have glossed over, as in the fairy-story
   of 'The Emperor's new clothes';
5. localities need to be defined on the basis of subjective experience,
   rather than administrative convenience;
6. participation demands an informed public, which means that local
   people will need access to information and education;
7. initiating community involvement is likely to require an informal or
   personal approach, building on local leaders and networks: formal
   meetings are not enough to overcome a long history in which people
   have been excluded from decision-making;
8. for the same reasons persistence will also be required, and appropriate
   administrative support available which avoids bureaucratic procedures
   and professional jargon;
9. effective participation requires genuine dialogue, and demands that
   professionals learn to listen to local people;
10. finally, success breeds success—first steps in participation need to be
    built around projects where visible outcomes are likely to be created
    sooner rather than later (Hoggett and Hambleton, 1987; Beresford and
    Croft, 1986).

## Working with conflict

Bringing many different 'stakeholders' into a single planning forum will
introduce significant differences in interests, perspective and ideology.
Indeed making conflicts explicit at the planning stage is an intentional part
of the strategy to avoid plans being undermined during implementation.

In planning a future service which depends on involvement from a
broad spectrum of groups these differences need to be recognized and
understood. Small planning groups often function quite comfortably for
their members, precisely because they have excluded any dissenting
voices. However, the price of this exclusion is subsequent opposition.
There seems to be much to be gained from identifying and exploring
differences at an earlier stage in the process.

Conflicts are often embodied in the varying perspectives which derive
from different therapeutic models. The classic expression of such conflicts
is the difference between the 'medical' and 'social' models of distress,
epitomized by tussles between doctors and social workers.

Some of these conflicts relate to fundamental differences in approach to people with long-term psychiatric disabilities, their 'human nature' and the place they deserve to take in the world. Underlying these differences, however, are often other agendas concerning providers' interests, and the relative influence of different groups in changing patterns of services.

Amongst the professions represented within psychiatric service teams, doctors have been recognized as having a legitimate role in service development for the longest time. As services move out of the site of medical focus, and into a more social arena, other professional groups—psychologists, social workers, occupational therapists—come to play a more central role, and begin to assert rights as independent practitioners. Involvement of voluntary groups, consumer representative bodies such as CHCs and service users themselves, presents a new range of challenges. There are no easy ways to resolve these conflicts. A first step is to recognize them. A second step may be to identify areas of shared aspirations and areas of difference—and to accept that differences may form the basis of alternative approaches.

## BRINGING IN SERVICE USERS

Users are key stakeholders in planning and providing new services. The development of participative planning provides a major opportunity to increase the contribution which service users make to decisions about future patterns of provision, and to tailor specific services to their needs. The direct experiences and lives of people who use the service are powerful tools. Individuals do not fit neatly into service packages, particularly where rigid boundaries exist between organizations and professions. Breaking out of conventional patterns of thinking about services can generate a range of alternative ideas for future services. One way to achieve this is to use individuals and their experiences as the focus and starting point for planning new services.

One persuasive example of the way in which plans changed when individual needs became the focus is provided by a 'getting to know you' exercise carried out with five elderly men, each with a long history of residence in a large psychiatric hospital (Braisby, 1984). Working backwards from detailed knowledge of the five individuals, rather than forwards from residential places most easily available, suggested that the five would be better suited to a group home than the local authority 'Part III' home previously suggested. This is by no means a revolutionary solution, and in this case did not require a major re-think of local service provision. What the exercise did do was to challenge the conventional assumptions held about the individuals, and through getting to know them open up other—existing—service options which would much more effectively meet their needs for accommodation and support.

While starting out by considering individual needs can provide a source of creative tension it has also led to frustration and feelings of impotence in other situations. There seem to be three key points which anyone intending to design a service development process around individuals needs to be aware of. First, concern to meet individual needs must itself be rooted in a set of values and principles, established and agreed locally, which can subsequently provide reliable guidelines for the practical stages of the project. Second, the methodology needs to be well planned in advance: this will sustain activity and provide a means for organizing and sharing complex information. Finally long-term success can only be achieved through ensuring that innovative projects like this are integrated into the formal planning machinery.

People involved in other 'getting to know you' projects have devoted considerable time to familiarizing themselves with the day-to-day lives, and histories, of small groups of mental hospital residents, identifying similarities and differences in the residents' experiences, and ambitions for their futures. Using concrete terms and everyday language for these descriptions enabled staff and volunteers to get beyond the restrictive categories of existing service provision. This helped the groups to consider very specific needs, so that rather than thinking in terms of 'dependency levels' they spoke of needs for food, shelter, friends and so on. Moving on from specific individual needs they were able to hypothesize a range of alternative service designs. From these they drew out the service framework which needed to be created in order for the individuals to leave hospital and resume their lives in the community. Similar approaches are equally important in the design of services to support people with psychiatric disabilities already living in the community (North Manchester District Health Authority, 1987).

Service users can be brought into the planning process in a number of different ways. They may be asked to participate directly in a service planning group; their views may be represented through a user group; advocates could be appointed to seek out and represent service users' interests; views and experiences can be sought through interviews and discussions with service users (see Peck and Barker, 1986; Beresford and Croft, 1986). In addition to these direct methods there are numerous published accounts and collations of users' experiences of the mental health system, many of which provide an important stimulus for change (see for example, Barnes and Berke, 1971; Berke, 1979; Raphael, 1977; Women in MIND, 1986. There are also a number of video films, e.g. 'Speaking from experience' (ESCATA); 'We're not mad, we're angry' (Multiple Image); 'Living with schizophrenia' (Dialogue 4 projects).)

## DEVELOPING A VISION

If these participative methods are to be used to go beyond the familiar pattern of planning which reproduces old services in new places, a continuing investment will be needed in creating a shared *vision* of future services as a basis for subsequent action. Visions are not blueprints: rather, they entail seeking agreement on the values and principles which should underpin service design and starting to sketch the forms of provision most likely to ensure that these principles are realized in practice. Such principles need to be concerned both with the experience of the service as it will be delivered, and with ensuring the conditions for such a service to flourish. They also need to encompass both individual and community interests in the service (see Table 4.1).

Table 4.1    Some principles defining quality in psychiatric services.

| Focus on | Provision: conditions for quality service development | Output: ensuring quality experience for users |
|---|---|---|
| The individual | Clear service principles<br>Focus on individual users<br>Multi-agency network<br>Stakeholders involved in development<br>Support and training for staff<br>Evaluation and review process | Community presence and participation<br>Individual programme with continuity<br>Access to appropriate professional help<br>Opportunities for personal development<br>Protection of rights and citizenship<br>Enhanced self-respect, reduced stigma |
| The community | Adequate specialist resources<br>A range of general community services<br>Capacity to check for unmet and new needs<br>Value for money— economical delivery | Comprehensive services meeting a range of needs<br>Meets priority needs and needs of different groups<br>Provides access to primary and specialist care<br>Accessible and available when and where needed<br>Community education to reduce prejudice<br>Supports unpaid relatives carers |

There is an increasing number of sources from which principles for psychiatric service development can be drawn. Of particular interest is the MIND document *Common Concern* (MIND, 1983), and the work on normalization which is increasingly being adapted from its North American origins to fit a UK context (Wolfensberger, 1972; Braisby *et al.*, 1987; Echlin *et al.*, 1987; Independent Development Council, 1986; Kingsley *et al.*, 1985; O'Brien and Poole, 1983; O'Brien and Tyne, 1981).

However, service principles are only likely to have a significant impact in informing policy and initiating action if the development group itself has been involved in identifying those principles to which they are committed locally. There are a variety of procedures for doing this, the most powerful of which start from the experiences of service users. An exercise for large groups which has been developed for King's Fund workshops asks the group to identify, from users' experiences of current services, experiences which they would like to see more of—and experiences which should be avoided. This material is then grouped so that common aspirations fall together, and from these generalizations are drawn in the form of principles. An alternative approach, also based on the idea of users' experiences of service provision, adopts a card-sort technique to identify service goals and the principles underpinning future development (Brown and Alcoe, 1984).

Exploring the principles which could form a basis for future services both brings fundamental differences out into the open, and identifies areas of common ground. Our experience is that such common ground is often broader than anticipated—areas of disagreement about how services should develop have often obscured common aspirations for the service. In particular ideological differences about the nature, appropriateness and qualitative experience of different therapies have masked agreements about the quality of everyday life which we aim to ensure for people with psychiatric disabilities.

Generating principles provides the basis for further detailed work. In order to use them in developing the service it will be necessary to consider how different aspects of the service will operate in order to reflect the principles, and to write operational policies which express this at the level of daily practice.

## Planning from the vision

Charismatic leaders are often people who have clear and influential vision—yet to change reality or create an organization to deliver the vision, leaders have to find ways of translating the long-term goal into short-term steps and activities.

Traditionally planning groups have worked forwards from their present position, asking the question at each stage 'and then what happens next?' (Emery, 1981). This method assumes that the route, as well as the destination, are known to someone, or are at least knowable, and the task is simply to identify the best path (thus 'option appraisal' has come to be fashionable). Consequently the focus for planning is on the means rather than the ends. By contrast, in attempting radical changes the path is uncharted, each step needs to be invented as we travel, and the destination is often obscure. A 'vision' of how the future service might look provides a marker for our destination. The question which can then be asked is 'and what conditions should prevail for this to become the case?', and in this way questions about the product of planning can continually be raised. 'Backward mapping' is a technique which progressively identifies the elements which enable these outcomes to be achieved (Elmore, 1982). Starting with the ultimate goal and working backwards to the present position each step back generates a new intermediate objective. This provides a skeleton chart of targets to be achieved along the way—and then looking forwards an action framework can be identified (see Figure 4.2).

An example may make this procedure and its application clearer. In Hackney the psychiatric service experienced a shortage of acute beds some years after admissions to a distant long-stay hospital had ceased. On examination it was found that patients were remaining on the acute ward, because there was no alternative accommodation for them. These patients were of different ages, experienced different conditions and had different requirements. To solve the service problem, and to improve the patients' experience, a choice of alternative accommodation, together with appropriate support services, was needed. Choice required that a range of different sorts of housing be identified and made available. Finding these different sorts of housing would mean developing links with a number of agencies providing different forms of accommodation, together with identifying any direct provision which might be available. To make these links would require skill and a considerable investment of time: consequently the key to development, and the first step in terms of action, was getting approval for a new post of housing development officer. The planning, however, had started not from funding a new post, but from consideration of key issues which offered potential for real improvement in the patients' lives (Lovatt, 1985, 1987).

## Making the most of creativity

Since there is no single correct answer to the question about future services, which can be uncovered through a technically competent search,

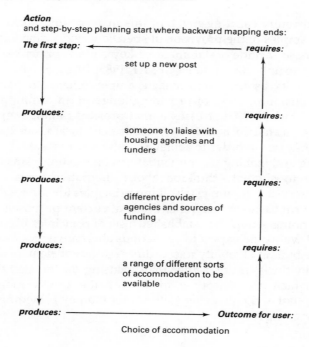

**Action**
and step-by-step planning start where backward mapping ends:

*The first step:* ← *requires:*

set up a new post

*produces:* *requires:*

someone to liaise with
housing agencies and
funders

*produces:* *requires:*

different provider
agencies and sources of
funding

*produces:* *requires:*

a range of different sorts
of accommodation to be
available

*produces:* → *Outcome for user:*

Choice of accommodation

*'Backward mapping'*
starts by considering what is to be achieved in the end.

Figure 4.2   An illustration of the 'backward mapping' process.

it will be important for the planning group to spend time generating and exploring alternatives and possibilities. Exercises like this, which do not produce an immediately practical result, are often experienced as 'time-wasting' and consequently avoided by planners. Their value, however, lies in the opportunities they offer to consider new approaches. Looking at alternatives brings fresh ideas into a group and helps to develop its ability to work creatively.

Alternative approaches to service provision can be identified through a variety of different routes. We have already described one powerful procedure for generating new ideas about service delivery through identifying the needs of individual service users—the 'getting to know you' exercises (Brost and Johnson, 1982.)

Finding out about services and projects in other places can provide useful sources of ideas. The Good Practices in Mental Health information service, for example, has accounts of innovative psychiatric service initiatives all over the UK, and including a few examples from North America.

They are currently collating much of this material into packs focusing on different examples of the provision of specific services (housing, advocacy, alcohol). These include a statement of key service principles and a brief introduction to important issues (GPMH, 1985, 1986a,b). The project is also able to call on its resources to provide examples relevant to particular client needs—for instance, ways of providing longer-term community support. One point which GPMH stresses is that projects cannot simply be transferred or replicated in a new site: a different local context will require different strategies in order to achieve similar outcomes.

Criticizing and making recommendations on existing plans can also be a useful way to simulate thinking about alternative ways of providing psychiatric services. Again, establishing principles for service development provides a firm basis for looking critically at current proposals.

If the planning group has established a set of principles like those set out in Table 4.1 we would expect to see serious alternative proposals emerging which have built in an ability to coordinate different elements of provision around individuals' needs rather than focusing on the elements in isolation; and which are concerned to develop the service mainly through supporting staff and enhancing skills rather than by providing buildings.

SEEKING INFORMATION

One of the major failures of conventional planning for future service provision is the assumption that individual needs can be met through services designed on the basis of information about populations. As a consequence of this approach people who need specific forms of help—for example, support in daily living activities—are slotted into mass-produced packages on a 'take-it-or-leave-it' basis. One of the most immediate problems faced by people leaving hospital is finding accommodation, and consequently housing is an aspect of community care which has received great attention. However, simply being housed in the community is not enough to constitute an acceptable life. The person who lives alone may require help with shopping and cooking; will be unused to housework; probably needs encouragement to go out, and someone to go with them—at least until the other members of the club or centre are familiar. Such help could be provided easily and regularly by a coordinated combination of home-help, CPN and social work services—without it self-neglect produces a situation in which 24-hour hospital care seems the only option.

Planners and other participants in the design process will need a number of different sorts of information gathered from a variety of sources, using a wide range of methods. Conventional techniques based on population estimates cannot produce the detailed information to design services which are tailored to meet individual needs: however, population estimates are important in creating an overall framework of provision from which individual needs can be fulfilled. Thus both sets of information are necessary, and neither excludes the other.

If local services capable of meeting individual needs sensitively and appropriately are to be designed, then much more attention should be given to the needs of individual users, and information about these individual needs should be integrated into the process of developing new services. Broad parameters for a local service can be developed from assumptions based on research and epidemiological data (McCarthy, 1982; Hirsch, 1986). These provide estimates of how many people are likely to suffer from dementia, to become severely depressed, or to have other psychiatric breakdowns requiring major assistance, each year. In the same way information about current patterns of service use can be employed as rough indicators of likely patterns of need. While these data provide estimates of the range and scale of service likely to be required, they should be supplemented with other information about the style and content of specific services (e.g. detailed accounts of individual needs and experience, and how these might be met). In addition to generating information about the aspirations and principles which will inform service development, planning groups should be clear about the constraints on development, particularly limits on the financial and human resources. There are also alternative resources which might be brought in to supplement the service. These include additional finance (Housing Corporation funding and payment by clients themselves from supplementary benefit entitlements, for example) and facilities—leisure centres, adult education provision, voluntary groups and so on.

McAusland *et al.* (1986), emphasized the importance of designing a strategy for relocating patients from large hospitals which paid attention to both the statistical parameters of the patient population (age, sex, borough of previous residence, estimated functional capacity, etc.) and took account of detailed individual needs for services (specific abilities and disabilities, friendships, patient's preferences). This required two distinct stages of information gathering and assessment. Firstly strategic planning in which the framework of different agencies and services is created; and secondly project planning which could meet individual needs of particular patients.

Similar distinctions will need to be drawn in developing other local services. It is not sufficient to design services for individuals on the basis of broad categories of need derived from whole populations. However, nor can services which adequately meet the spread of different needs found within a population be developed entirely on the foundation of the needs and experiences of existing service users. Indeed in service planning there may be three main targets for an information-gathering strategy: individual experiences, project design and population indices. The first target of individual experiences can be achieved through focusing on creating service packages for individual users, based on information about the needs, experiences and ambitions of those particular individuals. These 'packages' are likely to include elements drawn from a number of different projects which together make up a district service. Secondly, information about project design will require people to seek out ideas from other districts about how similar services have been set up, as well as (and as a stimulus to) creating local visions of the future. Thirdly, population indices will be necessary to ensure that the service is capable of meeting the range of needs across the district. This includes information about the size, age and ethnic structure of the population; and the incidence of needs for service in the district and in other similar populations. The process of service design will need to ensure that each level of information is scanned and rescanned as development progresses (see Figure 4.3).

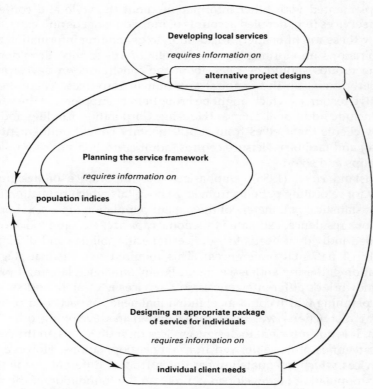

Figure 4.3   Information for planning new services.

## LINKING PLANNING AND IMPLEMENTATION

A further weakness in traditional centralized planning methods which this approach is designed to overcome is the disjunction between planning and implementation. At best, 'top-down' planning is vulnerable to alteration of purpose as middle managers and providers adapt the planners' ideas in putting them into practice. At worst planning divorced from implementation fails to make use of a most important resource—local practitioners who often have a wealth of good ideas for service development and ways of meeting specific local needs which do not figure in central planning assumptions.

Locality-based staff may know of underused community buildings and small-scale voluntary associations which might make useful contributions in support services for at least a few local people. Involvement in planning strengthens the prospects for effective implementation. It also provides an immediate test through local experience of whether intentions are being realized in practice as different aspects of the service are developed.

For example, progress was held up in one North London district by initial failure to involve front-line staff in plans and consultation for change. This meant that the Region's proposals to close a large hospital lacked credibility and were not taken seriously. Staff who had not been drawn into thinking through the issues of service development saw new ideas as 'pie in the sky'. It has taken a long time and much hard work to move away from this position, and to develop a climate in which real change is now a possibility. Many staff in the psychiatric service have a long experience of radical proposals which are frustrated by practical realities, and this increases their scepticism. However, without their commitment and energy major service changes will be impossible. At most what will happen is some shift in the site of service delivery, with little change in philosophy or style.

### Learning from experience

Planning for change recognizes that the future, although predictable in some respects, always involves uncertainty. It is not like a simple puzzle, where application will identify the answer, and a little more work will reveal how to fit it into place. Planning should be a continuing process of generating and testing ideas, with review and feedback mechanisms built into the system as key features.

There are numerous ways in which the experience of service development can be used as learning for subsequent initiatives. Creating a task force which identifies problems and possibilities, and also has resources to try out some local solutions, is one way to link planning, implementation and review. Another possible mode is the use of 'vanguard projects', or 'vanguard areas'. Identifying one area or aspect of service in which a new approach can be tried is one way of testing out the appropriateness of the approach, and offers valuable learning about the problems of implementation locally. In this way a district might try out some new ideas, without risking full commitment in an uncharted area.

Service principles of course have an essential role in monitoring and service evaluation by creating standards against which the service can be assessed. It is, of course, vital that such monitoring leads to change where it is indicated, and this further reinforces the point made earlier in this chapter of gaining broad commitment to the directions and development of the service. Setting standards requires careful consideration of the different ways in which principles may be operationalized; and this will need to be considered from the point of view of individual service users, projects and the district service as a whole. For instance where the service has set a broad objective of enhancing the rights and citizenship of people with psychiatric disabilities different questions could be asked of different levels of the service 'system'. At individual user level the operation of the principle might focus on the ways in which patients' money and access to their money was dealt with. At project level concern could focus on ensuring that at least some attention was paid in each service to ensuring that people on welfare benefits received advice and help where necessary; and that service users were aware of mental health legislation as it affected them. Considering the district service it might be important to support these activities with an advice and advocacy service; and to ensure that procedures for involving the Mental Health Act Commission and ensuring access to tribunals and representation were established and effective (Independent Development Council, 1986; Kingsley et al., 1985).

Such activities depend on the development and maintenance of appropriate information bases. There is not yet a large body of experience in psychiatry in keeping routine information, apart from hospital case notes. However, there are examples of psychiatric case registers, in Camberwell, Nottingham, Salford, Waltham Forest, Hackney and Southampton (Wing and Bransby, 1970; Baldwin, 1971; DHSS, 1971; Wing and Hailey, 1972; Martindale, 1986). Case registers aim to track all patients across a service, or a district, providing a continuing record of their psychiatric state and contacts with services.

Information which can be used to monitor the extent to which a service is fulfilling its aims can also be collected in other ways. Interviewing users to find out the extent to which the service is meeting their needs is a valuable exercise; similarly the views of relatives and carers can indicate the extent of satisfaction and dissatisfaction with the service. User surveys which concentrate on previous history are valuable in determining which group or groups are making most use of the facility, and in identifying whether the service is reaching its intended target group. Identifying other agencies also likely to be used by a similar target group, and discussing with them the service's impact on their activities, is a further valuable source of information providing context for the development of the service (Tessler and Goldman, 1982; Scott and Black, 1986; Wing and Hailey, 1972).

In establishing quality assurance procedures as a means of sustaining service standards it may also be necessary to identify priorities. In particular when resources for review and evaluation are in short supply it is important to concentrate on the quality of service provided for those clients who are least 'attractive' and consequently most vulnerable. These would include people with long-term needs who demonstrate little enthusiasm for personal growth; elderly people, and especially those suffering from dementia; and minority groups (e.g. from the black and ethnic minority population) where the challenge is to rethink existing services to respond to different experiences and perceptions. There are clear warning signals from experience in other countries, especially the USA and Italy, where reform has neglected some of these groups, and in failing to respond to their needs has been seriously undermined as an effective strategy (Tessler and Goldman, 1982; Chu and Trotter, 1974; Jones, 1985).

## PUTTING PSYCHIATRIC SERVICE PLANNING IN CONTEXT

All planning activity occurs, of course, in a wider political, organizational and economic context which shapes both the processes of change and the interests which are likely to be most influential. In particular the model of service development we have described needs to be situated in the administrative context of established health and local authority decision-making arrangements.

It is especially important that creative processes of development are linked to the formal planning and resource allocation procedures of the public agencies. Whilst these procedures may not seem to be the best way to plan for major changes in service delivery they remain the keys to generating action. Thus service principles will need to be developed at the same time as resource bids are being made—especially in areas where long lead times are typical. There may be either dialogue or struggle with managers who have to allocate resources across a wide range of service areas. These exchanges should indicate the resources likely to be available, and may be useful as a foundation for negotiating the nature of the service and the volume of resources with higher tiers of management. Political allies will be valuable at this point, but may need to have been identified and fostered earlier in order to make full use of their potential.

As well as linking activity up and down different tiers of the same agency the development process needs to take account of planning being carried out in parallel—in large institutions, in local authorities, and in the voluntary sector, for example. Since services are interdependent, planning needs to find ways of recognizing mutual impacts and to create a continual process of mutual adjustment.

Inevitably the implementation of new services will also require that priorities be identified: these might take the form of experimenting with new forms of provision focusing on underserved groups, or developing high-quality services which may provide a model for subsequent initiatives.

Financial advice from treasurers and others responsible for regulating the resource framework will be vital in these activities. Funding new services is increasingly a sophisticated entrepreneurial task, both because of the need to develop policies which enable funds to be shifted from old to new services (including various 'bridging' arrangements) and because of the increasing dependence on dispersed sources of funding (including from the NHS, local authorities, housing agencies, Manpower Services Commission, Social Security and special government project initiatives) for the local psychiatric service programme budget.

A further important component in the wider strategic framework (Towell and Kingsley, 1987) which influences the process of service development, is the manpower and staff development policies established by the NHS and local authorities. In many areas manpower plans and training strategies are being formulated which are at best only loosely associated with the kind of detailed service planning we have proposed. If these processes remain in separate channels then staff support for change is likely to be undermined, and the implementation of new services damaged by the lack of appropriately trained staff. What is required instead is that service planning coordinators maintain a continuing dialogue with personnel managers about the staffing implications of emerging plans, and ensure that a significant investment is made in training and support for the people who will be delivering the future pattern of services.

## CONCLUSION

Meeting the challenge of creating effective community-based services will require commitment and imagination. Several other contributors in this collection demonstrate what this might mean within particular aspects of local provision. We have tried to outline some ideas about the process of development which we believe have a greater chance of producing genuinely community-based psychiatric services than the traditional approaches to planning distilled through bureaucratic structures. Working through the complexity of existing organizations and systems we have argued that service development requires a continuous process of:

1. building networks of concerned people;
2. developing shared views of the present state of services and the trends which provide the pressure for future changes;
3. creating shared images of desirable futures for individuals in the light of a real appreciation of their current life experiences;
4. identifying a wide variety of constructive actions, large and small, which people in these networks can undertake in their own situations to increase the prospects of these desirable futures being realized.

We have also argued for a dynamic approach characterized by a commitment to learning: learning about better ways to plan and manage services; learning about the impact of services on the individuals and communities they are designed to serve; and learning about the real potential of people with serious psychiatric disabilities when given appropriate opportunities and support.

## ACKNOWLEDGMENT

The authors would like to thank the National Health Service Training Authority for supporting the work on which this chapter is based.

## REFERENCES

Audit Commission (1986). *Making a Reality of Community Care*, HMSO, London.
Baldwin, J. A. (1971). *The Mental Hospital in the Psychiatric Service: a case register study*, Nuffield Provincial Hospitals Trust, Oxford University Press, London.
Barclay Report (1982). *Social Workers: their role and tasks*, Bedford Square Press, London.
Barnes, M., and Berke, J. (1971). *Mary Barnes: two accounts of a journey through madness*, Hart-Davis MacGibbon, London.
Beresford, P., and Croft, S. (1986). *Whose Welfare: private care or public services?* Lewis Cohen Urban Studies Centre, Brighton Polytechnic, Brighton, Sussex.
Berke, J. (1979). *I Haven't Had to Go Mad Here*, Penguin, Harmondsworth.

Braisby, D. (1984). On the road to self-reliance, *Social Work Today*, 6 August, pp. 16–17.

Braisby, D., Echlin, R., Hill, S., and Smith, H. (1987). *Changing Futures: developing housing with support services for people discharged from long-stay psychiatric hospitals*, King's Fund Centre/GPMH, London.

Brost, M., and Johnson, T. (1982). *Getting to Know You—One Approach to Service Assessment and Planning for Individuals with Disabilities*, Wisconsin Council of Development Disabilities, Madison, Wisconsin.

Brown, H., and Alcoe, J. (1984). *Lifestyles for People with Mental Illness. A staff training exercise based on normalisation principles*, ESCATA, Brighton, Sussex.

Butts, M., Irving, D., and Whitt, C. (1981). *From Principles to Practice: a commentary on health service planning and resource allocation in England from 1970 to 1980*, Nuffield Provincial Hospitals Trust, London.

Chu, F. D., and Trotter, S. (1974). *The Madness Establishment: Ralph Nader's study group report on the National Institute of Mental Health*, Grossman, New York.

Collin, T. (1985). Transition in mental illness services—creativity in planning, *Hospital and Health Services Review*, September, pp. 235–7.

Court, M. (1984). Grassrooting for better health services, *NAHA News*, November, p. 6.

DHSS (1971). *The Nottingham Psychiatric Case Register Findings 1962–1969*, Statistical Report Series No. 13, HMSO, London.

DHSS (1980). *Organisational and Management Problems of Mental Illness Hospitals. Report of a Working Group (Nodder report)*, DHSS, London.

Elmore, R. F. (1982). Backward mapping: implementation research and policy decisions. In W. Williams (ed.) *Studying Implementation: Methodological and Administrative Issues*, Chatham House Publishers Inc., New Jersey.

Emery, F. E. (ed.) (1981). *Systems Thinking*, Vol. 2, Penguin, Harmondsworth (see especially F. E. Emery, 'Planning for real but different worlds', pp. 57–79).

Etherington, S., and Bosanquet, N. (1985). *The Real Crisis in Community Care: developing services for mentally ill people*, Good Practices in Mental Health, London.

Glennerster, H., Korman, N., and Marslen-Wilson, F. (1983). *Planning for Priority Groups*, Martin Robertson, Oxford.

GPMH (1985). *Housing Information Pack: ordinary housing for people with major long-term psychiatric disabilities*, Good Practices in Mental Health, London.

GPMH (1986a). *Advocacy Information Pack: advice and advocacy services for people with psychiatric disabilities*, Good Practices in Mental Health, London.

GPMH (1986b). *Alcohol Services Information Pack*, Good Practices in Mental Health/Alcohol Concern, London.

Hirsch, S. (1986). *Psychiatric Beds and Resources: factors influencing bed use and an approach to service planning*, A Report of the Working Party on Bed Norms and Resources, Royal College of Psychiatry Section for Social and Community Psychiatry, Royal College of Psychiatry, London.

Hogget, P., and Hambleton, R. (eds) (1987). *Decentralisation and Democracy*, Occasional Paper 28, School for Advanced Urban Studies, University of Bristol, Bristol.

House of Commons (1985). *Second Report from the Social Services Committee, Session 1984–85. Community care: with special reference to adult mentally ill and mentally handicapped people*, vol. 1, HC 13-I, HMSO, London.

Independent Development Council (1986). *Pursuing Quality*, IDC, King's Fund Centre, London.

Jones, K. (1985). Lessons from Italy, the USA and York. In T. McAusland (ed.) *Planning and Monitoring Community Mental Health Centres*, pp. 3–8, King's Fund Centre, London.

King, D., and Court, M. (1984). A sense of scale, *Health and Social Services Journal*, 21 June, pp. 734–5.

Kingsley, S., Towell, D., and McAusland, T. (1985). *Up to Scratch: Monitoring to Maintain Standards* (available from King's Fund College, 2 Palace Court, London, W2 4HS).

Lovatt, A. (1985). Community Psychiatry Research Unit, Hackney. In *Housing Information Pack: ordinary housing for people with major long-term psychiatric disabilities*, Good practices in Mental Health, London.

Lovatt, A. (1987). Independent living in the city, *Health Service Journal*, 15 January, p. 65.

McAusland, T., Towell, D., and Kingsley, S. (1986). *Assessment, Rehabilitation and Resettlement*, Psychiatric Services in Transition Paper No. 2, King's Fund College, London.

McCarthy, M. (1982). *Epidemiology and Policies for Health Planning*, King Edward's Hospital Fund for London, London.

Martindale, D. (1986). *The Psychiatric Service Register*, Working Note No. 1, National Unit for Psychiatric Research and Development, Lewisham, London.

MIND (1983). *Common Concern*, MIND Publications, London.

North Manchester District Health Authority (1987). *All our Futures: a report of a study group on services for elderly people prepared for the Joint Care Planning Team in North Manchester*, NMDHA, Manchester.

O'Brien, J., and Poole, C. (1983). *Planning Spaces—A Manual for Service Planners*, CMH (Campaign for Mentally Handicapped People), London.

O'Brien, J., and Tyne, A. (1981). *The Principle of Normalisation: a foundation for effective services*, CMH/CMHERA, London.

Peck, E., and Barker, I. (1986). Power to the patients, *Health Service Journal*, 3 April, p. 457.

Raphael, W. (1977). *Psychiatric Hospitals viewed by their Patients*, King Edward's Hospital Fund for London, London.

Scott, W. R., and Black, B. L. (eds) (1986). *The Organisation of Mental Health Services: societal and community systems*, Sage, London.

Tallis, P. A. (1981). *Planning in the NHS*, Working Paper No. 55, Health Services Management Unit, Department of Social Administration, University of Manchester, Manchester.

Tessler, R. C., and Goldman, H. H. (1982). *The Chronically Mentally Ill: assessing community support programs*, Ballinger, Massachusetts.

Towell, D., and Kingsley, S. (1987). Developing psychiatric services in the welfare state. In S. Ramon and M. Gianichedda (eds) *Psychiatry in Transition* (forthcoming) (also available from King's Fund College, 2 Palace Court, London, W3 4HS).

Towell, D., and McAusland, T. (1984). Psychiatric services in transition, *Health and Social Services Journal*, 25 October, Centre 8 Supplement.

Wing, J. K., and Bransby, B. R. (eds) (1970). *Psychiatric Case Registers*, DHSS Statistical Report Series No. 8, HMSO, London.

Wing, J. K., and Hailey, A. M. (1972). *Evaluating a Community Psychiatric service: the Camberwell Register, 1964–1971*, Oxford University Press, London.

Wolfensberger, W. (1972). *Normalisation*, National Institute for Mental Health, Toronto.

Women in MIND (1986). *Finding our own Solutions*, MIND, London.

**Video material**

'Speaking from experience', ESCATA, 6 Pavilion Parade, Brighton, Sussex.
'We're not mad, we're angry', Multiple Image, Faringdon House, Faringdon Road, Swindon, Wiltshire.
'Living with schizophrenia', Dialogue 4 projects, 11 Richmond Terrace, Bristol, BS8 1AB.

Chapter 5

# Finance and Government Policy

## JOHN MAHONEY

Government involvement in the process of closing the large psychiatric institutions and developing alternative community services can be traced back to a Royal Commission Report of 1957. This recommended a shift away from institutions and stated that the 'aim of hospital treatment or training is to make the patient fit to return to life in the general community'—at which stage the provision of residential care in the community would become the responsibility of the local authority. Since then tens of thousands of people have been discharged into the community. In addition more patients have been dying in hospital than have been admitted for long-term care. The result has been vast reductions in the size of psychiatric institutions. In the South West Thames Regional Health Authority area alone, the population of mental illness hospitals fell from 11,000 in 1960 to just over 4000 in 1985. Nationally there has been no corresponding increase in community provision.

In the early 1970s the government saw the need to coordinate this process of deinstitutionalization and successive policy documents have subsequently been issued. National policy was stated most comprehensively in *Better Services for the Mentally Ill* (DHSS, 1975), which remains the clearest statement of policy on the development of new patterns of service. The mentally ill form one of the 'priority groups' identified in the government handbook *Care in Action* (DHSS, 1981a). Authorities were expected to give priority to the needs of the elderly, mentally handicapped people, physically and sensorily handicapped people and the mentally ill. Co-operation between health and local authorities was seen as vital to the development of community care, and joint consultative committees were set up in 1974 with a remit to 'establish a joint approach to planning and make recommendations on priorities for joint planning'. As a further inducement to cooperation special 'joint finance' monies were made available to health authorities (DHSS, 1977). Following a consultative document

*Care in the Community* (DHSS, 1981b), these joint finance arrangements were extended to facilitate the movement of people out of hospital (DHSS, 1983).

The thrust of government policy has been to improve services for the priority groups and to develop community care. However, the recommendations and priorities contained in these successive documents have not been implemented by regional and district health authorities. A major reason is the difficulty of financing these new services. Quite simply, current funding levels are not sufficient. Some notable initiatives have been taken, but these are the exception rather than the rule. As will be shown, these developments have tended to occur in services that have higher than average costs.

## THE NATIONAL HEALTH SERVICE FUNDING

Health services worldwide are faced with a fiscal crisis. The extent of the crisis in Britain has been subject to intense public debate (Smith, 1988), and the staggering size of the under-funding documented in a series of reports (Social Service Committee, 1986; Office of Health Economics, 1987; Bosanquet, 1986). The financial crisis has been concentrated on the cash-limited hospital service. An increasing share of spending has gone to primary care and services for the physically handicapped, whilst the share of total NHS spending devoted to the mentally ill has actually fallen (Bosanquet, 1986). Community care is being developed in very troubled times.

In the late 1970s the Resource Allocation Working Party (RAWP) opened the debate about resource allocation to the fourteen regional health authorities within England. There were considerable differences in the level of expenditure per head of population within the country, with the highest-spending regions being within the south-east, particularly in the Greater London area, which has a concentration of teaching hospitals. The original intention was to maintain the level of revenue spending in the 'over-provided' regions whilst at the same time increasing the resources to the 'under-provided' regions to bring them up to similar levels. The situation subsequently changed when it was decided to take money away from the 'over-provided' regions and to reallocate it to the 'under-provided' regions. Four regions have been classified as major RAWP losers and these are North-West Thames, North-East Thames, South-East Thames and South-West Thames.

The suggested changes to revenue funding at regional level to equalize spending are not large in comparison with overall budgets. However, each region has introduced what is termed subregional RAWP, which makes changes between districts within the same region significantly greater. For example, the Islington district within North-East Thames is calculated as being 25 per cent over its target revenue allocation, whereas the Southend district within the same region is considered to be almost 20 per cent under its target allocation. The Islington Health Authority will therefore have to lose almost one-fifth of its revenue allocation over the next 10–15 years. Generally, district health authorities in London suffer the most from this policy. A major concern for these health authorities will be their capacity to contribute to the new community services for priority care groups, which can only be funded by reducing the demand on their acute hospital services.

It is extremely difficult to disentangle recent effects of RAWP redistribution policy on the development of services to the mentally ill. Firstly, it is doubtful whether most districts have received any real increase in funding. Districts are therefore probably using extra RAWP growth monies to fend off cuts in existing services. Secondly, the RAWP losing districts would be arguing for RAWP gaining districts to increase their acute services to take the pressure off their own services. Thirdly, it is extremely difficult to establish new priority care services from scratch. The requirement to develop new methods of working and recruit and train appropriate staff, combined with the capital lead in time for new developments, means that it can take three or four years to open the first components of a new service. Additional resources (if indeed there have been any) are therefore easily consumed by existing services and lost for the development of priority care services. Recent trends in the south-east regions indicate that nearly every district, including the RAWP gaining districts, is over-spending. In this climate priority care developments will almost certainly suffer, either through their postponement or abandonment for the time being.

Perhaps the major problem with RAWP is the failure to make sufficient allowance for deprivation in calculating funding for psychiatric services. To determine RAWP allocation the regional health authority calculates the spending of individual district health authorities according to the needs of its population. Some regions do make some allowance for deprivation, but it is rarely sufficient when calculating the district's level of spending on mental health services. The calculation is usually based on the size of the population, weighted by age, sex and marital status. It ignores the large body of evidence that shows a strong correlation between psychiatric morbidity and indices of social deprivation including social class, employment status, housing conditions, ethnicity, the proportion of single parents and pensioners living alone (Hirsch, 1987). In addition the general movement out of inner cities has resulted in the less able being left behind.

The policy of RAWP also ignores the location of hostels for homeless people, which are situated mainly in the inner areas of larger cities. For example, 'large old hostels in London are both the resource and the problem' (SHIL, 1986). They provide shelter for more than 10,000 single people at any one time. Studies of this homeless population consistently show that between 20 and 35 per cent (and sometimes up to 50 per cent) will have a severe psychiatric illness (Baxter and Hopper, 1984).

Many of the old ex-long-stay population of the large institutions will at the time of their discharge have lost all contact with their original areas of residence. Having been discharged many have received inadequate support and follow-up, and have tended to drift to areas such as inner cities, where they represent a severe drain on already overstretched services. Failure to give sufficient weighting to social deprivation flies in the face of common sense and accumulated evidence, and has left RAWP creating more problems than it solved.

## LOCAL AUTHORITY FUNDING

The lack of growth in financial resources devoted by the health service to the mentally ill would not be so critical if there had been a commensurate rise in local authority spending. Nationally local authorities spend about 4 per cent of the total money allocated to services for mentally ill people, although there are massive variations in the levels of provision throughout the country. The mentally ill represent a very low priority for local authorities, compared with other groups such as children, the elderly and people with a mental handicap. The recent changes in local authority funding can only exacerbate the problems. The present system for distributing rate support grants to local authorities acts as a deterrent to the expansion of community-based services. Under the present block grant system local authorities stand to lose between £3 and £4 in grant for every additional £1 they spend.

Another immediate problem is the implications of rate-capping. This is the procedure whereby the government estimates what the appropriate local government spending should be (i.e. grant-related expenditure assessments) and assesses, after taking all central government grants into account, what the shortfall is and therefore how much can be raised locally through the rating system. As an example, for inner London central government calculations allow for only 72 per cent of planned expenditure. This very bleak climate greatly affects those who are resonsible for trying to plan and improve community care. This certainly affects the joint planning process with health authorities. Local authorities threatened with rate-capping are extremely reluctant to enter into negotiations about the development of new services, whilst having to make contingency plans to cut their own services. Similarly they are often unable to guarantee to voluntary organizations continued funding, which creates an air of desperation amongst some voluntary workers. This affects their ability to run their part of the service. Although there seems to be some scope for improved efficiency within these rate-capped authorities, it is doubtful whether efficiency savings would be able to bring about the savings required in the time available. Almost certainly the services that will be most at risk for rate-capping will be the personal care services, which account for almost half of the local authorities' expenditure (i.e. residential care, day care and domiciliary and community support services, such as meals-on-wheels, home help, social work and rehabilitation services). The Department of the Environment's formula for estimating the grant-related expenditure assessments is very complicated, but fails to take into account the increased demand for services in the inner city areas with their high levels of social deprivation. Unfortunately it is these areas that are most at risk from rate-capping.

The recent Audit Commissions Report, *Making a Reality of Community Care* (1986), points out the absurdity of local government finance in relation to community care policies. Virtually all authorities that provide social services lose grant if they increase spending in real terms. Those authorities that wish to develop community care policies must either make equivalent cuts elsewhere in their budgets, or transfer a disproportionately high burden of cost to local ratepayers.

## JOINT FINANCE

The first major step forward to encourage the development of locally based services in partnership with the local authorities and voluntary organizations began in 1977 with the introduction of joint finance funding (DHSS, 1977). This was meant to encourage local statutory and voluntary organizations to help the movement of people out of hospital and to meet the additional costs of developing new services, while at the same time maintaining existing services. Regional health authorities are responsible for allocating joint finance funds to districts, and for ensuring that joint finance programmes accord with national and regional policies and priorities. Under a subsequent initiative, district health authorities may offer lump-sum payments for continuing grants to local authorities or voluntary organizations for as long as necessary in respect of people to be cared for in the community (DHSS, 1983). It is intended that these arrangements will eventually be put on a permanent footing by means of a central transfer of resources.

Health and local authorities are required to set up Joint Care Planning Teams of officers to support the Joint Consultative Committees, whose membership consists of local councillors and members of the health authorities. The use of joint finance has undoubtedly helped to improve understanding between health and local authorities, although the funding mechanism has only had a very limited influence, for a number of reasons.

Firstly, joint finance is still marginal in relation to the total level of expenditure by health and local authorities. Furthermore the amount of new joint finance money available annually is estimated at only £200,000 per social services authority. Given that the cost of purchasing and converting a home for five people in areas where housing is expensive would be in the region of £150,000, it is quite clear that joint finance can only play a very limited role in facilitating patient transfers, or indeed in improving services to people in the community. It is important to remember that joint finance is aimed at all of the priority care groups, including services for people with a mental handicap and the elderly. The proportion of joint finance spent on these care groups varies considerably from authority to authority. A postal survey to London DHAs revealed that the proportion of joint finance devoted to the mental health services was a mere 18.7 per cent in 1985/6 (Kay and Legg, 1986).

Secondly, local authorities are becoming increasingly reluctant to accept the long-term commitment to pick up the costs of joint finance schemes. Such schemes are normally tapered over a 7-year period (full funding being for 3 years). If payments are made for the purpose of enabling the transfer of patients from hospital into the community, the tapering period can be extended to 13 years (full funding for 10 years). Social service participation in the programme has fallen significantly over the past 10 years, from an average of 92 per cent in 1976/7 to 75 per cent by 1985. One of the major reasons for this is that the long-term revenue commitments made by the local authority may in turn lead to a loss of grant from the Department of the Environment. In contrast, health authority take-up of joint finance has more than doubled since 1981, and a significant proportion is now being spent either on health authority schemes (18 per cent of the total joint finance expenditure 1985) or the voluntary sector (7 per cent).

A third common criticism of joint finance within the health service is that local authorities use it to fund schemes of only marginal benefit to the health service. It is understandable that local authorities, which must pick up the costs, wish to ensure that schemes are in support of their own policies and priorities. It is not surprising therefore to find that in a survey carried out by the National Association of Health Authorities in 1983 only a minority of health authorities supported the case for the further expansion of joint funding, even in more favourable financial circumstances. All this led the all-party Parliamentary Social Services Committee (1985) to conclude that 'as a means of transferring further responsibilities from the NHS to local authorities joint finance is virtually played out'.

It is not surprising, with hindsight, that the system has not had the benefits originally envisaged in terms of developing community services. Generally the priority for local authorities is to improve services for people already in the community, whereas the health authorities in the main are anxious to establish schemes to move people out of hospital. A further major hindrance is the inbuilt resistance to change and mutual suspicion between health and local authorities, and the naive expectation that the provision of central funds would result in professions and organizations working together. There have been a few notable successes, but as Green (1986) points out, 'on the larger issues affecting the size of the budget, the demand for more staff, or where different professions took different views about what type of care was appropriate, then officials acted more as negotiators or protagonists than as colleagues'.

## FUNDING THE NEW SERVICES

Additional funds for the development of services for the mentally ill are at best marginal, and the major resources available for a change are those tied up in the provision of existing services. These costs are very difficult to release because such a high proportion are taken up with the non-direct patient care costs, which includes maintaining crumbling institutions. By 1981 the government accepted that about one-third of mental hospitals had reached the end of their life as viable buildings, and the total cost to the health services as a whole on maintenance and repairing existing buildings is estimated as £2 billion (Davies, 1982).

There are just over 100 large psychiatric institutions within the fourteen regional health authorities in the country. Many of the 192 district health authorities are served by a remote mental hospital. There are massive variations in resources tied up in these institutions. For example, in the South-East Thames region the difference between the average patient costs in Hellingly Hospital, which is the highest-cost hospital, and Cane Hill Hospital, which is the lowest, is 54 per cent. The average cost per patient per year in Hellingly is over £14,000 and the average cost in Cane Hill Hospital is £9000 (at 1983 prices). If the average cost per patient per year at Hellingly Hospital were applied to Cane Hill Hospital an additional £4 million per year would need to be invested at Cane Hill.

Community-based services appear to have developed most rapidly in areas served by hospitals that have historically been expensive to run. The well-publicized Exeter experience has been based on the releasing of resources from the run-down of high cost hospitals. For example Digby Hospital, serving Exeter City, had an average patient cost of £16,800 per year (1983 prices). This contrasts sharply with the task faced at Brookwood Hospital in Surrey, where the average patient cost is a mere £8500 (1983 prices).

Differences in funding are reflected in differences in staffing levels between regions and hospitals within regions. Those best provided (Wessex and the South-Western RHA, which contains Digby) have 0.75 and 0.74 nurses per available mental illness bed. The worst-provided region, South-West Thames, has only 0.58 nursing staff per bed (DHSS, Performance Indicators, 1984/5). Lack of nursing staff has a direct effect on patient care: poorly staffed hospital wards may be left unattended at night, whilst on long-stay wards it may be barely possible to do the minimum of attending to patients' physical needs. Where staffing levels are very low the prospects of releasing resources to develop alternative community services is remote.

Regional health authorities' plans again differ quite significantly. Some are planning to increase expenditure considerably, and are making allowances for the double running costs relating to the run-down of the large psychiatric hospitals and the development of new services, whilst others have different priorities.

The only way to develop new services is to release as much of the existing hospital resources as possible. Nearly all regional health authorities have adopted a policy of transferring the average hospital costs (or the average regional costs) directly to the agency that takes responsibility for the patient transferred. This is known as the dowry system. This is a most important funding initiative, as it provides a financial incentive for the development of district services. The success of this system is, however, dependent upon releasing the costs tied up in the institutions. This is not easy. Health authorities need to spend money to develop community services, but cannot derive financial savings from hospitals that are running down until they are substantially reduced in size or are completely closed. It is simply not possible to reduce costs in line with bed reductions. A hospital would need to transfer substantial numbers of patients before it would be able to make the savings on the scale required. For example, reducing ward sizes by a few patients in each would not result in less staff being required on those wards (which are staffed to the bare minimum anyway, in most cases). The major costs associated with heating, lighting and fuel and maintenance of buildings would not be affected, whilst the numbers of support staff such as domestic and catering personnel could not be reduced proportionately and savings are marginal. (Given the huge economies of scale domestic, catering and provisions costs are extremely low.) There is in any case extreme pressure in the long-stay hospitals to increase substantially the staffing and resources devoted to many sectors but particularly to services for long-stay patients. (Staffing accounts for 70 per cent of hospital costs.) Existing staffing levels are still not adequate to begin the process of rehabilitation of patients who have spent many years, if not most of their lives, in hospital.

It is worth repeating some of the criticisms of the dowry system mentioned by the Audit Commission (1986) and the National Federation of Housing Associations (1987).

1. Some health authorities have linked transfer payments to a particular individual and have told the agencies providing the community based service that the payment will only continue so long as the service is provided for that particular person.
2. A few authorities have adopted the unacceptable practice of deducting board-and-lodging payments from their calculation of the transfer payment.
3. The dowry is often too low, it should not provide just for the person discharged but for others who might otherwise have had to come into hospital but who are now cared for in the community.
4. Transfer payments are only made after a transfer has taken place.
5. Many residents of long-stay hospitals will not be discharged into the community and in this event no finance is transferred at all.
6. Where people are placed by health authorities directly into private or voluntary sector accommodation, funded by supplementary benefits, no money is transferred although day care services may be required.
7. Many local authorities are now refusing to develop services without a transfer of funds from health authorities.
8. An average dowry makes no allowance for differing dependencies among patients.

A major problem associated with the dowry system is that there has been a tendency throughout the service to develop facilities for those in hospital who are least handicapped. The 'difficult-to-place' patients requiring resettlement are often left till last, putting increasing strain on the declining institution and compromising the viability of successor services.

There has been an expectation amongst managers and clinicians that the new services developed will reduce admissions to psychiatric hospitals. However, this has not been proven. The new services will provide a more accessible and acceptable local community service to a wider range of patients than would have been previously possible: this may well lead to increased pressure on hospital beds. These services may also provide for the first time a service to a previously unsupported, untreated group of people in serious need, whilst former long-stay hospital residents will require more resources as they become old and frail.

There is a view that district health authorities should not develop services on a shoestring, but should wait until the costs tied up in the hospital are sufficient to develop community services at no extra cost. This is achieved because the number of people requiring long-term care in institutions is declining rapidly as staff succeed in keeping patients out of hospital. Assuming the cost of the hospital remain about the same, then the amount spent on each patient will increase significantly. The major problem with this approach, apart from leaving people in decaying institutions, is that thousands of people already in the community requiring further support will continue not to have access to the new services. The outcome of such a policy would be a much smaller and less adequate service.

A further argument for delay in implementing hospital closure has been that health authorities should await the evaluation of the 'Care in the Community' projects that have been set up using DHSS funding. Unfortunately there have been considerable delays in setting up these projects. To date (October 1987) only 47 per cent of the initial 353 identified patients have been discharged to the community. These projects are, in any case, doubtful as models of the future services, not least because they are likely to be more costly than other initiatives. Additionally, it is doubtful whether these projects will have the scope that will be needed if the estimated 20,000 inpatients who require alternative forms of provision are to be discharged.

The Audit Commission (1986) point out that bridging finance is inadequate, and argue that the costs of providing community-based care for ex-patients, and possibly more importantly for those discharged from hospital before becoming long-stay patients, would cost an additional £220 million a year.

The scale of capital financing required to develop the new services is enormous. As a rough estimate it would cost each district health authority with a population of 300,000 about £15 million to provide the necessary buildings. This money would obviously be a first charge against any additional expenditure, and could not be recouped until the land and buildings of the existing institutions are sold. Some may be sold in piecemeal fashion as and when the institution reduces in size, although a major problem forecast is that many of these institutions are in green belt land and therefore would be unlikely to attract planning permission from the local planning authorities. In this case their land value would be substantially reduced. The availability of capital is obviously in the short term as crucial as the availability of additional running costs. Community services just cannot operate without a substantial range of accommodation for both residential and day care needs.

The vast majority of people in the service would totally concur with the House of Commons Social Services Committee's conclusion that health authorities at present spend scarcely enough per capita on mentally ill or mentally handicapped patients to enable decent community services to be provided at the same price, even if immediate and full transfer of patients or cash or both were possible. Only central funding over a period of several years can help the development of genuine community care over the hump (Social Services Committee, 1985).

## OTHER SOURCES OF INCOME

Given the constraints of the health and local authority financing outlined earlier, many authorities are seeking to attract other sources of finance to supplement the income they receive. In working with the voluntary sector and housing associations they are able to develop schemes that can charge residents fees or rent which can be met by DHSS payments or housing benefit. It is possible by using the welfare benefit system to raise between £1000 and £7500 per resident per annum. The Secretary of State at the DHSS asked the district health authorities in September 1987 to restrict the use they make of such revenue until the major review of community care funding, by Sir Roy Griffiths had been completed. No clarification was issued following the publication of the report, which recommended decreasing social security benefit for those in residential care while allowing social service departments to pay the balance of the cost when such care was deemed necessary (DHSS, 1988). However, many health authorities are already committed to plans for community care which depend for financial viability on income generation from these services. The use of additional funds raised in this way will increase substantially over the next few years unless present legislation is changed. Such a change is likely to prove difficult to implement, since the government must be reluctant to restrict access to this money from the voluntary sector whilst at the same time allowing the private sector to continue to have their charges met through social security payments. The massive growth in the care offered by the private sector since 1979 has already been discussed by Ramon in Chapter 2.

Charges to residents operate in the following way. Residents will either be regarded as living in their own housing or in receipt of board and lodging. For those living in their own housing, whether it is owned by a housing association or is rented privately, the source of income is derived from rental charges paid for by housing benefit, which is administered by the local authority housing department. A proportion of this rental income will go towards the cost of managing and maintaining the property, and the balance will contribute towards repayment of a mortgage. This income, however, cannot contribute towards the costs of providing support and care staff.

For those resident in board and lodging schemes (shared housing) the income generated is substantially more, since residents can claim whatever charges are levied on them up to a maximum figure laid down by the DHSS. For people with special care needs lodging charges can be supplemented by Attendance Allowance. The money available for residential care may result in a perverse incentive for organizations to provide an unnecessary level of care: no similar finances are offered to encourage 'home care' schemes (Audit Commission, 1986). Such perverse incentives favouring institutional solutions operate throughout the Western world (see Chapter 3).

Homes registered under the 1984 Act attract higher payments: criteria for registration state that the house should accommodate more than four people; the scheme provides personal care; the residents are categorized as being dependent; and finally the project must provide board as well as lodging. The Social Service Department of the local authority are required to register these properties, and often set fairly high standards of accommodation. Many local authorities will require all schemes to have night cover, and therefore given economies of scale it is cheaper to provide much larger accommodation than might otherwise be desirable or necessary. Similar regulations exist governing the registration of nursing homes, which is a health authority responsibility.

One other source of finance that is payable only to housing associations (i.e. those registered under the 1985 Housing Association Act) is hostel deficit grant. Housing associations can claim between £1000 and £1500 per year per resident if they can prove they are providing a housing scheme with higher levels of care than would normally be the case. The maximum level of staff is one professionally trained person to two and a half residents. There are schemes where this limit is being circumvented by organizing staff so that those staff employed over and above the ratio are employed by another organization.

These financial incentives lead to planning with income generation in mind, rather than looking primarily at the needs of each individual. However, this is inevitable unless adequate funding (particularly bridging finance) is provided (see Appendix).


GENERAL MANAGEMENT — THE MANAGEMENT OF CHANGE

General management in the NHS is a product of a previous report by Sir Roy Griffiths. It is hoped that the advent of general management will bring leadership and initiative to the development of local services. Its success depends crucially on the individual in post, the effective general manager being the person who will be able to argue the case for additional resources to foster new developments. However, the general manager for the priority care services is often isolated since the majority of district health authority resources, and therefore management, will be tied up in the acute hospital sector. Concentration on 'acute' care is not unique to the general medical/surgical and specialist high-tech. services. It is undoubtedly the case that most training, research and indeed status within psychiatry lies within the acute sector.

It is important that district health authorities have a commitment to develop a comprehensive service that gives priority to the needs of the most seriously psychiatrically ill. In reality it is those patients with chronic mental illnesses who make the greatest demands on acute services: inevitably paying attention to their needs must be a cost-effective policy. The chronically disabled and the elderly have historically been ignored in favour of more glamorous recipients of health care, despite the blandishments of central government.

Service planning in the past was highly unsatisfactory. Comparatively recently, however, management and planning has been linked with the management of financial resources. This gives the new breed of general managers much greater potential to devise and implement new services. The new general managers will be assessed by their ability to meet stated objectives. Unfortunately these objectives are often set on the premise of unrealistic assumptions about the availability of capital and revenue. Managers may then be forced to push through the deinstitutionalization programme without the necessary resources, or risk termination of their Contract. The current 3-year time span of the General Manager's contract is also unhelpfully short, placing a premium on quick results.

The development of community mental health services presents managers with a very demanding challenge. There is a lack of readily available models on which to base new services, and there is therefore a pressing need for innovative solutions. In particular, managers need to work in partnership with many other statutory and voluntary organizations. At the same time, there is an enormous challenge in managing the declining institution with all the problems associated with funding, staffing and morale that this brings. A further task is the development of appropriate systems for monitoring service activity. In the acute hospital sector the traditional view is that good managers are able to control expenditure, increase productivity and efficiency whilst maintaining the same quality of care. The priority care manager must, however, concentrate on the quality and scale of the service. Productivity can be usefully applied to the acute sector where it is fairly easy to identify; for example, the number of patients treated or operations undertaken per year. However, it is dubious if the indicators developed for the acute sector have any value in measuring services for mentally ill people. The mental illness service is labour-intensive and 'quick throughput' is probably detrimental to the outcome of patient care. Managers must therefore develop measures that concentrate far more on quality and evaluation, rather than assess productivity and use spurious measures of efficiency.


## THE FUTURE

In an excellent review of the problems of developing community-based services the Audit Commission (1986) argue that it is 'not tenable to do nothing about the present financial, organisational and staffing arrangements. This will have serious consequences'. Even if authorities decided not to develop alternative services for long-term patients their quality of life is bound to deteriorate. Acute psychiatric services will in the main be transferred to district hospital sites, and services for the elderly confused patients (suffering from dementia) can more easily and more appropriately be provided in non-institutional settings. This will lead to a worsening atmosphere of decline (and neglect) within psychiatric hospitals, which will become even more difficult to staff and maintain. The vast majority of long-stay patients are, however, capable of functioning in a non-hospital setting. Also a high proportion of people with long-term mental health problems in the community (including ex-patients) will have very similar needs. New services must aim to meet these needs.

A major current problem is that, in general, no agency accepts responsibility for funding the various components of the new services, particularly for people with long-term mental health problems living in the community. The situation is further complicated by the fact that there are huge discrepancies in local authority and health authority provision (and resources) throughout the country.

There are two major reasons why the development of mental health services has been neglected. First, and perhaps most important, is the inadequate level of funding, particularly bridging finance and capital. The issue of funding has to be tackled. The King's Fund College (1987) is correct in arguing for

> the construction centrally, from all available sources, of a single national budget for community care. This would involve the recognised annual earmarking of proposed expenditure from all of the departmental budgets concerned . . . central Government may need to institute some form of interdepartmental community care policy and expenditure review group. This group would ensure adequate and equitable distribution of funding across the country.

Community care funds have to be protected, and in this respect health authorities should be specifically prevented from siphoning off funds to fend off further cuts in acute services.

Additionally, it is crucial that the government and regional health authorities recognize that sufficient additional 'bridging' funds are essential for districts that manage the large psychiatric hospitals to cover the double running costs in the period of transition from hospital- to community-based services. If not, the development of new services will be substantially delayed. Lastly, many health authorities are using, or have specific plans to use, social security benefits to top up the costs of their new services. This should be explicitly recognized and protected.

Concerning capital funding, it is important for district health authorities to be clear about the likely level of resources over the next ten years. Regional health authorities will generally favour the accelerated closure of hospitals with high site values as substantial funds can be released to other districts to enable them to develop alternative schemes. These funds should be specifically earmarked. Capital is available from other sources but is negligible when measured against the scale of resources required. Few local authorities make their own capital available and the Housing Corporation have stated that they would not consider schemes to enable the closure of hospitals as a priority, which is perfectly understandable given the scale of other needs. Many more organizations are now looking towards private finance to raise capital, but this is clearly a false economy, as private investors will obviously want a return on their investment. This in turn will reduce the amount of revenue available to each project (unless, of course, these costs can be met by board and lodging payments).

The second major impediment to service development is a lack of clarity over where the responsibility for change lies. This has resulted in endless unresolved discussions over responsibilities and resources. Four solutions have been proposed: to leave arrangements as they are but clarify financial responsibility and provide more of a central lead; establish a joint board of health authorities and local authorities; give the NHS the lead responsibility for services for mentally ill people; or transfer responsibility for non-hospital care to the local authorities. Griffiths favours the final option (DHSS, 1988).

It is a fact of life that nearly all of the resources and staff are still vested with the Health Service. The current expenditure on mental health services is approximately £1 billion (at 1984/5 prices). The current spending by local authorities on services for mentally ill people is £42 million! In contrast local authority spending on services for mentally handicapped people is more than 50 per cent, the level of health spending, and perhaps more significantly local authorities spend more on services for the elderly than the total cost of the 'geriatric' services of the NHS. In reality health authorities have to take a lead in developing new services, and this should be formalized. Service development should, however, remain a joint enterprize, and the use of consortia or joint boards deserves encouragement.

It is becoming increasingly clear that previous guidelines for service provision are no longer adequate. High-quality community-based services that have no access to large psychiatric hospitals are likely to require much greater provision than that envisaged in *Better Services*.

In conclusion, unless the issues of funding, organizational responsibility and level of provision are addressed at a national level, adequate services for continuing care clients are unlikely to develop.

## REFERENCES

Audit Commission (1986). *Making a Reality of Community Care*, HMSO, London.

Baxter, E., and Hopper, K. (1984). Troubled on the streets: the mentally disabled homeless poor. In J. A. Talbot (ed.) *The Chronic Mental Patients, Five Years Later*, Grune and Stratton, Orlando.

Bosanquet, N. (1986). *Public Expenditure on the NHS: recent trends and outlook*, Centre for Health Economics. University of York.

Davies, C. (1982). *Underused and Surplus Property in the NHS*, HMSO, London.

DHSS (1975). *Better Services for the Mentally Ill*, HMSO, London.

DHSS (1977). *Joint Care Planning: health and local authorities*, DHSS, London.

DHSS (1981a). *Care in Action: a handbook of policies and priorities for health and personnel social sources*, HMSO, London.

DHSS (1981b). *Care in the Community: a consultative document on moving resources for care in England*, DHSS, London.

DHSS (1983). *Health Service Development: care in the community and social finance*, DHSS, London.

DHSS (1985). *Performance Indicators—Mental Illness Nursing Manpower (M47) 1984/85*, DHSS, London.

Green, D. (1986). Joint finance an analysis of the reasons for its limited success. *Policy and Politics*, **14**, 209.

Hirsch, S. R. (1987). Planning for bed needs and resource requirements in acute psychiatry, *Bulletin of the Royal College of Psychiatrists*, **11**, 398–407.

Kay, A., and Legg, C. (1986). *Discharged to the Community*, Housing Research Group, The City University.

King's Fund College (1987). *Making a Reality of Community Care: a response to Sir Roy Griffiths and his review team*, King's Fund College, London.

National Federation of Housing Associations (1987). *Housing, The Foundation of Community Care*, NFHA, London.

Office of Health Economics (1987). *Compendium of Health Statistics*, OHE, London.

SHIL (1986). *Single Homelessness in London*. Report of a Working Party.

Smith, T. (1988). New year message. *British Medical Journal*, **296**, 1–2.

Social Services Committee (1985). *Community Care with Special Reference to Adult Mentally Ill and Mentally Handicapped People*, HMSO, London.

Social Services Committee (1986). *Public Expenditure on the Social Services*, HMSO, London.

Community Care in Practice
Edited by A. Lavender and F. Holloway
© 1988 John Wiley & Sons Ltd

Chapter 6

# Evaluation and Service Planning

## GEOFF SHEPHERD

This chapter is concerned with issues of assessment and evaluation in the context of planning and monitoring services for people with long-term mental health problems. 'Assessment' and 'evaluation' are fashionable terms; everyone likes to argue that their service is based on a careful—and preferably scientific—assessment of needs, but to what extent is this really possible? Can planning of new service developments be based on assessment data? In these days of general managers and performance indicators there are pressures to demonstrate that services are providing a good quality of care in an efficient and cost-effective manner. How can this be done? How can 'quality of care' be measured? How can the quality of care be weighted against costs? This chapter attempts to address these questions. It begins by reviewing the contribution that assessment methods might make to the planning of new services.

## ASSESSMENT IN SERVICE PLANNING

In a technical sense, assessment refers to measurement. Thus, when discussing the assessment of the needs for a particular kind of service, what is actually being discussed are attempts to 'measure' these needs in some way or another. Now, measurements in science should be both reliable and valid, i.e. when different observers make the same measurement they should come to roughly the same conclusion and, more importantly, assessments should measure accurately whatever it is that we are actually interested in. When assessing the need for service, it is this latter criterion that may be particularly difficult to meet. This is because there are a number of different ways of assessing service needs, and it is often extremely difficult to decide between the validity of differing approaches.

91

Methods of assessment can be grouped into two main categories: *quantitative*, and *qualitative*. Quantitative approaches attempt to provide simple 'head counts' of the number of people requiring services and then estimate the level of specific kinds of provisions by applying some set of general norms or standards. Qualitative methods attempt to construct a model of service needs based on a much more detailed analysis of individual's strengths and difficulties.

## Quantitative methods

The first question that has to be answered is: 'How many people are there requiring a particular kind of service?'. Where the population is fairly static, for example a group of long-stay patients in a mental hospital who have to be resettled in the community because the hospital is closing, this may be relatively straightforward. However, if the numbers depend upon the development of services beyond a single health district, then the situation is more complicated and other districts' plans may need to be considered. If the region's plans are that each district will become self-sufficient, when is this meant to be occurring? When will it actually occur? What is meant to be happening to the long-stay patients in the meantime? What will happen to them if the region's plans do not materialize? Answers, however approximate, to these kinds of questions, are necessary before one can begin to make decisions about numbers and the likely scale of demand. If one is trying to plan a service to meet the mental health needs of a complete community then a different set of problems arise. Thus one has to decide who should the service really be aiming at, and what it should be aiming to do. Should it confine itself to traditional psychiatric service users, or should it be aiming to reach people who would not usually present to services? Should it be aiming to 'treat' people in the conventional sense, or should the emphasis be on 'prevention'? These 'philosophical' questions often generate considerable debate.

Deciding who the service should be aiming at, and identifying the priority groups, demands some understanding of basic epidemiology and a grasp of the prevalence of disorders of different severity. Community surveys have found that approximately 250 out of every 1000 people experience an episode of a recognizable psychiatric disorder in a year. Of these, some 230 are likely to present to their general practitioners, who are likely to recognize about 140, but who will refer on to specialist psychiatric service just seventeen. Only six out of every 1000 will actually be admitted to hospital (Goldberg and Huxley, 1980). These figures demonstrate the 'filtering' effect of different levels of service. A major factor determining the passage of individuals through these 'filters' is the severity of their disorders. Thus, most of the people with psychiatric symptoms who present to their GPs are suffering from relatively minor and transient mood disorders. Serious psychiatric conditions like schizophrenia are much less common. (At any one time three per 1000 in the population suffer from schizophrenia.) However, people with a diagnosis of schizophrenia occupy more than half the long-stay beds in psychiatric hospitals.

If direct access to specialist services were encouraged, it is therefore likely that these 'filters' would soon become 'clogged' with large numbers of people suffering from relatively minor disorders. (This is exactly what happened in the United States when the new Community Mental Health Centres first opened; see Mollica, 1983.) We should therefore be very cautious about broadening the traditional definitions of psychiatric disorder, especially in the name of an attempt to respond to new populations or 'unmet needs'. Apart from 'medicalizing' the ordinary stresses and strains of life, the concept of 'unmet need' is often a myth perpetuated by those who wish to justify the diversion of resources to new problems, rather than concentrating them on correcting deficiencies in existing systems for the delivery of care (Richman and Barry, 1985). Clearly, it is not acceptable to have a service which caters well for the least severely impaired clients at the expense of those who have the most serious problems.

But would dealing more effectively with relatively minor disorders help reduce the prevalence of more serious problems? This is often the argument put forward for shifting the balance from traditional treatment services towards efforts aimed at 'prevention'. The answer is probably 'no'. Little is known about the prevention of serious psychiatric disorders, and one suspects that even if we did have the knowledge, the implications would be socially and politically unacceptable. (For a discussion of the feasibility of 'primary' prevention in psychiatry, see Shepherd, 1984, pp. 141–6.) A more realistic approach is to concentrate effort on 'secondary' and 'tertiary' prevention; for example, identifying those 'at risk', trying to intervene as early as possible with effective treatments and minimizing the harmful effects of treatment itself. 'True' prevention—in the sense of being able to intervene so as to reduce the incidence of serious mental disorder, remains a desirable, but unrealistic, dream.

Assessing the total numbers requiring services may not therefore be as easy as it seems; however, it is only the beginning. For planning purposes, what is really important is not total numbers, but changes in numbers over time. Planning is ultimately about making predictions, and an understanding of the dynamics in a population is therefore crucial. Without this it is possible to make some spectacular mistakes. For example, Tooth and Brooke (1961) predicted that there would be no long-stay patients left in mental hospitals by the mid-1970s. Of course they were wrong, but what they illustrated was the difficulty of making predictions where the factors affecting outcome are not stable. Where the conditions which affect predictions (e.g. concerning the rundown of the mental hospital) are themselves subject to changes—social, political, economic—then it is not possible to extrapolate from previous experience as to what might happen in the future. That was certainly the case 20 years ago in relation to the future of the mental hospital, and it is still the case today.

Predicting future needs in terms of long-stay provision means trying to understand the factors which affect the growth or decline in numbers of long-stay patients over time. Some of these factors are very difficult to predict (e.g. changes in government policies and sources of funding). However, some simply demand good local data which describe the population and its characteristics. For example, a major factor affecting the rate of decline of 'old' long-stay patients is death. Knowing the age structure of a given sample of patients, and their age-specific mortality rates, it is then possible to predict reasonably accurately the rate of decline of this sample (or at least to give estimates and ranges). Similarly, knowing the annual rate of incidence of 'new' long-stay inpatients from a given geographical area, and their rates of discharge, it is possible to predict their rate of accumulation. Putting the two figures together gives the total need for long-stay provision (see Moore, 1985, and Shepherd, 1987, for an example of this kind of calculation). It should be stressed that the data on which such predictions are based must be based on local information. This is because the existing age structure may differ from hospital to hospital and the rates of accumulation of new long-stay inpatients may vary considerably from area to area (Gibbons et al., 1984). Of course, such predictions only refer to the numbers of people likely to need a particular kind of service. They do not specify how such needs are to be met. That requires recourse to some set of standard formulae or norms.

'Norms' embody the judgments of some set of outside experts or professionals regarding the levels and types of service provision required by specific numbers of the population, e.g. $x$ hostel places per 100,000; $y$ day centre places; etc. The widely quoted DHSS norms contained in *Better Services for the Mentally Ill* (DHSS, 1975) or the guidelines for comprehensive psychiatric service given in MIND's manifesto *Common Concern* (MIND, 1983) are examples of such estimates. The obvious problem with relying on norms is that they may not be applicable across different geographical areas or, indeed, across time. Thus, many of the norms given in *Better Services* now look sadly out of date given the major changes in funding residential provisions which have occurred, and the effects of high levels of unemployment on the need for day care and community services in many areas. As the House of Commons Select Committee noted: 'There cannot be precise or binding national norms of any value. Local circumstances will always affect the local needs for particular services' (House of Commons, 1985, para. 213). They further recommend the preparation of national 'guidelines' for levels of service provision, and suggest specific help for districts in the collection and interpretation of local data to assist in the planning process.

Normative planning may also restrict people's ingenuity, and stifle attempts to provide more creative solutions to the problems of service delivery. An over-emphasis on norms is therefore not likely to be helpful. However, norms sometimes do have their uses. They provide 'benchmarks', minimum guidelines below which levels of service provision should not be expected to fall. Since successive governments have failed to meet even these basic guidelines, perhaps we should not be too eager to abandon them. Nevertheless, most people would argue that we should try to construct models of service not based on some abstract set of formulae, but on a careful, qualitative assessment of people's needs. This sounds attractive, although qualitative approaches are also not without their problems and limitations.

## Qualitative methods

The first question to be answered here is: 'From whose perspective should we be making the assessments?'. There are at least three possible independent sources: the user, the relative, and the staff or professional involved. Each may have rather different, and possibly conflicting, viewpoints.

The involvement of primary service users in the planning process has been discussed in a previous chapter (see Kingsley and Towell, Chapter 4). Clearly the users of the service have a central role in defining what these needs are. This has been recognized for some time, although the popularity of 'consumer participation' in psychiatry is something that has waxed and waned. At the turn of the century, the 'Mental Hygiene Movement' was probably the first example of an organization where patients and professionals worked together in a common cause (Leighton, 1982). Similarly, the 'Therapeutic Communities' of the 1950s and early 1960s attempted to try and reduce the status differentials between staff and patients and give users a direct 'say' in what went on (Clark, 1974). Consumer views are now beginning to be taken seriously again, and developments such as the North Derbyshire Mental Health project (Hennelly and Milroy, 1984) and the Nottingham Patients' Council (Weare, 1986) reflect some of the efforts currently being made. These projects tend not to use formal assessments, and so it is not possible to judge the reliability of the information they collect. It is also not clear to what extent those who are most influential in such settings validly represent the full range of users' views. However, some attempt to consult consumers is clearly preferable to no attempt, and these projects show that it is possible to involve users directly in service planning if an effort is made and appropriate channel of communications are set up.

Some specific problems may arise when attempting to consult long-stay patients in hospital (e.g. in the context of running down large institutions) since they may lack the verbal or reasoning skills necessary to give informed replies. Long years spent in an institution may have made them accustomed to a very poor physical environment and amenities, and they may then have difficulties in conceptualizing what community-based options are being offered. They may therefore choose to stay where they are simply because it is familiar and secure. In some of the studies where the preferences of long-stay patients have been formally assessed less than 50 per cent of those questioned gave a clear answer, but of these just under half indicated a wish to remain in hospital (Mann and Cree, 1976). These assessments may not be considered to be truly valid, and probably the fairest thing to do in such circumstances is to give the patient a chance to sample one or two community options on a trial basis. After a period of time, providing that they are not subject to undue pressure, their 'true' preferences should emerge. Nevertheless, obtaining good assessments of the motivation and preferences of users is vital, and there is now some evidence that this is being attempted (McCarthy et al., 1986).

Relatives also have an important and legitimate stake in the shape of future services, and their views must also be considered. There are examples in the literature of quite formal attempts to do this, which have yielded some interesting results. For example, the relatives of schizophrenic patients living in the community seem to attach greatest importance to the availability of services which would actually give them a break from looking after their mentally ill offspring, e.g. day care, holiday relief, etc., and they are not particularly interested in additional domiciliary services (Community Psychiatric Nurses, home helps) or permanent changes in the patients' accommodation (Creer et al., 1982). These ideas may contrast sharply with those of the service planners or the professionals.

Relatives may also have quite a different perspective from the patients themselves, and this is perhaps most apparent regarding the question of the future of the mental hospital. Organizations such as the National Schizophrenia Fellowship generally seem to favour the retention of the mental hospital—at least until it is quite clear that there is something better to put in its place (National Schizophrenia Fellowship, 1986). In contrast, patient organizations such as the Campaign Against Psychiatric Oppression (CAPO) tend to take a more radical, anti-institutional, stance. It is not easy to reconcile these opposing views, but neither is it possible to pretend that such differences do not exist. Both are surely 'valid', in the sense of being legitimate and reasonable, and both sets of interests must be adequately represented.

Just as it is vital to obtain the views of the user, it is important to take account of the relatives' perspectives. Again, this can be done in formal or informal ways (e.g. with standard questionnaires, open meetings, etc.) and care must be taken to ensure that the information collected is reliable and valid. Of course, if relatives can be genuinely involved in service planning it may pay considerable dividends in the long run, as they often not only have very good ideas on what should be included in service provisions, but they may also be in a unique position to see that these ideas are implemented.

The most widely used methods to assess service needs are those based on the collection of 'objective' data by care staff, researchers or service planners. There are basically two different kinds of approach: (1) standardized rating scales which aim to assess individuals' levels of functioning and then compare these with a number of 'criterion groups' in a number of different settings; (2) instruments which present staff directly with a number of service options (e.g. types of residential care with different levels of supervision; different kinds of day programmes; etc.) and ask them to indicate the suitability of each option for individual patients. Examples of the former approach are scales such as the CAPE (Pattie and Gilleard, 1979). This scale classifies elderly people according to five levels of dependency from 'independent living in the community' to 'psychogeriatric ward in hospital'. The REHAB scale (Baker and Hall, 1983) classifies long-stay patients into three groups, 'Severe dependency', 'Moderate dependency' and 'Discharge potential'. Examples of the second approach are to be found in reports such as Mann and Cree's (1976) survey of the needs of new long-stay inpatients, and Clifford and Szyndler's (1986) study of the needs of long-stay patients in Bexley Hospital.

Both these approaches have advantages and disadvantages. The use of standardized rating scales should improve the reliability of the information. Standardized scales, if they are well constructed, should be quick, convenient and easy to use. The involvement of direct care staff in making judgments about patients' needs also has a certain 'face' validity. They presumably know the patients well, and should therefore be in a good position to suggest appropriate services. There may also be other 'spin-offs' in terms of enhanced involvement and commitment to the process of change, especially if staff are allowed to follow their judgments through. On the negative side, standardized scales may lack validity. Thus they may not actually assess the most important aspects of patients' functioning. For example, Kingsley et al. (1985) argue that networks of social support are just as important when considering the resettlement of long-stay patients as their self-care or social skills. Similarly, the patients' views regarding their future, their motivation to change, etc., are often not well covered in standard rating scales. 'Objective' methods can give a distorted picture if they are used in isolation, and should therefore be supplemented with information from other sources.

Another disadvantage of asking staff to choose between options is, of course, that they will be limited by the range of options present (or range of criterion groups used in the standardization) and by their knowledge and familiarity with these options. Thus, if one wants to explore new options, then the available instruments may not be appropriate. Similarly, one may be asking judges to give opinions on services they know very little about. The validity of such opinions is then clearly questionable.

Staff-based assessments also have only a limited predictive value. Whether it is ratings of functioning in hospital, or judgments of what alternative services people might need, it is actually very difficult to predict behaviour accurately from one setting to another. Behaviour is often 'situation-specific' (Shepherd, 1983) and, without knowing all the factors that affect performance in a particular setting (e.g. social networks, motivation, perceived support) it is unlikely that assessments will generalize from one setting to another. They can therefore only be taken as very broad indications of need, and certainly cannot be expected to give precise numbers requiring specific types of provision. Determining individual needs can really only be done on an individual basis, by a process of trial and error. There is really no alternative to trying to develop as wide as possible a range of different settings and then offering people the opportunity to sample one or two until they find the one that suits them best. This may sound overly pragmatic, perhaps even unrealistic, but it is how most 'normal' people choose their homes, jobs and friends, and it certainly stands in sharp contrast to the seemingly endless series of assessment settings that people sometimes have to go through in order to get out of hospital.

We have looked at a number of different assessment methods and their advantages and disadvantages. We have seen that it is not really possible to plan a service based on a 'scientific' assessment of needs because there is no one 'scientific' way of assessing needs. For each method we may have to choose between increasing the reliability of the information obtained, at the expense of decreasing its validity (and vice-versa). No single approach can provide a totally adequate or comprehensive picture of the needs experienced by a particular population. Thus,

the guiding principle found throughout the needs assessment literature is that, to the extent that time and budget permit, combinations of complementary approaches should be used either simultaneously or in tandem, with the various methods selected so that the strengths and weaknesses compensate for one another (Jaffee, 1982).

Whatever method we choose, we should be sceptical of attempts at 'blueprint' planning, i.e. the idea that you can specify in advance the kind of service required to meet a given set of needs. Services are seldom planned in this way; rather they 'grow', almost organically, influenced by opportunism, pragmatism and expedience. They reflect what can be done, rather than what should be done, and it is therefore important that there are mechanisms built into the process whereby one can monitor what is going on. Although it may not be possible to control it precisely, one can then at least tell whether or not the system is going generally in the right direction. This brings us to questions of monitoring and evaluation: how can we keep a check on the operation and quality of service provisions?

## MONITORING AND EVALUATION

The process of internal monitoring and evaluation of services has become increasingly important in recent years, as both the public and politicians have demanded much greater accountability from the various agencies providing care. In the United States, 'quality assurance' programmes were developed specifically to meet the demands of a 'third-party' payment system where they constitute, 'the promise or guarantee made by mental health care providers to funding sources . . . [that] certain standards of excellence in mental health care are being met' (Lalonde, 1982). In this country, although we cannot ignore these questions of cost, there are not quite the same pressures to demonstrate the cost-effectiveness of every element of care on an item-by-item basis (as least not yet!). In the UK, where costs become important, it is usually in the context of comparing the overall benefits of two services. This is a complex undertaking (for an introduction to cost–benefit analysis in a service context, see Goldberg, 1985). However, before beginning to weigh costs against benefits it is necessary to have some factual information about how the service is performing. This section concentrates on these non-financial aspects of quality assurance. If what is happening within a service is known, it is possible, at least in principle, to decide whether or not it is worth it.

The other main reason for wanting to monitor and evaluate services is, of course, to promote change. Evaluation should ideally always be linked to action, i.e. there should be 'positive' monitoring with a real commitment to use the results to improve the service in some way. Evaluation is of little use in isolation. This has clear implications for the way in which evaluation and monitoring projects are set up. Thus, the methods and outcomes employed should be meaningful and useful to the clinicians responsible for delivering the services (preferably they should also be involved in designing the system and collecting at least some of the data) and there should be a commitment from senior managers to provide whatever resources are deemed necessary to implement the recommended changes. If this is not the case, then the process of evaluation and monitoring can become an empty exercise.

## What to evaluate?

The question of what constitutes adequate measures of quality of health care is one that has long concerned evaluators. On the basis of a thorough historical review, Donabedian (1985) argues that we need assessments of quality that are both socially more relevant and scientifically more valid than those that have generally been used. He argues that our technical concerns must also be supplemented by 'attention to the interpersonal, social, even moral dimensions of quality' (p. 259). He notes that what we really require is a much better understanding of the process of health care, and how differences in outcome are influenced by the various interventions that different services provide. Deciding what to evaluate is therefore not just a matter of deciding what we would like to see happen—although that is difficult enough in itself—it is also a matter of being able to identify what is needed to achieve these aims. This requires a scientific understanding of the process of care itself.

Lavender (1985) makes a similar point where he suggests that much of the confusion surrounding the concept of 'quality of care' stems from the fact that different clinicians, with different theoretical models, have different conceptions of what constitutes a good-quality service; e.g. behaviourists will want to look at the reinforcement contingencies; analysts will want to look at the nature of the relationships between staff and patients; 'normalizers' will want to look for socially valued service elements. There is really no way of resolving these theoretical disputes without trying to collect some data on how the presence or absence of these different features affects outcome. Since very little of this kind of data exists, and data collection is difficult, much of what we decide to measure in terms of 'quality' of care will actually be based on assumptions about what is desirable, rather than established empirical relationships. This should be clear at the outset.

After Lalonde (1982), we can make a distinction between 'quality assurance' and 'programme evaluation'. Quality assurance is oriented towards assessing the outcome of specific programmes in relation to individual clients. The data obtained are therefore usually concerned with the day-to-day process of care, and are most likely to be relevant to direct care staff. Programme evaluation, on the other hand, is much more concerned with aggregate data relating to the overall operation of a programme or service. This information is more likely to be used by administrators and managers to plan services and to make decisions about the allocation of resources. Lalonde suggests that, in either case, quality of care can be assessed from three different perspectives: input, process and outcome. 'Input' refers to the physical characteristics of the setting and the resources (staffing, technical, etc.) that are provided. Obviously, a certain level of physical and other resources is necessary to provide and maintain an adequate standard of care, but the precise nature and level of these resources will vary from setting to setting depending on the specfic aims of each project and peoples' subjective views as to what constitute appropriate levels. There are few 'objective' criteria relating resource allocation to quality of care, and thus it is important when projects are set up that the various levels of the necessary resources are agreed. For example, how many staff are required to run a particular kind of new hostel provision? What kind of staff? (grade, professional training, etc.) What other facilities are necessary—laundry, cleaning, transport. Once agreed, the provision of these resources can then be monitored as part of the overall process of evaluation. As already indicated, the precise relationship between these physical characteristics and a good quality of care is uncertain, but they can be regarded as necessary, although not sufficient, conditions.

'Process' refers to the actual nature of the service provided. Does it meet the client's needs? Are effective treatments being offered? Are resources being deployed in an efficient and cost-effective manner? These questions are often very difficult to answer. In the first place we have already seen some of the difficulties of making reliable and valid assessments of need. Secondly, the whole issue of treatment effectiveness is a minefield of controversy, with bitter disagreements about whether or not a particular procedure can be said to be of demonstrable value and therefore should be present in a service which is of a high quality. Thirdly, if a number of treatments—physical, psychological, social—are used in combination (and, of course, this is extremely common) how can we tell if it is being done efficiently and effectively? What we require to cut through this uncertainty are some fairly simple principles concerning organization and practice in long-term care settings which are generally agreed to reflect a good quality of care. Fortunately, such principles do exist, and their central theme is the recognition of the uniqueness of each individual and their right to an individualized programme of care.

Support for these principles comes from a variety of sources, for example, normalization theory (O'Brien and Tyne, 1981) and the 'nursing process' (Yura and Walsh, 1983). Perhaps most importantly, it comes from a considerable body of empirical research. Starting with Goffman's (1961) classic description of the 'total' institution and Wing and Brown's (1970) early work on *Institutionalism and Schizophrenia*, a body of research has grown up which attempts to relate management practices in long-term care settings to the quality of care provided (see Shepherd, 1984, Chapter 4 and Lavender, 1985, for reviews). This work has focused on a number of dimensions of practice, 'autonomy' vs. 'restrictiveness', 'personalization' vs. 'depersonalization', 'staff integration' vs. 'segregation'. It is now generally agreed that a good quality of care should offer opportunities for choice and personal expression, the retention of personal possessions, privacy and contacts with everyday life. Care should be provided in as 'normal' a setting as possible, by staff who are not remote and segregated and who do not see everything in clinical or pathological terms. Thus, we do have some conception of what might constitute the 'process' of good-quality care, and these ideas have some basis in research. However, it has to be acknowledged that the connection between some of these factors and positive outcome has still to be clearly established.

This raises controversial questions concerning the definition and measurement of outcome. Outcome indices should reflect what happens to people as a result of their being involved in the service. But it is necessary to decide not only according to what criteria, but also according to whom. In the context of the assessment of needs it is not easy to say exactly whose needs should be assessed. A similar problem arises when considering outcome. Is it only outcome as judged by the user? (self-ratings, client-satisfaction questionnaires, etc.). Or should the judgments of professional staff (using rating scales, case reports, etc.) be relied on? What about the relatives' opinions? What about the views of the wider community? All these sources of information should be brought together, since they are all likely to have rather different perspectives. This may sound like a 'counsel of perfection', but the unfortunate fact is that health care—particularly psychiatric health care—is a complicated commodity and must be evaluated from a number of different viewpoints. It is simplistic to pretend otherwise, and it may also be extremely misleading.

So, what measure might be used to assess the three levels of quality of care discussed above? The choice of a suitable measure will always depend upon the particular circumstances and purpose for which it is to be used. As far as possible, measures should also be both reliable and valid. These basic criteria must be borne in mind.

## Assessing 'input'

Much of the information on staffing and other resources may be collected routinely, for example staffing ratios, levels of support services. It is then a matter of ensuring that this information is regularly fed back to those who are responsible for maintaining adequate support to the project, that is the service managers. Regarding the physical environment, a number of publications contain guidelines on the adequate provision of space and facilities for residential accommodation, for example the Annexe to the 'Nodder' report (DHSS, 1979); *An Ordinary Life* (King's Fund Centre, 1980); *Home Life: a code of practice for residential care* (Centre for Policy on Aging, 1984). They all share a common theme of trying to provide an environment which is as domestic and 'homely' as possible. This is important not only in contrast to the rather bleak, impersonal character of many of the old institutions, but also in terms of the messages about social value that the use of ordinary housing conveys (its 'normalizing' value).

It has recently been argued that ordinary housing may even be provided on an institutional site and still offer a good quality of care (Wing and Furlong, 1986). This may sound unlikely, but until the data evaluating the project are available, perhaps we should keep an open mind. Regarding physical guidelines for other facilities such as day services and social centres, there is little formal advice available. However, the informal feeling is that one should shy away from 'purpose-built' buildings. Wherever possible the aim should be to use ordinary buildings in the community (houses, schools, industrial units, etc.) sharing these with other groups where appropriate.

A more sophisticated monitoring service input is possible through the use of 'tailor-made' information systems based on microcomputers (Gibbons, 1986; Fagin and Purser, 1986). These systems enable one to keep track of basic data on client characteristics such as numbers of referrals, source of referral and presenting problem. They can also be used to improve the process of individual care planning and to review outcomes (see below). Of course, it is not necessary to set up a complicated computer system to collect some simple data on how the service is operating. Providing adequate records are kept, staff can do their own monitoring. Indeed, there are advantages in them doing so, since they are more likely to pay attention to data they have helped to collect. The process of collecting such data can also serve to remind staff of the original intentions of the project, what it was set up to do, and who it was set up to serve. Without these prompts, these initial aims can easily get forgotten.

## Assessing 'process'

There are a number of alternative approaches to the measurement of the process of care. As indicated earlier, what constitutes a good-quality service is still a matter of controversy; nevertheless there are a range of features which are generally accepted to be of positive value. For example,

Table 6.1    The essential ingredients of a psychiatric rehabilitation programme,
(from Anthony *et al.*, 1982).

| Ingredient | Examples of how observed |
|---|---|
| 1. Functional assessment of client skills in relation to environmental demand. | 1. Client records show a listing of client skill strengths and deficits in relation to environmental demands; strengths and deficits are behaviourally defined and indicate client's present and needed level of functioning. |
| 2. Client involvement in the rehabilitation assessment and intervention. | 2. Record forms have places for client sign-off and comments; percentage of clients who actually sign off; sample of audio tapes of client interviews indicate client understanding of *what* programme is doing and *why*. |
| 3. Systematic individual client rehabilitation plan. | 3. Written or taped examples of objective, behavioural, step-by-step client plans; a central 'bank' of available rehabilitation curricula; client records specify on which plans client is working. |
| 4. Direct teaching of skills to clients. | 4. Practitioners can identify the skills they are capable of teaching, describe the teaching process, and demonstrate their teaching techniques. Programme's daily calendar reflects blocks of time devoted to skill training. |
| 5. Environmental assessment and modification. | 5. Practitioners can describe characteristics of client's environment to which client is being rehabilitated, and how the environment may be modified to support the client's skills level. Functional assessment should have assessed unique environmental demands. |
| 6. Follow-up of clients in their real life. | 6. Client records indicate a monitoring plan and description of monitoring results; audio tapes of practitioner and client feedback assessions; record-keeping forms provide space for changes in the intervention plan. Percentage of clients whose plans have changed; number of appointments for 'follow-along' services. |
| 7. A rehabilitation team approach. | 7. Team members can verbally describe each client's observable goals and the responsibilities of each team member in relation to those goals (may refer to client records for this information). |

Table 6.1 *continued*.

| Ingredient | Examples of how observed |
|---|---|
| 8. A rehabilitation referral procedure. | 8. Client records indicate referral letters requesting specific outcomes by specific dates; telephone referrals demonstrate these same rehabilitation referral ingredients. |
| 9. Evaluation of observable outcomes and utilization of evaluation results. | 9. Agency records show the pooled outcome data for all clients; agency directors can verbally describe their setting's most significant client outcome. |
| 10. Consumer involvement in policy and planning. | 10. Administrators can list the number of joint meetings with consumers; consumer ratings of satisfaction with the rehabilitation programme. |

Anthony *et al.* (1982) have attempted to list the essential ingredients of a good rehabilitation programme, and this is reproduced in Table 6.1.

It can be seen that there is an emphasis on individual planning, client involvement, observable outcomes and transfer of skills to 'real life'. This list could be used as a checklist against which the overall adequacy of the rehabilitation being practised in a particular setting might be evaluated.

More specific measures are to be found in the research mentioned earlier concerning management practices in long-term care settings. This identified a number of dimensions which can be classified under the general heading of 'client-oriented' vs. 'institutionally oriented' practice. Building on Goffman's (1961) original work, King *et al.* (1971) developed a number of scales to assess management practices in residential settings for mentally handicapped people, and these were further developed by Raynes *et al.* (1979) to include staff perceptions of the extent to which they felt involved in decision-making within the units. Client-oriented management practices were found to be correlated with higher levels of staff–client interaction and a more positive quality to the interaction. Both client-oriented management and high levels of positive staff–client interaction were correlated with staff involvement in decision-making. Similar results were obtained by Shepherd and Richardson (1979) and Garety and Morris (1984) using modified versions of these scales in day and residential settings for long-term mentally ill adults.

An alternative approach to studying management practices is contained in the 'Hospital-Hostel Practices Profile' (HHPP) developed by Wykes *et al.*

(1982). This is based on Wing and Brown's (1970) work, and measures the 'restrictiveness' vs. 'permissiveness' of the setting. It has been used by Hewett *et al.* (1975) and Ryan (1979) to study hostels for the long-term mentally ill, and by Wykes *et al.* (1982) to study both day and residential settings. It measures many of the same dimensions as the King *et al.* scales, and produces essentially similar results. For example, it was used to study the same unit which Garety and Morris had found to be relatively 'client-oriented' in its management practices and, according to the HHPP, the unit was less restrictive than comparable hospital wards and staff considered more of the residents' problems as requiring intervention. There is therefore probably very little to choose between the two approaches.

A comprehensive approach to assessing both input and process variable has been described by Lavender (1987) with his 'Model Standards Questionnaire'. This is also derived from the research discussed above on the importance of individualized care and active skills-based treatments, together with the guidelines on physical space from the 'Nodder' report (DHSS, 1979) and a separate section on 'Contact with the Community'. It has good content validity and has been shown to possess high inter-rater reliability. Lavender has described how it can be used to improve practice by giving specific feedback to wards regarding their assessments. It seems like a useful instrument, although before embarking on the complete questionnaire—which is rather long—one might consider whether individual sections could be used to monitor specific aspects of quality of care. A limitation of the scale is that it is really only suitable for assessing hospital environments.

A new procedure designed to improve the process of care for the long-term mentally ill has recently been described by Brewin *et al.* (1987). This is known as the 'Needs for Care Assessment' and is based on an individualized assessment of need linked with a schedule that prescribes appropriate actions. The assessment of need is achieved by examining functioning in certain key areas such as symptoms, behaviour problems, and personal and social skills (including the appropriate exercise of choice). A need is said to be present if functioning falls below some minimum specified level, this judgment being made by the staff most directly involved with the patient's care, if possible in collaboration with the patient him or herself. An unusual feature of the needs assessment is that a need can only be judged as present if an intervention exists which is appropriate and potentially effective. If a need is present, but no intervention is possible, then, unless there is a danger to the patient's safety or those close to him/her, Brewin *et al.* argue that there is a problem or deficit, but no need; for example, in the case of an apparent 'need' for neuroleptic medication due to the presence of active psychotic symptoms, but where the patient is refusing medication. Since no intervention is possible, no need exists. This slightly peculiar situation arises directly from the attempt to relate the concept of need to the process of intervention—that is the attempt to link the treatment plan with the assessment.

If needs are deemed to be present, then they can either be 'met' or 'unmet'. 'Met' needs are defined as those that have attracted some, at least partly effective, interventions when no other interventions of greater potential effectiveness exist. 'Unmet' needs are defined as those that have attracted only partly effective interventions, or no interventions at all, when other interventions of greater potential effectiveness exist. Brewin *et al.* provide a sample list of possible interventions for patients with positive psychotic symptoms, and a scale for classifying interventions according to their actual or potential effectiveness, their appropriateness, and their acceptability to the patient. There are also guidelines as to how long interventions should be maintained before they are deemed to be ineffective or not worth continuing (usually about three months). Finally, there is a system for rating if an intervention is regarded as superfluous, that is the patient is still receiving an intervention even though their functioning is not impaired and there is no danger of relapse if the intervention is withdrawn.

The 'Needs for Care Assessment' is an interesting and ingenious procedure, but is still in the early stages of development. The strength of the approach is that it attempts to specify in a systematic and standardized way which of a patient's symptoms and problems are receiving appropriate treatment and where there may be areas of under- or over-provision. It thus offers an explicit model of clinical practice which can be used to examine the quality of care being given in a particular setting and to compare one setting with another. The authors also stress that the judgment of 'no need'—which is based on the non-availability of an effective treatment—must always be provisional and dependent upon current knowledge. They express the hope that it will not stop the search for innovative types of care and service delivery.

However, the system is based on a series of judgments—first about the presence or absence of problems, and secondly about the effectiveness or not of interventions. The reliability and validity of these judgments are still in doubt, although some data are presented to support the general validity of the range of problems and interventions, and very little data are available as yet on the judgments concerning need in individual cases. Given the scope for potential disagreement both regarding the appropriateness of different interventions and their effectiveness, it is important to collect more reliability data. The controversy alluded to earlier concerning the effectiveness of different interventions certainly suggests that a degree of unreliability would be expected. It is also a little disappointing to note that, in the data which are presented, there is a very low rate of 'unmet need' (less than 3 per cent). Since presumably this is one of the primary objectives of the procedure, one has to ask if unmet need, as defined by this system, is so uncommon, then why does one need such a complicated procedure to identify it? The 'Need for Care Assessment' is thus an interesting new approach which has considerable potential for improving the quality of care for people with long-term problems, but there are still a number of outstanding questions concerning its scientific basis and practical utility. At the current stage of development there may simply be insufficient 'hard' data on which to base a truly scientific model of good clinical practice in rehabilitation. Nevertheless, this schedule stands out as the best attempt so far.

We noted earlier that some of the 'mini' information systems developed to monitor specific new services may also be used to monitor the process of care. For example, in Fagin and Purser's system a range of demographic and personal data is collected in order to produce an initial formulation which is then recorded and may be updated every six months until the case is closed. Similarly, in Gibbons's system there is a simple format for recording individual care plans which also contains other important information such as the names of the key-worker and consultant, who to contact in an emergency, whether the patient is maintained on depot medication and when it is due, the date of next review, etc. These systems, based on the new generation of cheap, widely available and relatively easy-to-use microcomputers, thus have enormous potential both in monitoring process and evaluating outcome in service development.

## Assessing 'outcome'

At the level of overall 'programme evaluation' if one wishes to assess outcome, then one option is to set up a comprehensive 'case register'. This is a data-linkage system, usually based on a large, mainframe computer, which records contacts with the service by the population from a given geographical area (for an introduction to the use of case registers, see Walsh, 1985). Case registers provide a means for evaluating the total service being offered (e.g. Wing and Hailey, 1972) and they can also act as a 'sampling frame' to look at specific client groups or sets of services (e.g. Sturt et al., 1982; Wooff et al., 1983). Such systems have provided an enormous amount of important evaluative and epidemiological data; however they are difficult (and expensive) to set up and maintain. It is unlikely that many new registers will be created in the future and, as indicated above, with the current developments in computer technology, the trend will probably be towards smaller, more 'tailor-made' systems.

Outcome at an individual level must be considered from a number of different perspectives. From a consumer point of view the aim must be to collect information which is as reliable and valid as possible. This may be difficult, not only because of the communication problems of some long-term patients, but also their general tendency to report high levels of satisfaction almost irrespective of the situation (Cox, 1982). Careful interviewing is required in order to counteract this bias towards placing a 'rosy glow' on the results. Wykes (1982) has described a simple scale to measure residents' attitudes to a new 'hospital–hostel' compared with a group who remained on a traditional hospital ward. The hostel-ward residents gave generally more favourable replies, but they also expressed some dissatisfaction. Wykes suggests that these expressions of dissatisfaction might suggest a less passive and apathetic attitude. Thus, even where self-reported outcomes are apparently negative, the results may need to be carefully interpreted. However, these kinds of studies are rare and there has been very little systematic attempt to measure client satisfaction, particularly in the context of the rundown of the mental hospital (see also Mann and Cree, and Clifford and Szyndler's, work cited earlier). It is therefore important to direct more attention to obtaining good assessments of client satisfaction in the future.

Regarding observer-rated outcome, a number of measures are available. One of the best is probably the REHAB scale (Baker and Hall, 1983). This assesses deviant behaviour, social and clinical functioning; it is simple, reliable, quick and easy to use. It has good content and discriminant validity and has been specifically designed for chronic patients. It is particularly suitable for evaluating change. An alternative is the Social Behaviour Scale (SBS) developed by Wykes and Sturt (1986). This covers a similar range of deviant, social and clinical behaviours; it is also short, and has good reliability and validity. The SBS has also been widely used and there is now quite a large amount of comparative data. REHAB and SBS are both good instruments and there is little to choose between them; SBS has the merit of being less expensive.

There has been little systematic research into the family's perspective on outcome. Creer et al.'s (1982) work stands out as one of the best examples. What is striking about the data available is the relatively high rate of satisfaction expressed by relatives, despite the precedence of quite severe problems. (In Creer et al.'s study, around two-thirds of relatives declared themselves as 'content' with the support given, and Johnstone (1987) reports a similar figure from her study of schizophrenics discharged to the community.) This is clearly an area which deserves further research.

RESEARCH DESIGNS

It is important to look briefly at the question of research design. Formal evaluations of the quality of care must begin with the formulation of a clear question about the relationship between one (or more) of the variables concerned in the process of care, and the selection of reliable and valid measures to assess outcome. It is then necessary to examine the relationship between these different variables, particularly their causal status. The means by which this can be achieved constitutes the research 'design' and a number of different kinds of design are possible.

The most common is probably the 'random controlled trial'. Thus in the evaluation of the effectiveness of a particular service in producing a particular kind of outcome (e.g. a new hostel in producing enhanced satisfaction or improved functioning compared with a traditional hospital ward) one would begin by taking a group of potential residents, randomly dividing them into two so as to produce matched samples, and then placing one group (the experimental) into the new hostel, while the other (the control) remained on the traditional ward. After a period of time if there were changes in measures of satisfaction and/or functioning in the experimental group, but not in the controls, one could infer that moving to the new hostel actually caused these changes. The experimental design permits one to reject a number of other possible explanations which might also account for the results. For example, 'maturation' (i.e. it would have happened anyway); pre-existing differences between the groups (they weren't matched beforehand); or measurement error (providing that the measures used were reliable). Different designs have different 'power' according to the extent to which they permit the rejection of alternative explanations. The random controlled trial is a particularly powerful design and has been widely used. However, in the context of service evaluation it presents some difficulties.

Firstly, it may not be possible to recruit sufficient numbers of subjects to provide two matched groups. If the sample sizes are very small—say less than six—then randomization is unlikely to be successful in producing equivalent groups. Secondly, randomization (or the inferior process of attempting to match subjects 'a priori') will only work if the variables likely to affect outcome, which the matching process should take into account, can be specified beforehand. If they are not known, then neither randomization nor matching will produce equivalent groups. Thirdly, there may be practical or ethical reasons why it is not possible to deprive one group of some new facility or intervention. For these kinds of reasons there has been interest recently in 'quasi-experimental' designs (Cook and Campbell, 1979). These do not employ conventional control groups, but rely instead on taking repeated observations from the same group of subjects (or a single individual) over a longer period of time. The simplest design of this kind is known as an A–B (where A = the baseline period before the intervention and B = the period following it). Providing that a stable baseline is secured, then if the measure shows reliable change after the intervention, compared with before it, one can be reasonably sure that exposure to the intervention has caused the change. (Of course, it is still not possible to be sure what element of the intervention is responsible for the change.) Control is obtained by using repeated measurements to establish a stable baseline and each subject thus acts as his/her own control. This removes the need for a conventional control group. Such 'single-case' designs offer a simple and flexible method for evaluating a number of complex problems of service delivery.

They can be used prospectively or retrospectively, although the former is usually to be preferred because of the possible unreliability of retrospective data. If good records are kept it may be possible, for example, retrospectively to evaluate the effectiveness of some new community facility on reducing admissions to hospital simply by examining the records of a series of referrals before and after admission. Prospective data, with repeated measures over a period of time before and after admission, might answer more subtle questions concerning the effect of attendance on functioning, self-reported satisfaction, or relatives' satisfaction. With prospective assessments outcome measures can be chosen more carefully. This is just one example of a 'quasi-experimental' design and there are several more (see Owens et al., 1988, for further examples). Evaluating quality of care therefore does not necessarily depend upon performing classical 'experiments'. There is much that can be achieved with simpler, more 'rough-and-ready' methods, providing that reliable and valid data are available.


## POSTSCRIPT

I hope that I have not made the process of monitoring and evaluating the quality of services sound too technical. It is important to try to be clear about what you think the service should be aiming to do, and what measures might best reflect outcome. However, the most important thing is that there is a group of people who are actually interested in looking at the service in a critical way, and that there is someone who will listen to, and has the power to act upon, their findings. One can dispense with all the technical sophistication if, at the end of the day, no-one ever bothers to visit patients in the community, to look at how they are spending their days, and to ask them—and their families—whether they are happy or not. In a sense it does not matter who does this (researchers, health authority members, citizen advocates) or how they do it, just so long as it gets done. It is certainly not good enough simply to point to the run-down of the mental hospitals and know that this means we must have achieved something positive. The mental hospitals were set up partly because people were concerned about abuses occurring in a dispersed, and larely unregulated, private system. It would be a tragic irony if we were to replace them with a system which did not contain effective mechanisms for dealing with exactly the same concerns.

## REFERENCES

Anthony, W. A., Cohen, M. R., and Farkas, M. (1982). A psychiatric rehabilitation treatment program: can I recognize one if I see one?', *Community Mental Health Journal*, **18**, 83–95.

Baker, R., and Hall, J. N. (1983). *REHAB: Rehabilitation Evaluation*. Hall and Baker, Vine Publishing: Aberdeen.

Brewin, C. R., Wing, J. K., Mangen, S. P., Brugha, T. A., and MacCarthy, B. (in press). Principles and practice of measuring needs in the long-term mentally ill: the MRC Needs for Care Assessment. *Psychological Medicine* (in press).

Centre for Policy on Ageing (1984). *Home Life: a code of practice for residential care, CPA*, Nuffield Lodge Studio, Regent's Park, London NW1 4RS.

Clark, D. (1974). *Social Therapy in Psychiatry*, Penguin Books, London.

Clifford, P., and Szyndler, J. (1986). *Bexley Hospital Patients' Needs Survey*. Available from National Unit for Psychiatric Research and Development, Lewisham Hospital, Lewisham High Street, London, SE13 6LH.

Cook, T. D., and Campbell, D. T. (1979). *Quasi-experimentation—Design and Analysis Issues for Field Settings*, Rand McNally, Chicago.

Cox, G. B. (1982). Program evaluation. In M. J. Austin and W. E. Hershey (eds) *Handbook on Mental Health Administration*, Jossey Bass, San Francisco.

Creer, C., Sturt, E., and Wykes, T. (1982). The role of relatives. In J. K. Wing (ed.) *Long-term Community Care: experience in a London borough, Psychological Medicine* Monograph Supplement 2, Cambridge University Press, Cambridge.

DHSS (1975). *Better Services for the Mentally Ill*, Cmnd 6233, HMSO, London.

DHSS (1979). *Organisation and Management Problems of Mental Illness Hospitals: report of a working group*, DHSS, London.

Donabedian, A. (1985). Twenty years of research on the quality of medical care. *Evaluation of the Health Professions*, **8**, 243–65.

Fagin, L., and Purser, H. (1986). Development of the Waltham Forest Local Mental Health Case Register. *Bulletin of the Royal College of Psychiatrists*, **10**, 303–6.

Garety, P. A., and Morris, I. (1984). A new unit for long-stay psychiatric patients: organisation, attitudes and quality of care, *Psychological Medicine*, **14**, 183–92.

Gibbons, J. (1986). '*Co-ordinated Aftercare for Schizophrenia: the community care information unit*, University Department of Psychiatry, Royal South Hants Hospital, Southampton SO9 4PE.

Gibbons, J., Jennings, C., and Wing, J. K. (1984). *Psychiatric Care in Eight Register Areas, 1976–1981, Psychiatric Case Register*, Knowle Hospital, Fareham, Hants., PO17 5NA.

Goffmann, E. (1961). *Asylums: essays on the social situation of mental patients and other inmates*, Anchor Books, Doubleday, New York.

Goldberg, D. (1985). Cost-effectiveness analysis. In T. Helgason (ed.) *The Long-term Treatment of Functional Psychoses*, Cambridge University Press, Cambridge.

Goldberg, D., and Huxley, P. (1980). *Mental Illness in the Community*, Tavistock Publications, London.

Hennelly, R., and Milroy, A. (1984). Exploring infinity: ways out of dead ends. Paper presented at MIND Conference 'Life after mental illness: opportunities in an age of unemployment', MIND, London.

Hewett, S., Ryan, P., and Wing, J. K. (1975). Living without the mental hospitals, *Journal of Social Policy*, **4**, 391–404.

House of Commons (1985). Second Report from the Social Services Committee: Community Care with special reference to adult mentally ill and mentally handicapped people, HMSO, London.

Jaffee, B. (1982). Assessing community mental health needs. In M. J. Austin and W. E. Hershey (eds) *Handbook on Mental Health Administration*, Jossey Bass, San Francisco.

Johnstone, E. (1987). The frequency and distribution of mental illness. Paper presented at a Consensus Conference on 'The need for asylums in society for the mentally ill or infirm', King's Fund, London.

King, R., Raynes, N., and Tizard, J. (1971). *Patterns of Residential Care*, Routledge & Kegan Paul, London.

King's Fund Centre (1980). *An Ordinary Life*, King's Fund, London.

Kingsley, S., McAusland, T., and Towell, D. (1985). *Managing Psychiatric Services in Transition: designing the arrangements for moving people from large hospitals into local services*, King's Fund Centre, London.

Lalonde, B. I. D. (1982). Quality assurance. In M. J. Austin and W. E. Hershey (eds) *Handbook on Mental Health Administration*, Jossey Bass, San Francisco.

Lavender, A. (1985). Quality of care and staff practices in long-stay settings. In F. N. Watts (ed.) *New Developments in Clinical Psychology*, The British Psychological Society/Wiley, Chichester.

Lavender, A. (1987) Improving the quality of care on psychiatric hospital rehabilitation wards: a controlled evaluation, *British Journal of Psychiatry*, **150**, 476–81.

Leighton, A. (1982). *Caring for Mentally Ill People*, Cambridge University Press, Cambridge.

McCarthy, B., Benson, J., and Brewin, C. R. (1986). Task motivation and problem appraisal in long-term psychiatric patients. *Psychological Medicine*, **16**, 431–8.

Mann, S. A., and Cree, W. (1976). 'New' long-stay psychiatric patients: a national sample survey of fifteen mental hospitals in England and Wales 1972/3, *Psychological Medicine*, **6**, 603–16.

MIND (1983). *Common Concern*, MIND Publications, London.

Mollica, R. F. (1983). From asylum to community: the threatened disintegration of public psychiatry, *New England Journal of Medicine*, **308**, 367–73.

Moore, A. T. (1985). Long-stay psychiatric rehabilitation bed requirements in Cambridge: a planning model. Unpublished MFCM thesis, Cambridge Health Authority.

National Schizophrenia Fellowship (1986). *Short Report—Short Change*. NSF, 78 Victoria Road, Surbiton, Surrey KT6 4NS.

O'Brien, J., and Tyne, A. (1981). *The Principle of Normalisation: a foundation for effective services*, Campaign for Mental Health, London.

Owens, R. G., Slade, P. D., and Fielding, D. M. (1988). Patient series and quasi-experimental designs. In G. Parry and F. N. Watts (eds) *Skills and Methods in Mental Health Research*, Lawrence Erlbaum Associates, Brighton (in press).

Pattie, A. H., and Gilleard, C. J. (1979). *Clifton Assessment Procedures for the Elderly (CAPE)*, NFER–Nelson, Windsor.

Raynes, N., Pratt, M., and Roses, S. (1979). *Organisational Structure and the Care of the Mentally Handicapped*, Croom Helm, London.

Richman, A., and Barry, A. (1985). More and more is less and less: the myth of massive psychiatric need, *British Journal of Psychiatry*, **146**, 164–8.

Ryan, P. (1979). Residential care for the mentally disabled. In J. K. Wing and R. Ilsen (eds) *Community Care for the Mentally Disabled*, Oxford University Press, London.

Shepherd, G. (1983). Planning the rehabilitation of the individual. In F. N. Watts and D. H. Bennett (eds) *Theory and Practice of Psychiatric Rehabilitation*, Wiley, Chichester.

Shepherd, G. (1984). Quality of care, Chapter 4 in *Institutional Care and Rehabilitation*, Longmans, London.

Shepherd, G. (1987). Needs in the community: a district model. Paper presented at Consensus Conference on 'The need for asylum in society for the mentally ill or infirm', King's Fund, London.

Shepherd, G., and Richardson, A. (1979). Organisation and interaction in psychiatric day centres, *Psychological Medicine*, **9**, 573–9.

Sturt, E., Wykes, T., and Creer, C. (1982). Demographic, social and clinical characteristics of the sample. In J. K. Wing (ed.) *Long-term Community Care: experience in a London borough*, *Psychological Medicine* Monograph, Supplement 2, Cambridge University Press, Cambridge.

Tooth, G. C., and Brooke, E. (1961). 'Trends in the mental hospital population and their effect on future planning', *Lancet*, **i**, 710–13.

Walsh, D. (1985). Case registers for monitoring treatment outcome in chronic functional psychoses. In T. Helgason (ed.) *The Long-term Treatment of Functional Psychoses*, Cambridge University Press, Cambridge.

Weare, P. (1986). Discussion group bridges gap between patients and staff. *Social Work Today*, 12–13.

Wing, J. K., and Brown, G. W. (1970). *Institutionalism and Schizophrenia: a comparative study of three mental hospitals, 1960–1968*, Cambridge University Press, London.

Wing, J. K., and Furlong, R. (1986). A haven for the severely disabled within the context of a comprehensive psychiatric community service. *British Journal of Psychiatry*, **149**, 449–57.

Wing, J. K., and Hailey, A. (eds) (1972). *Evaluating a Community Psychiatric Service: the Camberwell Register, 1964–1971*, Oxford University Press, London.

Wooff, K., Freeman, H. L., and Fryers, T. (1983). 'Psychiatric service use in Salford: a comparison of point-prevalence ratios 1968 and 1978, *British Journal of Psychiatry*, **142**, 588–97.

Wykes, T. (1982). A hostel-ward for 'new' long-stay patients: an evaluative study of 'a ward in a house'. In J. K. Wing (ed.) *Long-term Community Care: experience in a London borough*, *Psychological Medicine* Monograph, Supplement 2, Cambridge University Press, Cambridge.

Wykes, T., and Sturt, E. (1986). The measurement of social behaviour in psychiatric patients: an assessment of the reliability and validity of the SBS schedule', *British Journal of Psychiatry*, **148**, 1–11.

Wykes, T., Sturt, E., and Creer, C. (1982). Practices of day and residential units in relation to the social behaviour of attenders. In J. K. Wing (ed.) *Long-term Community Care: Experience in a London borough*, *Psychological Medicine* Monograph, Supplement 2, Cambridge University Press, Cambridge.

Yura, H., and Walsh, M. B. (1983). *The Nursing Process*, Appleton Century Croft, Connecticut.

Community Care in Practice
Edited by A. Lavender and F. Holloway
© 1988 John Wiley & Sons Ltd

Chapter 7

# Staff Training

## A. LAVENDER and A. SPERLINGER

The development of community-based services for long-term clients has brought into sharp focus the question of how adequately the staff within these services are trained. For community-based services to succeed, staff need to adopt very different roles from those traditionally held by hospital and social services staff. The quality of training which staff receive to prepare them for these new roles will, in a large part, determine the quality of treatment and care provided for consumers.

The success of training is dependent on moving from a model based on single learning experiences, only marginally related to the workplace, to an adult experiential learning model (Knowles, 1978; Cross, 1982; Kolb, 1984) which addresses the attitudes, skills and knowledge which staff are required to possess in their particular setting. Thus, as Mittler (1987) points out: 'there is a sense in which the number of people needing training is as great as the number of people in the service'. Given this, training should be designed to reflect the philosophy, goals and type of staff recruited to, or found within, a particular service or project.

Training should not be a passive process. It must allow staff to make plans and policies as to *how* to apply new skills and principles within their services. Training must address the gap between 'teaching week/days' and the real work situation through an integration of work and training and the setting of achievable goals for staff. Training should be seen as a *process* that is continuous, dynamic and takes account of changing staff and client needs. Thus a dynamic approach is important for staff both in existing community- and hospital-based services and in new services where fresh ground is being broken and there is uncertainty about the precise nature of the training needs.

Staff training will only happen if individuals involved in the development of services produce and implement well-thought-out strategies which are part of the structure and process of service provision. These strategies must be given priority and appropriately resourced. When producing such strategies, planners and managers need to take into account three related tasks. Firstly, to take the opportunity which the development of new services provides to offer a much improved and different type of service. Secondly, to ensure that a high-quality service is maintained in the existing hospital-based services, and thirdly, to care for staff and clients in the process of transition. Districts/units involved in changing existing services and creating new services must balance these three tasks and resolve the conflicts between them.

There is a current tendency to respond to the urgent need for staff training in one of four ways. The first response involves a uniform approach or package which is offered routinely to all staff regardless of their place of work. The rationale behind this approach appears to be that, since services are changing, it is as important for staff in hospitals to learn the skills required of staff in community settings as it is for those actually working in community settings. The second response involves a frantic search for external courses on which staff can learn the new skills in the hope that they will return trained for current and future roles. The rationale is that if the skills do not seem to exist locally we need to send people to learn from the experts. The third involves an uncoordinated combination of the first two, and the fourth a paralysis brought on by the overwhelming nature of the task.

There is clearly a need for a more thoughtful and planned response to staff training. There is no point in teaching staff skills which they are not able to put into practice and which are not valued or expected in their place of work. If staff are unable to practise what is taught, training will lead to bitterness, frustration and low staff morale. The end-point in this cycle of frustration is difficulty for the service in recruiting, motivating and retaining staff.

Training must therefore be one of the key tasks which service planners and managers address when planning the development of services. Training should be an integral part of the planned process of change and not a reaction to crisis. This chapter attempts to explore what strategies might be adopted, what attitudes, knowledge and skills need to be learned and how these might be taught. In the development of continuing care services it is important to develop separate but related strategies for the following three groups of staff:

1. Staff within new services.
2. Staff within existing services (hospital- and community-based).
3. Staff involved in the process of service planning and development.

## STAFF TRAINING WITHIN NEW SERVICES

There are many initiatives currently being taken to establish community-based services for continuing care clients. Some of these initiatives are concerned with helping long-stay hospital patients back into the community and some with providing support for those continuing care clients currently living in the community. Staff in these new services usually face completely new roles. Thus, those working in many new residential facilities will not have the range of ancillary staff found in hospital and Part III homes to cook and clean whilst they function as 'direct carers' (Durward and Whatmore, 1976). Indeed, many services are developing, and have developed, for people with a mental handicap, in which one group of staff perform the total range of tasks required within the residential establishment (Felce *et al.*, 1985; Tyne, 1981). These staff could be doing everything from cleaning the toilets to going to the cinema with a client. Similarly, staff in 'day care' facilities are likely to be required to provide clients with treatment and support within the community, that is within clients' homes, educational and leisure centres. Such provision requires the development of new therapeutic skills. Similarly, in the area of employment, staff are likely to be required to deal with local industrial firms and the Manpower Services Commission, as well as initiating small businesses.

Preparation for these new roles is the cornerstone of training for new services. Clients who move from hospital need help to find, in the community, substitutes for a whole range of hospital activities, such as a social life, evening and weekend activities and formal and/or informal jobs. Staff and clients can easily feel isolated and miss the support that the networks within large institutions provide. Just as clients must be prepared for the new settings, so staff must be helped to develop these new roles.

When setting up a new service, or a component of a new service, it is essential for successful training that there is fundamental agreement at the highest level on the principles around which the service is to develop. Principles such as those described in *A Common Concern* (MIND, 1983) have frequently been used in services. These principles need to be used and understood by staff organizing the training *and* by staff working in the services if they are 'really' to shape what is being provided, rather than be a collection of platitudes with which everybody agrees. Similarly, the aims of services and of staff training need to be clear in order to be evaluated. If there are no clear aims it is difficult to see against what evaluations would be based.

In training staff for new services it is useful to adopt a cyclical model of training, which has three phases: (1) Induction, (2) Operational and (3) Review. In the Induction phase the staff are prepared to work in the new setting through a period of training which precedes the opening of the

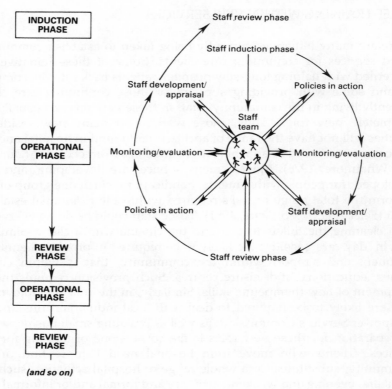

Figure 7.1   Model of training.

setting. In the Operational phase—that is, between induction and review, or between successive reviews—methods of ensuring the continued development of individual members of staff and the staff group are utilized. In the Review phase the staff have the opportunity to reflect on how the setting is working, to use any formal or informal evaluations, to revise current policies and to have access to further training tailored to meet the needs which staff and/or service evaluations have identified. Following this review phase a new operational phase begins, and is followed by the annual or bi-annual review and so the cycle of training is initiated and continued indefinitely. This model is illustrated in Figure 7.1 and described below.

## Induction phase

In the development of a new setting it is essential to prepare staff not only as individuals, but as a group or staff team, for the job in hand. This phase is best organized in a place which has access to training materials (teaching equipment, flip charts, etc.) and can be used for both formal and informal teaching methods. The phase needs to be organized by a single individual or, preferably, a small group who are both familiar with the roles required of the new staff and have experience of a variety of teaching methods. It will be important to organize recruitment so that the Project Leader, or first line manager, is in post prior to the remaining staff. He/she may then get to know the setting and the potential clients and assume responsibility for parts of the training. This is vital not only in affirming his/her role as a skilled and knowledgeable manager, but in ensuring commitment by key staff to training and policy-making from the start of the service.

It is important that *all* staff connected with this setting, from managers to direct care workers, are fully involved in the whole training and that outside groups who are only marginally connected with the unit are involved in the induction phase in some planned way. Experience has shown that a period of between one and four weeks is the optimal length for the induction period. It is also known that it is much more useful to have the induction training in solid blocks of weeks, rather than 'one off' days, as the latter system often leads to dilution of training and dissipation of energy of all involved.

An essential prerequisite of these induction training weeks is that the staff know, prior to the actual teaching days, the clients with whom they are to work. This is facilitated by having the first line manager in post in advance of other staff and arranging for staff to get to know some clients briefly, to find out their strengths, needs, interests and desires. There are a variety of 'getting to know you' exercises and profiles useful for staff and clients in learning about each other (see Chapter 4).

The induction phase should involve considerably more than the usual round of meeting the relevant people that is often arranged when an individual moves into a new post. The aims of such periods, for teams or groups of staff working in particular settings, should be to begin the process of enabling staff to understand and respect the clients with whom they will work, to provide staff with the knowledge and skills necessary for their work, to help staff establish detailed operational policies and to build group cohesion.

What follows is a description of the content and methods likely to prove useful in such induction training.

1. Presentation and discussion of the principles of the service and how these relate to the service and setting.
2. Presentation and discussion of the consumers' view of services; a typical day in the life of a consumer; the needs of the client group involved and 'getting in their shoes', i.e. understanding and respecting them as people.

3. Presentation and discussion of the place of the particular setting or teams in that service currently and in the future service.

4. Identification of the aims of the setting; producing clear goals against which the service may be evaluated. This is best achieved in task-oriented small groups.

5. Identification of skills and knowledge required to meet these goals. These will obviously vary considerably, but the identification can be achieved through brainstorming, small and/or large group discussions followed by poster presentations.

6. Exploration of personal values and the way these affect views of, and interaction with, clients. Useful methods include: small-group discussion, 'getting to know you' exercises involving particular clients (using videoed teaching tapes, or better still, the information collected by staff prior to the teaching days on the real clients), lifestyle exercises (ESCATA, 1985), and other value-based exercises (O'Brien and Tyne, 1983).

7. Discussion of the skills, strengths and needs of the (known) client group who will use the setting; how to ensure that consumers' views are made known and continuously heard, and how to enable the clients to function as a group.

8. Clarification of operational policies. Small (four to six people) and/or large (all staff) groups should establish how to implement particular policies and, in the light of the discussions, reformulate the existing policies. A list of the policy issues which other groups have found it useful to discuss is presented in Table 7.1. Amongst the most important of these are; establishing the referral and acceptance procedure (i.e. how and who should carry out an assessment, what should be assessed and how decisions will be made), the function of a key worker/case manager, record-keeping and confidentiality procedures.

9. Completion of the 'Working Day' exercise. This involves large- or small-group work establishing what a typical day in the life of the setting/project will be like as a means of deciding where and when particular tasks will be undertaken, and by whom. For example, if one of the tasks is to help clients integrate into the community through using community facilities, staff need to work out how this might be accommodated within staff working hours and staffing ratios.

10. Skills and knowledge teaching. Presentations which attempt to help staff develop their knowledge and skills need to take account of two factors. Firstly, the skills and knowledge must be relevant to the job in hand. Secondly, the teaching must tackle the problem of generalization directly (Shepherd, 1977), by dealing with the difficulties likely to be experienced in implementing the skills in the 'real' settings (Milne, 1986). It is in this context that the training described in the operational

Table 7.1 Operational policy checklist.

| 1. Acceptance procedure | What criteria for clients? Are existing clients involved in filling vacancies? |
|---|---|
| 2. Staff recruitment | What criteria for shortlisting?; Are clients involved in interviews? Who selects? |
| 3. Choosing decor, etc. | Are clients involved? When and how? What if there is disagreement? |
| 4. Moving in | How will clients 'get to know' unit and staff? Neighbours? Will key staff know them? |
| 5. Relatives/advocates | Are relatives involved? When? How? What if conflict of views? Citizen advocates? |
| 6. Financial | Will clients hold own allowance books? Who arranges with Post Office? |
| 7. Day facilities | Will clients have choice? Do they require staff to escort? What are the options? |
| 8. Privacy rules | What rules for visitors?/access to bed and bathrooms?/locking rooms?/staff records? |
| 9. Client records | Confidentiality?/storage?/security?/accessibility to clients?/who records and what? |
| 10. Record-keeping | What will be recorded, by whom, where, when and why?/storage?/requirements locally? |
| 11. Housekeeping | What rules for recording food, etc. purchases?/clothing and personal items?/receipts? |
| 12. Keys/security | Will each client/staff have front door key?/are keys held by each shift? (drugs?) |
| 13. Meetings | What will staff/clients attend and why?/residents meetings?/what decisions are made? |
| 14. Relationships | May clients' friends stay overnight?/clients go out overnight?/share bedrooms? |
| 15. Risk-taking | Is there an agreed policy for supporting staff and clients taking calculated risks? |
| 16. Transport | What local trains/buses? What rules for staff taking clients in own cars? |
| 17. Medicines | Can all staff give them? May clients take own? Drugs cards/prescriptions? Records? |
| 18. Household | What rules for clients taking own furniture/decorating/gardening/wiring plugs, etc.? |
| 19. Replacement staff | What induction and by whom? Where? Before starting work? What about Bank staff? |

phase is so vital in encouraging the regular use of these skills. The skills and knowledge likely to be useful in such settings have been presented elsewhere, (Watts and Bennett, 1983; Shepherd, 1979; Watts and Lavender, 1987a and b).

11. Clarification of the roles of staff members and the development of effective multidisciplinary teamwork. Most new services for long-term

clients involve working in multidisciplinary teams and, indeed, Watts and Bennett (1983b) point out 'Because successful rehabilitation needs to take a broad comprehensive view of patients' problems, it is necessary for a number of different professions to share the work that needs to be done with each individual patient.' Thus, during the course of any induction period, the staff need to spend time working in a group, preferably led by a non-staff member, on issues which include defining individuals' roles (i.e. where they are different and where they blur), examining leadership issues (i.e. not so much who, but what model of leadership to adopt—see Watts and Bennett, 1983b), and identifying and resolving conflicts. Some workshop input on group processes, particularly the destructive processes known to operate in groups, are likely to be especially helpful (Roberts, 1980). The aim of such an enterprise is to create a cohesive and effective multidisciplinary team.

12. Discussion, clarification and agreement on the role of various meetings involving staff (and consumers) within the service. It is important to establish, for each meeting: who should attend; who should lead the meeting; what the business of the meeting should cover; what decisions the meeting is empowered to make; who should follow up such decisions; what records should be kept and who should have access.

In any induction period, obviously all the issues described above may not be resolved, but it remains important that the group attempts to tackle them from the beginning. Having started to examine them, the group is then in a position to establish which issues will need continued work and how these might be tackled during the operational phase.

### Operational Phase

The operational phase refers to the training which occurs as an integral part of the everyday work of staff and is vital to the maintenance of a high quality service. The operational phase training can take a variety of forms and is, perhaps, more usually referred to as staff development. Systems for ensuring the continued development of staff are discussed later in the chapter. However, it is helpful to describe some of the forms which this operational training can take.

The most common is regular supervision, either by peers or a senior member of staff. This supervision can occur in a multi-professional and/or uni-professional context and is relevant to all styles of work. The detailed nature of this supervision will vary according to the nature of the work being supervised, but it is important to make two general points. Firstly, all staff should receive some form of supervision regarding their work with clients. Secondly, there is a tendency for the more senior members of staff to be unsupervised, which conveys some implicit message that they have been 'trained' and no longer require much supervision. This is a particularly serious problem in a service where the relevant attitudes, knowledge and skills are constantly changing. It is, however, important to emphasize that the most effective supervision is that which can identify and encourage the strengths of supervisees as well as identify and discourage weaknesses.

Other types of formal within-setting training include the running of staff seminars and discussion groups. These can include presentations by outside agencies or experts followed by discussion. Involving clients in these experiences is often extremely helpful. Less formal training, but often important learning experiences, are staff meetings aimed at reviewing staff's work with clients. These include policy meetings at which the organization and running of the settings are reviewed, client review meetings in which staff's work with clients is reviewed and planned, and staff support groups where staff can look at the interpersonal issues (Bion, 1966) that are affecting the functioning of the team. All these are important training opportunities which, if taken advantage of, ensure that the setting or team will be both a stimulating one in which to work, and one which offers a high quality of care.

The evidence on this latter point of the relationship between training, as it is discussed here, and high quality care is compelling. Training involves providing staff with the opportunity to develop new skills and the autonomy to put these into practice within a supervised and supportive framework. A substantial body of work has indicated that, when decision-making is delegated to the direct care workers, it produces not only better-motivated staff, committed to implementing change, but better quality of care for clients (Raynes et al., 1979).

Finally it is necessary to mention the role of external courses within the operational phase. One drawback of the approach to training described so far is that it can produce a very insular group of staff. External courses do have a role to play in providing the outside stimulus to staff to ensure that the setting or team system remains 'open' (Bridger, 1980). The important point with external courses is that they should occur in the context of the planned development of individual members of staff (perhaps as a result of the appraisal meeting described later), or of the staff group as a whole. In addition, it is useful for the Project Leader to consider how individual members' training experience can be shared.

In summary, the aim of the operational phase is to create a setting/staff team which offers continuous training for staff and provides clients with a consistently high quality of care.

**Review Phase**

The review phase involves a period briefer than the induction phase in which staff reflect on their own performance as individuals and the performance of the team/setting, using the formal and informal evaluations at their disposal. This structured review then becomes the focus for revising policies, responding to identified changes in clients' needs, and planning future staff development. Ideally, such a phase should involve a period of a week, or single focused days, in the setting in which the induction phase was conducted. This is likely to be difficult in many residential or day care settings, for practical reasons. However, it is important that the difficulties are tackled and that alternative arrangements, such as conducting review days within the settings and/or organizing a series of half-days, are considered.

As with the induction phase, it is important that *all* staff are involved in this review phase, and that it should be convened by a small group who are familiar with the experiences of staff, and are skilled at using a variety of teaching methods. The tasks which need to be addressed in these review phases include:

1. Review of the aims of the setting/team and the goals identified during the induction phase. This can include the presentation and discussion of any evaluative research conducted and small group discussions about the existing aims and goals of the setting/team. Task-oriented small groups can then be used to produce revised aims and goals.
2. Review of operational policies in the light of above. Again, small task-oriented work groups can be used to discuss and produce revised operational policies.
3. Skills and knowledge teaching. The success of such sessions is dependent on staff being able beforehand to identify what they require. The convenors may facilitate such identification through discussions with staff, but the key point is that the content of teaching is not only pertinent to the work of the staff team, but has been identified by staff themselves. Such teaching sessions can draw on a variety of methods, including seminar/tutorials, formal dyadic presentation, workshop-style formats which use video, small group work and role play. These teaching sessions are essential to provide the balance, within the review period, with the more insular reviews described in (1) and (2).
4. Review of roles of staff members and the functioning of the multidisciplinary team. The issues and methods described in the Induction Phase are useful in these review tasks. It must be noted that it is inevitable that there will be replacement staff who have joined since the Induction Phase. A review of the roles of staff members will be particularly

important for the staff group where there have been changes in membership of the staff team.

The review phase should be part of the continued life of the staff team and be repeated at regular (six-monthly or yearly) intervals. These review phases provide the opportunity for the team to evaluate its performance using all the information at its disposal. Feedback from empirical evaluations is useful during this phase (Lavender, 1987), as are the statistical data (DHSS, 1984a) collected by the Health Authority or Local authority about service users. In addition, the informal evaluations and observations of staff provide further vital information. The review phase is the context in which the feedback from a variety of sources is used by the team to evaluate their performance and to make specific plans/goals for the future.

## Summary

A cyclical model of training has been presented for staff in continuing care settings. This model provides staff with a stimulating environment in which learning is continuous, and provides clients with a team that offers a high standard of care that is responsive to their changing needs. Such a model requires a more elaborate definition of 'training' than is usually implied by that word, but is vital if the mistakes of the past (i.e. the creation of institutionalized settings and teams) are to be avoided in the new community-based services.

## STAFF TRAINING IN THE ESTABLISHED SERVICES

A comprehensive staff training strategy needs to take account of the staff within the established service, particularly as new models of care and community-based services are developed. The established services usually include day care provision (e.g. day hospitals, day centres), hostels and other residential facilities in the community as well as hospital-based wards, social and employment areas. Staff within these services face many problems. Often the services around them are in transition and there is little communication about new developments, the roles of various agencies and the changing roles of staff within the new services. Many of the staff in existing services feel threatened, and quite rightly so, because often how they will fit into the new services has not been, or does not appear to have been, considered. Many of the established services see the high-status, highly resourced, and relatively luxurious physical settings of the new services growing whilst their own remain static. This leaves staff feeling increasingly devalued. In addition, it is not uncommon for new projects to be developed in close proximity to existing services, which for staff only serves to heighten the inequality of staff conditions, rather than to 'serve as a model for them'. The cumulative effect of these problems is to create a highly anxious and envious group of staff who feel demoralized and without a future. This clearly runs the risk of creating a group of staff resistant to change, who are reluctant to make a positive contribution to the development of services and who find it difficult to provide a high quality of care in their own setting (Georgiades and Phillimore, 1975).

These dangers are not easy to avoid. As Cullen (1983) notes: 'There is little point in trying to change the quality of life of those who live in an institution by focusing on only one aspect of the organisation. Too many components are inextricably linked together to make this a sensible approach.' Those involved in planning and managing services need to take into account this complexity. Thus, when considering the introduction of training for staff, it is vital that much thought is given to the environment in which the training is to be applied, the constraints on the setting (and on the staff), and the existing practices of staff. In addition, before embarking on training, it is important that both planners and those involved in training have a clear understanding of how services are likely to be developed and a positive view of how staff in the existing services might contribute to those developments.

The training of staff in existing services should aim to create a staff group who are informed about changing attitudes to services for their client group, are informed about future developments, who can see their place in the developments and who are active innovators in that process of change. Mittler (1987) points out: 'Training should provide opportunities for learning to be a change agent in one's own work setting.' Clearly, one useful approach is to introduce the cyclical model of training with its Induction, Operational and Review Phases to these established services. During the process of transition from traditional hospital- to community-based services, this model of training simultaneously enables staff to improve the quality of care in their current setting and prepares them to take up new roles in the developing service. How such a model might be introduced requires further discussion. Introducing genuine training is difficult. Solutions to the problem will be dependent on local circumstances and the inventiveness of the staff involved. One way forward is the creation of a Training Team, either from staff within the existing services and/or new staff. It may be preferable if people from within and outside the service combine to form the Team. What is essential is that team members possess the organizational and teaching skills to introduce the cyclical model of training to the established services. This team needs to keep in close contact with management and those involved in planning new services, in order to gain new resources when required, or at least to be clear about the resource constraints.

Such a training team could target particular settings and, in close consultation with staff, develop individualized training programmes for that setting. The initial programme or series of programmes would be the Induction Phase. From this platform it is possible to develop the Operational and Review Phases, which could similarly, be facilitated by the Training Team.

## Induction Phase

Training must always be linked to the actual working conditions of the staff concerned. The team organizing the induction phase must assess the needs of staff and understand the goals of the existing setting, in the context of the developing service. It is important that all staff involved with the setting are included in the training, and that an agreed time limit is set on the induction phase. Involvement of all staff requires negotiation, so that nursing and auxiliary staff, for example, may all be involved simultaneously. If this is not done, there is a danger of perpetuating a 'two-tier' way of working and training. It also militates against 'team building' for the staff group as a whole. It will be important to involve the first line manager in the preliminary discussion of the content of training, and the organization of the induction phase. He/she will have substantial knowledge of the clients and staff in the setting, and could contribute to the teaching sessions, with support from the Training Team as required. This is vital, not only in affirming his/her role as a skilled and knowledgeable manager, but in ensuring, from the start, the commitment of key staff to training and policy-making.

The setting in which the training will take place is likely to require special negotiation, and the solutions will be dependent on the particular circumstances of the setting. It is probably best if the induction phase occurs away from the workplace. Easy access to training materials and space for formal and informal teaching sessions is required. It may, however, be necessary for the training to be carried out within the setting, and arrangements should then be made for bringing in the equipment. The problem of continuing to run the setting may arise, and it may then be necessary for members of the Training Team, or staff from other areas of the service, or Bank staff, to cover whilst training is in progress. It might be, for example, that the training period would need to be spread over a longer period (maximum two months), with shorter sessions, although there is evidence that the most productive arrangement is for a 'block' of time to be set aside

for training. If the practical problems seem insurmountable, it is likely that
someone or some group is sabotaging the training exercise and, in this
case, it would be better to find out who and why, rather than to continue to
seek solutions to an endless list of problems (Lavender, 1986).

The induction phase should, for established services, cover the same
issues as that for new services (see New Services Induction Phase, points
1–12) and could usefully employ similar teaching methods. These will not,
therefore, be repeated. However, some general points about the induction
phase for established services need to be made. Firstly, during this phase
the Training Team are likely to become aware of the setting's resource
deficits. The deficits might be of equipment and/or staff, and the Training
Team must have a relationship with planners and managers whereby they
can either help staff to gain these resources and/or be clear about what
cannot be gained, so that staff can set about the task of working within
their resources. There is nothing so frustrating as hoping to teach clients to
use a washing machine, for example, when it is continually promised, but
never arrives. Secondly, with each setting, the goals established and the
knowledge and skills conveyed need to be tailored to specific jobs required
of, and identified by, staff. Unless these issues are addressed, training can
easily turn into an abstract exercise which leaves the staff unaffected.

## Operational Phase

The operational phase for established services should closely follow that
described previously for new services, and so will not be repeated here.
Howevver, it is important to elaborate on the role that the training team, or
staff responsible for organizing training, can play. The team should act as
facilitators of training, rather than providers of training, in this phase. The
task is to enable staff to conduct their own systems of appraisal, supervision and teaching. Similarly, staff should be helped to develop both
methods of evaluating the progress of the setting and the means for
introducing change to improve its functioning. Once again, the commitment of the first line manager will be essential in this phase.

In all these enterprises the Training Team, or group of staff introducing
training, are essentially change agents and, as such, should be at least
knowledgeable of the difficulties in such a role (Towell and Dartington,
1976; Lavender, 1986). Ideally they should also have some experience of
working in this way. Clearly, this team or group are likely to become well
informed about the resources, physical and staffing, available to the
setting, and would need to feed this information into the planning system
to promote the continued development of staff and setting. Once again, it
is vital, if a high quality of care is to be maintained, that training becomes
an integral part of the everyday work of staff.

## Review Phase

The review phase is as essential for the established services as it is for new services. This should follow the process described for the review phase within new services in terms of arrangements, staff included, issues covered and methods employed (see 'New Services, Review Phase'). It is therefore unnecessary to describe this phase in detail again.

## Summary

Clearly, it is most important that the staff in the established settings move into the phased cycle of training in the same way as staff in new settings. Unless these established staff are engaged in training, which encourages them to develop as individuals, an embittered and ill-prepared staff group will be left behind in the old services. This is likely to present the new services with two significant problems. Firstly, unless the established staff are available and equipped for the posts in the new services, there will simply not be enough staff for the new developments. Secondly, the neglect will breed bitterness and sabotage from the established staff, which will hinder the development of good community-based services. These problems could be avoided if some energy and resources are put into training the established staff, whose skills and potential will be much needed in the new services.

## TRAINING IN SERVICE DEVELOPMENT

High-quality planning is crucial in the development of continuing care services, and it is vital that staff are trained for this task. Planning is concerned with creating a coordinated district-wide service which takes into account the specific needs of the locality (see Kingsley and Towell, Chapter 4). Planning usually involves clinicians, planners, works officers, service managers, financial advisors, service users and voluntary agencies, although only rarely are the people trained to carry out this activity. In most services, staff involved in planning are likely to have to arrange their own training. There is clearly a role for Regional Training Officers, the NHS Training Authority and establishments such as the King's Fund, to help with the provision of this training. However, more usually planning teams will need to identify and organize their own training using a self help model.

Most services have established planning groups to develop services. Members of such groups often begin planning before considering what is involved in this process, and whether they have the knowledge and skills to carry it out. In many ways the first task should be to consider their own training needs and to establish a training cycle, with Induction, Operational and Review Phases. For this training to be meaningful it should be linked directly to the planning tasks and, consequently, it is through a consideration of these tasks that the training needs of the group can be identified. The analysis below identifies the tasks in each of the phases, and suggested ways that training in these activities might be organized.

### Induction phase

When a planning team is established, it is important that time is set aside to consider the tasks of the group and to identify the skills, experience and training necessary for its members to carry out these tasks. This should be organized during an induction period, which could last up to six weeks, but should include the team spending at least a week together on identifying the tasks. The week is best conducted in a setting similar to that described for previous induction phases and organized collectively, or by delegated members of the planning team. There is a clear role for Unit General Managers and District General Managers in the health service and Directors of Social Services to ensure that planning teams are allowed the time and encouraged to organize such induction periods. In this section it is perhaps most useful to identify the tasks which many planning groups need to address.

1. Establish service principles. Discuss and decide upon what philosophy and principles the service is to be based (e.g. *A Common Concern*— MIND, 1983).
2. Establish ideas for the future service which are innovative and avoid the mistakes of the past (e.g. *Creating Local Psychiatric Services*—Kings Fund, 1983).
3. 'Get to know' the client group. This includes getting to know at least some clients at a personal level, as well as the numbers, needs, preferences and interests of the continuing care clients in general (see Chapter 6).
4. 'Get to know' the current services and how they are used by clients.
5. Identify the financial resources and constraints.
6. 'Get to know' the planning mechanisms operating within health, social services and housing departments, and the relevant housing and voluntary associations.
7. 'Get to know' the service district. This is information about the district in which the service is being planned and includes: (a) demographic characteristics of the population, (b) geographical distribution of the

population, (c) local employment and employment training opportunities, (d) local public facilities, e.g. public transport, education facilities,
local social and interest clubs, etc.

8. 'Get to know' the current policies relating to staff training and development.
9. Establish procedures for planning and making operational particular
   projects. This process involves the following tasks: (a) Consulting with
   consumer groups (i.e. service users, CHCs and other interested
   groups) and staff (unions) currently involved in the services. The
   process serves to inform staff and to discover problems with, and gain
   support for, the plan. (b) Establishing accurate capital and revenue
   costing for the projects. (c) Constructing detailed operational policies.
   (d) Detailing the use of rooms and the equipment requirements for
   each room. (e) Identifying an appropriate building or, in the case of a
   new building, identifying the appropriate site and architectural
   design. (f) Constructing job descriptions and organizing advertising.
   (g) Selecting staff. (h) Liaising and informing other staff involved in
   the service about how the project will relate to them and the project's
   place in the overall service. (i) Organizing the tendering of and building work on projects involving capital investment. (j) Organizing and
   implementing an induction training period for new staff. A more
   detailed analysis of these tasks can be found in the CAPRICODE
   planning documents issued by the DHSS (DHSS, 1984b).
10. Establish procedures for involving direct care staff in planning.
11. Clarify the functions of members of the planning group and establish a
    cohesive multidisciplinary group.
12. Establish procedures for monitoring and evaluating the effectiveness
    of the service.
13. Produce an outline strategic plan of the future of the service. The use of
    such a plan is described by Kingsley and Towell (in Chapter 4).
14. Clarify the roles of the planning group members and promote the
    development of effective, multidisciplinary planning (see 'New
    Services Induction Phase', point 11).

During an induction period it is likely that a combination of training
techniques will be required to identify the tasks and begin the process of
training. These techniques or methods include: dyadic presentation of
information (e.g. experiences of other services, planning procedures and
financial information); task-oriented small group work with poster exercises and collective discussion; 'getting to know you' assignments; seminar
and tutorial groups with guided reading and visits to other services and to
parts of the existing services. Those organizing the induction period must

choose the method which most suits the task in hand. It is therefore not possible to be prescriptive about which methods are appropriate for which tasks. Thus, the aim of the induction period is to *begin* the process of identifying the tasks of the group and acquiring the experience/training necessary to successfully undertake service planning.

## Operational Phase

As with all training described in this chapter, operational phase training must be closely integrated with the work in hand. The operational phase training is closely linked to staff development and any individual's planning activities should be considered within the context of their profession's system of appraisal and review. However, it is important to identify some specific forms of operational training which are likely to be useful for people involved in planning.

The most obvious is supervision, either by seniors or peers. At a practical level this is most easily organized through professional lines so that individuals involved in planning have the opportunity to have their work supervised by seniors or peers within their own profession. Alternatively, or in addition to this, the work can be supervised collectively or individually by outside consultants (Clifford, 1987), or by the group presenting regularly to Regional Training Officers, as has been developed with services involving people with a mental handicap (*Bringing People Back Home*, SETRHA, 1987).

During the course of planning, it is likely that new tasks are identified for which the members require training. These new training needs can be met in one of two ways. Firstly, by the planning group arranging training sessions (lectures, seminars, discussion groups, workshops, etc.), within the service. This might involve drawing on local and/or outside expertise. One useful experience is for planning teams to present their plans to other districts' planning teams for the purpose of sharing ideas, problems and solutions. Secondly the team may attend workshops and outside courses at which the identified tasks are tackled.

The operational phase ensures that training is not a series of events separate from the work, but rather an activity closely integrated with the work of the group. This means adopting an adult learning model of training, which increases the likelihood of the group producing high-quality service plans.

## Review Phase

This phase is similar to other review phases in that it involves a period, usually shorter than the induction period, during which the planning group can evaluate progress and plan future activity. Such a learning experience needs to include all members of the planning group and involves them spending a period of at least two to three days in a structured review. This should take place in a similar setting to other induction periods, once a year. It is useful if the review phase is organized collectively by delegated members of the planning group.

The review should include presentations of formal and informal evaluations, review of tasks identified in the operational phase, and the identification of new tasks. These latter two activities are best completed in task-oriented small groups where the results of the discussion are fed back to all participants. Clearly, it is vital that a written record of the group's work is kept. In addition to these essentially insular activities, it is helpful if external speakers and discussants can be brought in to help the group consider particular issues, for example consumer consultation or liaison with housing associations. Once again, it is important that the organizers of this phase ensure that the involvement of external speakers is closely linked with the needs of members of the planning group.

**Summary**

Planning involves a complex series of tasks. If multidisciplinary planning groups are to be asked to complete these tasks, the individuals involved must be trained for them. Although there is likely to be some blurring between the phases, the framework of induction, operational and review phases provides a useful structure within which training can be organized. Unless those involved in planning receive this training as an integral part of their work, service planning is likely to proceed in a haphazard and amateurish fashion.

SYSTEMS OF SUPPORTING STAFF DEVELOPMENT

A vital part of all operational phases is the system for ensuring the continued development of staff. Many services are presently suffering because systems of encouraging this development have not been used. The fact that so many staff currently need retraining is testament to this failure, as are the many reports of 'burn out' from staff working in continuing care services (McCarthy, 1985). The 'systems' which are being referred to are variously known as Individual Performance Reviews (NHS Training Authority, 1986), staff appraisal, and individual appraisal and review. These systems are very similar and are best organized within the separate professions so that a senior member of each profession appraises and reviews the junior staff. It is essential that this system is extended to all, including the most senior members of each profession.

These systems of appraisal and review are intended both to review past performance and to plan future action, in order to encourage the development of each member of staff. Most systems involve a senior member of staff reviewing the performance of staff at regular intervals (six months to a year), in an interview lasting at least one hour. It has been pointed out by Metcalf (1985) and Stratford (1985) that appraisal systems only work when:

1. There is an atmosphere in which both parties can communicate openly.
2. The appraisee is prepared to actively engage in self-appraisal, and the appraiser to appraise his/her ability to create the personal conditions in which this can take place.
3. A democratic negotiating style of appraisal is adopted.
4. The appraiser and appraisee maintain confidentiality (if confidential issues are to be raised outside the meeting, then this should be the subject of negotiation).
5. A problem-solving approach is adopted, in which goals and methods to achieve these goals are clearly identified.

Thus, the emphasis is on the appraiser and appraisee actively working to identify the appraisee's professional needs and how these needs can be met. Within the context of this meeting the training needs of the appraisee will emerge out of the overall review of performance. The task of the appraisee and appraiser is to identify specifically what training experiences (within or outside the unit) the appraisee needs. In terms of outlining what areas would be considered in this appraisal and review, it is important to state that the purpose of the meeting is to improve the appraisee's performance, and that the appraisal must consider both the precise nature of the appraisee's job and the appraisee as a whole person.

There are a number of systems of appraisal on offer. One example is the Individual Performance Review currently being introduced by the NHS Training Authority, which reviews three broad areas: strengths and weaknesses of current job, career interests and development needs. The problem with many of these systems is that it is rarely worked out, in any detail, who will appraise whom. The words appraiser and appraisee, or manager and subordinate, are not explicit enough. Given this difficulty, what is the solution? Two factors need to be taken into account. Firstly, each profession has different areas of expertise and, in making judgments about an individual's performance, and in helping them to identify their training needs, it is necessary for the appraiser to have a good grasp of the professional area of expertise. Secondly, the appraiser must have some knowledge and experience in the specific level of work (i.e. directly with clients, within particular units, or in service planning), in which the appraisee is working. Thus, it is most sensible if appraisal systems are introduced within particular professions and it should be the responsibility of the service manager to ensure that such systems exist.

Within the nursing profession, for example, such a system could operate whereby the enrolled nurses and staff nurses would be appraised by the sister/charge nurses who, in turn, would be appraised by the clinical nurse manager who, in turn, would be appraised by the senior nurse manager. Thus, within each profession, the existing hierarchy within that profession can be used as the basis for the systems of appraisal. At a certain point within each profession the top of the hierarchy is reached, and there is no obvious person to review the work (professional, administrative and planning) of that individual. This can be achieved in a number of ways. One is for a professional peer or group of peers from a neighbouring district area to review the professional work of that individual whilst the administrative and planning work of these individuals may be reviewed by a senior manager to whom they report, or are in some measure account- able. The only profession to whom this system would be problematic is the medical profession, whose lines of managerial accountability within dis- tricts have remained somewhat unclear. It is, perhaps, time that this apparent anomaly was reviewed.

In summary, during the operational phase it is necessary to institute a system which is likely to ensure the continued development of staff. The system suggested is one of appraisal and review organized within profes- sions, in which the specific training needs of each member of staff are identified and a plan drawn up to meet these needs. It is the responsibility of the service managers to ensure that such systems exist, and that adequate resources are available to meet these training needs. In conclu- sion it is important to add a note of caution. Appraisal is a sophisticated exercise, requiring considerable skills on the part of the appraiser if it is to help staff development rather than be used as an opportunity for 'mana- gers' to exercise punitive control.

## PRE-QUALIFICATION PROFESSIONAL TRAINING

There are rightly many professions involved in continuing care services and it is essential that these groups receive appropriate training at the pre-qualification stage. The most fundamental strategic point is that each profession should receive training specifically concerned with continuing care clients. Ideally, this should be an integrated combination of super- vised work experience in a variety of good-quality continuing care settings and a programme of formal and informal teaching. The focus for the teaching should be the client; the experience of long-term psychological/ psychiatric problems. This work with continuing care clients has traditionally been termed rehabilitation, which is probably something of a mistake because rehabilitation, as Watts and Bennett (1983a) have eloquently pointed out, is relevant for people with many other psychiatric problems.

The second strategic point is particularly important at the pre-qualification stage. Staff in training should be exposed to relatively few poor-quality settings. The majority of settings in which those in training are placed should offer a good quality of care where their work can be supervised by staff who will act as 'good models'. If pre-qualification staff are exposed to one poor quality setting after another, with 'poor' supervision by 'poor' role models, they are likely either to become trained staff offering poor care, or to leave the profession in frustration and despair. The fact that some staff battle through training and, by their own endeavours, remain innovative and thoughtful, is no reason to continue with the poor quality training frequently offered.

The third issue, which is also particularly important at the pre-qualification stage, is that of breaking down the barriers between different professions and different agencies. Mittler (1987) has stated that, whilst lip service is paid to multidisciplinary teamwork, the initial training of most professionals 'is carried out in largely watertight compartments, with the result that few students are provided with opportunities to learn about the work of colleagues in other disciplines'. He suggests a variety of ways in which it is possible to prevent the isolation of initial training; e.g. lectures by other specialists, work placements with other disciplines and common lectures for students from different disciplines. He argues that this is essential if we are to avoid the isolation of specialist staff from one another both in training and in subsequent practice.

It is important for organizers of pre-qualification training to address the following questions:

1. Is part of the course specifically concerned with training people to work with continuing care clients?
2. Is there supervised work experience as part of the training in continuing care settings?
3. Are the settings monitored by the organizers of training to ensure they offer a high quality of care and, therefore, offer examples of good practice?
4. Are the supervisors within those settings monitored by the organizers of training to ensure the staff in training are offered experienced and good role models?

5. Is part of the training programme specifically designed to provide staff in training with the necessary knowledge and skills to work with continuing care clients?
6. Are staff in training monitored in a way which enables the organizers of training to be sure that they have the appropriate knowledge, skills and experience to work with continuing care clients?
7. Are opportunities provided for staff in training to learn about the work of colleagues in other disciplines working with continuing care clients?

If any answers to these questions are negative for the broad range of professions involved in the care of people with long-term and severe mental health problems, then it is clear that staff are not being adequately trained to work in services for these people.


## CONCLUDING COMMENTS

'Staff are the key resource for community care. Sound manpower planning and effective training are, therefore, essential. But, unfortunately, both appear conspicuous by their absence so far as community care is concerned.' 'Community care needs a new impetus in training, if the needs of existing hospital staff and properly trained community staff are to be met' (Audit Commission, 1986). This chapter has attempted to describe strategies for training which could be introduced by health authorities, social services and each profession to begin to meet these training needs. Clearly, the introduction of such strategies is now a matter of great urgency if continuing care clients are to be offered high-quality community-based services.


## REFERENCES

Audit Commission, the (1986). *Making a Reality of Community Care*, HMSO, London.
Bion, W. R. (1966). *Experiences in Groups*, Tavistock Social Science Paperbacks, London.
Bridger, H. (1980). The implications of ecological change on groups, institutions and communities—reviewing a therapeutic community experience with open systems thinking. *Proceedings of VII International Conference of Group Psychotherapy*, Copenhagen.
Clifford, P. (1987). *Services for the Long-term Mentally Ill*: a one-year specialist course, National Unit for Psychiatric Research and Development, London.
Cross, P. (1982). *Adults as Learners: Increasing participation and facilitating learning*, Jossey Bass, San Francisco.

Cullen, C. (1983). *The Residents' Development Project*. Final Report to DHSS, Manchester, Hester Adrian Research Centre.
DHSS (1984a). Steering Group on Health Services Information, *Fourth Report to the Secretary of State*, HMSO, London.
DHSS (1984b). *CAPRICODE. Health Building Procedures*, HMSO, London.
DHSS (1986). *Individual Performance Review*, HMSO, London.
Durward, L., and Whatmore, R. (1976). Testing the measures of quality of residential care; a pilot study, *Behaviour Research and Therapy*, **14**, 149–57.
Felce, D., de Kock, U., Saxby, H., and Thomas, M. (1985). *Small Homes for Severely and Profoundly Mentally Handicapped Adults*. Final Report, Health Care Evaluation Research Team, University of Southampton.
Georgiades, N. J., and Phillimore, L. (1975). The myth of the hero innovator and alternative strategies for organisation change. In C. C. Kiernan and F. D. Woodford (eds) *Behaviour Modification with the Severely Retarded*, Associated Scientific Publishers, Amsterdam.
Kings Fund Centre (1983). *Creating Local Psychiatric Services: papers from the Long Term and Community Care Team*, Kings Fund Publications, London.
Knowles, M. (1978). *The Adult Learner: A Neglected Species*, Gulf, Houston, Texas.
Kolb, D. A. (1984). Experiential Learning: Experience as the Source of Learning and Development, Prentice Hall, New Jersey.
Lavender, A. (1986). Quality of care and staff practice in long-stay settings. In F. N. Watts (ed.) *New Developments in Clinical Psychology*, Wiley, Chichester.
Lavender, A. (1987). Improving the quality of care on psychiatric rehabilitation wards: a controlled evaluation, *British Journal of Psychiatry*, **150**, 476–81.
McCarthy, P. (1985). Burnout in psychiatric nursing, *Journal of Advanced Nursing*, **10**, 305–10.
Metcalf, B. A. (1985). Looking forward to performance, *Health and Social Services Journal*, August, pp. 101–2.
Milne, D. L. (1985). An observational evaluation of the effects of nurse training in behaviour therapy on unstructured ward activities and interactions, *British Journal of Clinical Psychology*, **24**, 149–58.
MIND (1983). *A Common Concern*, MIND Publications, London.
Mittler, P. (1987). Staff development; changing needs and service contexts in Britain. In J. Hogg and P. J. Mittler (eds), *Staff Training in Mental Handicap*, Croom Helm, Beckenham.
NHS Training Authority (1986). *Individual Performance Review: Guide and Model Documentation*, Training and Development Publications Ltd, Brentford, Middlesex.
O'Brien, J., and Tyne, A. (1983). *The Principle of Normalisation: a foundation for effective services*, CMH/CMHERA, London.
Raynes, N. V., Pratt, M. W., and Roses, S. (1979). *Organisational Structure and the Care of the Mentally Retarded*, Croom Helm, London.
Roberts, J. P. (1980). Destructive processes in a therapeutic community, *International Therapeutic Communities*, **1**(3), 159–70.
Shepherd, G. W. (1977). Social skills training and the generalisation problem. *Behaviour Therapy*, **8**, 100–9.
South East Thames Regional Health Authority (1987). *Bringing People Back Home: a programme of courses*, SETRHA, Tunbridge Wells.
Stratford, R. (1985). Evaluating staff performance, a procedural guide. Paper presented to Division of Clinical Psychology Research Interest Group, Kings Fund Centre, London.

Towell, D., and Dartington, T. (1976). Encouraging innovation in hospital care, *Journal of Advanced Nursing*, **1**, 391–8.

Tyne, A. (1981). Staffing and supporting a residential service. Paper given to European Conference on Habitat and Living Environment for Adult Persons with a Mental Handicap, CMH Publications, London.

Watts, F. N., and Bennett, D. H. (1983a). *Handbook of Psychiatric Rehabilitation Practice*, Wiley, Chichester.

Watts, F. N., and Bennett, D. H. (1983b). Management of the staff team. In F. N. Watts and D. H. Bennett (eds), *Handbook of Psychiatric Rehabilitation Practice*, Wiley, Chichester.

Watts, F. N., and Lavender, A. (1987a). Rehabilitation investigation. In S. Lindsay and G. E. Powell (eds), *Handbook of Clinical Adult Psychology*, Gower, Aldershot.

Watts, F. N., and Lavender, A. (1987b). Rehabilitation treatment. In S. Lindsay and G. E. Powell (eds), *Handbook of Clinical Adult Psychology*, Gower, Aldershot.

## Video Material

ESCATA, (1976) 'Lifestyles', 6 Pavilion Parade, Brighton, Sussex.

# Section C

# The Components of Community Care

Community Care in Practice
Edited by A. Lavender and F. Holloway
© 1988 John Wiley & Sons Ltd

Chapter 8

# Housing

## PHILIPPA GARETY

The provision of residential services for those with persistent and severe mental health problems (the long-term mentally ill) is, currently, a matter of earnest debate. The closure of mental hospitals, or at least a real reduction in bed numbers, is creating a housing shortage amongst the long-term mentally ill, and access to alternative accommodation must urgently be made available. The House of Commons Social Services Committee (1985) has noted that the build-up of 'community' alternatives is clearly inadequate compared with the speed of the run-down of hospitals. In the United States, where 'deinstitutionalization' is further 'advanced' than in the UK (Bachrach, 1978) homelessness among the mentally ill now presents a major social problem (Baxter and Hopper, 1984).

The debate currently being waged within health and social services in the UK centres on competing ideologies rather than the empirical examination of what has proved most successful. Furthermore there appears to be a rush to set up services, with little concern about their evaluation.


SERVICES IN THE 1970s

In 1971 there were 104,600 people resident in mental illness hospitals, while in 1983 this figure had dropped to 69,030 (Wilkinson and Freeman, 1986). While a proportion of the decline in numbers is accounted for by the death of 'old long-stay' patients, the increase between 1975 and 1984 of places in specialized community residential accommodation for the mentally ill from 4145 to 5564 clearly does not represent an adequate increase in the level of community provision.

In 1975 the government white paper *Better Services for the Mentally Ill* estimated that social services departments should provide four to six places

143

per 100,000 population in short-stay hostels, 15–24 places per 100,000 in long-stay hostels, plus a range of accommodation without resident staff including group homes, flats and boarding-out schemes (Pritlove, 1983). These norms have not been met. The types of accommodation for the mentally ill envisaged by the government, and largely accepted in the 1970s, consisted of staffed hostels for short and long stays, boarding-out schemes, group homes and, implicitly, living with family members. Which type of accommodation might be most suitable for which resident, and to what extent staffed hostels and group homes differed, was unclear. Broadly it appeared that group homes were largely serving an older deinstitutionalized clientele, while staffed hostels tended to serve younger clients with a wider range of problems, some of whom had not spent any long period in hospital (Ryan, 1979).

There was some debate about whether these new residential services, particularly group homes and hostels, were 'restrictive'. While Apte (1968) had warned that there was a danger of developing new 'workhouses', Hewett and Ryan (reported in Ryan, 1979) found, in a study of hostels, that generally 'permissive' environments were being created. During the 1970s some changes were noted in the population being served by specialized residential facilities. Pritlove (1983) identified the presence, in 'group homes' in a northern town, of a younger 'more disruptive' group of individuals, discharged from short stays in hospitals. He did, however, note that relatively few people gained access to specialized residential facilities directly from the 'community', despite the fact that large numbers of ex-patients were living in totally unsatisfactory accommodation.

One rather different type of specialized accommodation was developed in the 1970s. This was the 'hospital–hostel' or 'hostel–ward' recommended in the White Paper of 1975 for 'new long-stay' patients who could not be discharged from hospital in the foreseeable future. The first such was opened in 1977 at the Maudsley Hospital in Camberwell, London, and has been favourably evaluated (Wykes, 1982; Garety and Morris, 1984); other similar units have followed (e.g. in Manchester, Goldberg et al., 1985) which, unlike the Maudsley prototype, are located off the hospital site. Both the Camberwell and Manchester units serve a population of severely disabled 'new long-stay' patients. The off-site unit is more selective with respect to the level of behavioural disturbance or handicap in functioning.

SERVICES IN THE 1980s

The 1980s witnessed a gradual increase in residential services for the mentally ill provided by the health service, local authority social service

Table 8.1    Range of accommodation currently available.

| Type of accommodation | NHS | LASS | LAHD | VO | Private |
|---|---|---|---|---|---|
| | | | Provider | | |
| Hospital acute ward | × | | | | |
| Hospital long-stay ward | × | | | | |
| Hospital hostel | × | | | | |
| 24 hour staffed hostel | × | × | | × | |
| Core and cluster network | × | × | | × | |
| Less than 24 hour staffed hostel | × | × | | × | |
| Shared house/flat, visiting staff | × | × | × | × | |
| Individual flat, visiting staff | × | × | × | × | |
| Adult fostering | | × | | | |
| Boarding out in boarding houses or residential houses | | × | | × | × |
| Boarding out in private houses | | × | | | × |
| Housing association tenancy ('special needs') | | | | × | |
| Local authority tenancy | | | × | | |
| Living with family (parents, partner, children) | | | | | × |
| Private tenancy | | | | | × |
| Private ownership | | | | | × |
| Bed and breakfast accommodation | | | × | | |
| 'Common' lodging houses | | | | | × |
| Shelters for homeless | | | | × | |
| Prison | | | | | |

*Abbreviations:* NHS, National Health Service; LASS, local authority social services; LAHD, local authority housing department; VO, voluntary organization.

and housing departments, voluntary organizations and housing associations. (Table 8.1 lists the chief options available; such a list can be almost infinite in length.) Much greater emphasis is currently being placed on making accessible ordinary housing, through local authority housing departments, to those with mental health problems (Lovett, 1984). In many areas this represents a pious hope rather than a reality. The House of Commons Social Services Committee commented in 1985 'There is now no shortage of lists of all the varieties of possible housing arrangements. They read like a repetitive litany, often culminating in repeated references to the idea of "core and cluster". Unfortunately listing the options does not create the housing.'

Districts differ in the extent to which they are making a serious effort to create new housing options. In the London Borough of Hackney, for example (Lovett, 1984; Reed, 1984), the number of hospital beds available has been reduced and a range of residential facilities has been developed which includes conventional hostels and group homes, communal houses, a flat-share scheme using council flats and a specially supported block of ten flats. In Hackney a partnership has evolved between the health and social services, the local authority housing department and a housing association. The emphasis is on making use of 'ordinary' housing where possible. Other districts currently provide an inadequate number of places in a few group homes and hostels which were set up in the 1960s and 1970s largely for the less disabled 'deinstitutionalized' clientele.

The development of local services cannot of course be uniform across districts. Some districts, such as South Southwark, have developed services largely to meet the needs of a newly accumulating population of long-term mental health service users. Other districts, particularly those in which a large mental hospital is sited, have to meet the needs of substantial numbers of 'old long-stay' as well as those of the 'never institutionalized'. Additionally where influential staff have had special interests which resulted in particular districts accumulating groups of inpatients with special needs, such as the multiply disabled, this will influence the nature of new provision. This fact, together with social and demographic differences, renders the setting of national or even regional norms of provision a misleading endeavour (Wing and Furlong, 1986).

The 'core and cluster' system alluded to by the Social Services Committee is currently a popular method (in planning documents if not in practice) of providing a number of residential places in small and flexible units with minimal staffing. McAusland (1985) describes a network of cluster houses which are administratively linked to a 'core'. The cluster houses provide a range of housing options, for individuals, twos or threes or slightly larger groups, which are geographically dispersed. At the 'core' is the administrative centre, from which staff travel to visit the cluster houses, providing support as and when needed. McAusland states that the major objective for such a system is to provide services in the community which can meet the needs of individuals as they change over time. He lists two basic assumptions—firstly that individuals can learn to be more independent, regardless of the severity of their mental health problems, and, secondly, that a service can be designed to meet individual rather than group needs. McAusland strongly believes that in such a system the 'core' should be only an administrative centre and not, as is sometimes the case, a staffed hostel. Johnson (1986), however, takes issue with this view, and argues that a larger staffed residential unit at the 'core' of a cluster system has therapeutic as well as administrative advantages.

No description of what is currently available would be complete without reference to the growing concern about, and awareness of, the number of mentally ill people who are homeless or in prison. The House of Commons Social Services Committee (1985) comments on the rising proportion of mentally ill amongst the homeless, suggesting that a quarter to a half of the homeless in shelters or hostels may have been recently discharged from psychiatric hospitals. They suggest that while mental illness among the homeless antedates the reduction in beds in psychiatric services, it is probable that the problem is growing as a result of present policies. In the United States concern over the homeless mentally ill has been widely expressed, although here too there have been real difficulties in determining the size and cause(s) of the problem. Bachrach (1984) points to difficulties with defining and detecting mental illness, especially amongst those who are often reported to be shy and frightened and who frequently abuse alcohol and drugs. There are difficulties with gaining accurate information about the shifting subpopulations of mentally ill, who may be found in a variety of residential settings, and of the homeless who may find their way to hospitals not simply or primarily by virtue of their mental health problems. Scott (1986) comments on the paradoxical situation whereby mentally ill people may be rejected by voluntary organizations and local authorities as unsuitable for specialized housing, such as staffed hostels. They may then be discharged from hospital and become homeless. The local authority housing department becomes responsible, under the 1977 Housing (Homeless Persons) Act, for housing these individuals. They are often placed in totally unsuitable bed-and-breakfast accommodation, in which many do not survive, drifting on to night shelters, prison or the streets.

Districts differ not only in the range of services available, but also in the extent to which a particular type of service is emphasized. Although not the subject of this chapter, it should not be forgotten that the single most important type of residential accommodation for the long-term mentally ill remains living with family members. Second to this may come any one of a number of types of housing. In some districts 'group homes' may have developed as the principal form of specialized provision, while in others 'boarding out' or 'adult fostering' in private homes may be the first option. Anstee (1985) reports on the use of landlady-run homes of varying sizes, which has become a major element in the Salisbury district service. Some psychiatric services are making extensive use of houses in seaside towns, formerly holiday lodgings, now run as private registered homes (Davidson, 1984).

## PHILOSOPHIES INFLUENCING SERVICES

A number of different, and at times conflicting, philosophies or ideologies are influencing the planning and development of new residential services.

Firstly there remains an element of the anti-institutional protest movement so well described, in the American context, by Bachrach (1978). This movement places a strong civil libertarian emphasis on the rights of individuals and on the modification of the environment as the primary avenue to social change. It involves the assumption that community-based care is preferable to institutional care for most, if not all, psychiatric patients, and that communities not only can, but also are willing to, assume responsibility (and leadership) in the care of the mentally ill. In this context good care is care which occurs outside the institution (the psychiatric hospital) and which avoids the excesses of the institution, as, for example, described by Goffman (1961).

A modified and more empirically based version of anti-institutionalism stems from the social environmental research of King et al. (1971) and Raynes et al. (1979), and from the social psychiatric work of Wing and Brown (1970). This emphasizes 'resident-orientated' management practices, the development of positive staff attitudes and of a high level of staff–resident interaction (Garety and Morris, 1984). Such a model of 'client orientation' in management practices does not see the locus of care in itself as crucial (i.e. 'hospital' as bad and 'community' as good) but the type and quality of care provided, which includes an explicit attempt to remove or minimize the debilitating features of the institution as identified by Goffman, and by Wing and Brown.

A second long-standing philosophy has been the provision of environments which enhance the process of 'rehabilitation'. Both UK (e.g. Shepherd, 1984) and US (Anthony et al., 1984; Carling and Ridgway, 1985) writers have stressed the importance of the social environment in 'rehabilitation', a concept which invokes notions of improving and maintaining skills and functioning, in the context of individual assessment and planning and of adaptation to continuing disabilities. Thus residential environments are 'good' in so far as they offer opportunities for the exercise of (normal) social and domestic roles and skills, with the appropriate access to support to maintain any improvements in functioning. Rehabilitation has in the past been confused with 'resettlement', where the end-goal is simply resettling an individual out of the hospital. Linked with this view has been a 'ladder' model of service provision, in which a person moves from the most supported setting (the ward) through gradual stages, to other less supported staffed facilities and on to independent living. This system, when applied to housing, can be extremely disruptive. The notion of a residential ladder may be replaced by the idea of residential 'spectrum' in which a wide range of housing options are provided with differing and flexible levels of support. Here the expectation is not that the client moves through the system but that a variety of housing options are provided, to which more or less support is given as needed while, where possible, the client stays in the housing he or she prefers.

A third and major contribution to thinking about residential provision is the philosophy of 'normalization' or 'social role valorization'. Its influence is controversial, and therefore it will be discussed in some detail. Normalization has generated much controversy, perhaps because it is not so much a philosophy as a principle, which has been presented in many different ways and with different shades of emphasis by its many proponents. In 1970, when Wolfensberger published his first article about normalization and psychiatric services (Wolfensberger, 1970) he described the principle of normalization as 'deceptively simple'.

> Reduced to its essentials, it states that human management practices should enable a deviant person to function in ways considered to be within the acceptable norms of his [sic] society; by the same token, human management practices should enable a person who is not a deviant to continue to be able to function within the acceptable norms of his society. As much as possible, the means employed should be culturally normative ones. . . . Normalization means that deviant persons should be exposed to experiences that are likely to elicit or maintain normative (accepted) behavior. These experiences can be derived from one's physical activities and from one's interaction with the physical environment (such as one's residence and one's furnishings) and one's physical neighborhood. It can also be derived from one's interaction with the social environment.

In this early paper Wolfensberger argued that deviant persons should never be congregated in numbers larger than that which the surrounding 'community social system' can readily absorb and integrate. Normalization also dictates, Wolfensberger asserts, that a person should be as independent, free to move about and empowered to make meaningful choices as are typical citizens of comparable age in the community. A person should have reasonable control over the physical environment, and be subject to the minimum feasible number of restrictions.

In subsequent writings the principle of normalization has emphasized the use of 'culturally valued settings', rather than the originally phrased 'culturally normative (accepted)' ones, but more recently still Wolfensberger (1983) has offered a 'new insight'. Here he states that

> the most explicit and highest goal of normalization must be the creation, support and defense (sic) of *valued social roles* for people who are at risk of social devaluation. All other elements and objectives of the theory are really subservient to this end, because if a person's social role were a societally valued one, then other desirable things would be accorded to the person almost automatically at least within the resources and norms of his/her society [emphasis added].

The term 'normalization' is to be found liberally scattered through current policy documents. For example the House of Commons Social Services Committee Report on Community Care (1985) argues that:

(1) There should be a preference for home life over institutional care. (2) There should be a *pursuit of the ideal of normalisation* and integration and the avoidance, so far as possible, of separate provision, segregation and restriction (i.e. the least restrictive alternative). (3) A preference for small over large. (4) A preference for local services over distant ones [emphasis added].

This statement of principle is interpreted in the report (and indeed in the policy statements of other groups) as entailing that providing for the basic needs of people affected by mental disability should, so far as possible, be in ordinary domestic housing, in ordinary occupational settings and through the use of ordinary recreational amenities. Chris Heginbotham of MIND in a recent (1984) publication states 'We require principles of ordinariness and normalisation; services which consider individuals first.' He further states in a 1985 *Good Practices in Mental Health* publication that 'good ordinary decent housing should be provided for anyone regardless of their disability. . . . Ordinary housing is also a "valued setting" in which people with long-term disabilities can develop valued social relationships and valued life styles.' He adds that the term 'special needs' housing is stigmatizing and leads to the provision of special housing. He asserts that the sort of housing that people with long-term mental illness need is the sort of housing that most people choose to live in, and that housing should be integrated within the community in the normal way. Tom McAusland (1985) supports this view. He argues that in British psychiatric services what we most lack is experience of supporting people with major and long-term psychiatric disabilities in ordinary housing.

This concern with 'ordinariness' seems to stem from the notions of 'culturally normative (accepted)' and 'culturally valued'. While some proponents of 'normalization' would question that the use of *ordinary* settings is implied by the theory, it is the case that at present 'ordinariness' (perhaps because what is 'ordinary' is cheaper than what is 'valued') has become a central theme of policy documents. In these days, when so much housing is substandard, care must be taken in interpreting such terms. In addition, a number of subprinciples are given in such documents, including minimal restriction and segregation, local services, small units and consumer involvement in planning and decision-making. McAusland's description of the ideal core and cluster system, mentioned earlier, is an example of the expression of these principles: his guidelines for such housing include the use of 'ordinary' not purpose-built housing, that is inconspicuous, accessible, and dispersed for 'as small a number as possible'.

Finally, there are those who assert that individuals have certain basic rights, such as to decent stable affordable housing (Carling and Ridgway, 1985), preferably separate from the provision of specialized rehabilitation services or other psychiatric care. Added to this is the right of self-determination, where the notion of 'choice' replaces the notion of 'place-ment'.

## FINANCE

Before moving on to discuss evaluative studies, it should be noted that current developments are linked not only to philosophical stances, but also to certain policies, particularly of funding, which favour certain develop-ments. 'Joint finance' was introduced in 1976 to encourage joint planning and collaboration between health and local authorities and to promote a shift from hospital to community care (see Wilkinson and Freeman, 1986, for details of current regulations and expenditure), and indeed £520 million has been spent in the period 1976–85. However local authorities have recently become increasingly reluctant to commit themselves to joint finance projects because (a) after a specified number of years they are expected to pick up the bill, and (b), they have been experiencing severe limits on their expenditure. The future of 'joint finance' is thus in some doubt.

A more significant contribution to 'community care' appears to be the option, under social security regulations, for individuals to receive not inconsiderable sums from social security for board and lodging payments. For those residing in registered homes payments may be as high as about £140 per week; in unregistered establishments payments are currently (early 1987) limited to about £70 per week. It is proving quite possible for private individuals and voluntary organizations to run residential services entirely funded in this way, and thus the cost of residential care can simply be transferred from the health to the social security budget. Of course, day and leisure facilities and specialized staff services are not funded in this way, and thus a serious gap in provision may appear by default. Further, the stability of this form of funding is doubtful, as a recent circular (December 1986) from the Chief Executive of the NHS Management Board to Regional Health Authorities amply demonstrates. In his letter, Mr Peach informs health authorities that they do not have the powers to levy charges from ex-patients residing in health authority establishments, and that supplementary benefit is not, under social security legislation, payable for such charges. While it is by no means clear why this should be so, some health authorities are acting quickly to make alternative arrangements. The introduction of another agency is popular, be it an independent housing association, a local authority housing department, a voluntary organiza-tion or a health authority-controlled housing association, into which the ownership of the health authority property is transferred. It is of major concern that some other change or novel interpretation of the regulations could further jeopardize this whole system of residential care.


## EVALUATIONS OF EFFECTIVENESS

Given the pressing need for systematic evaluations of current and new residential provision, remarkably little empirical work is being undertaken on its effectiveness, or to determine whether the principles presently enunciated with so much conviction are associated with a positive 'outcome' for users. Part of the difficulty, of course, lies in determining what constitutes a good 'outcome' measure. No single measure can stand alone, and the best evaluations incorporate a wide range, including measures of client functioning, symptoms, quality of life and consumer views, staff attitudes and behaviour, cost, carer views, service use and the quality of the social and physical environment.

Ryan (1979) reported on two studies of short- and long-stay hostels and group homes conducted in the 1970s. These provide information about the selection processes, management practices, resident views, length of stay of residents and costs of the respective services. Ryan commented that the different types of provision appear to serve somewhat different populations, and also that as the years progressed a less stable, more disturbed group (the 'new long-term') appeared increasingly to be served. Although he identified different selection procedures and management practices, he noted that no strict evaluation of the effectiveness of procedures used in hostels had been undertaken.

Pritlove (1983) describes a study of eight group homes in the late 1970s, although again this was a descriptive survey rather than an evaluation of effectiveness. This survey identified two groups of residents; an older, more stable group of 'old long-stay' deinstitutionalized residents, and a younger, more disruptive and socially handicapped group who generally found it difficult to settle. Few were admitted to the homes from anywhere other than psychiatric hospitals. Pritlove also considered the appropriateness of the 'family' model, for a group home; while he found that there was a degree of cooperation and socializing among residents, he did not find any strong attachment between individuals or any feeling of common identity. There was, despite the efforts of visiting staff, little involvement with the local community. Pritlove concludes by suggesting that the days of the model of 'family' life for an elderly group of deinstitutionalized residents are numbered. He puts forward a model of sheltered housing in which regular practical supervision is more appropriate. This housing should be well integrated into the community without pretending to be 'ordinary' and allowing for the permanence of handicap.

A number of studies have been conducted on the hospital hostels described above (Wykes, 1982; Garety and Morris, 1984; Goldberg *et al.*, 1985 and, in the United States, Gudeman *et al.*, 1981). All of these conclude that a residence specifically designed for the 'new long-stay' with a greater emphasis on individually planned interventions (often with a behavioural element) relatively high staffing levels and a more stimulating social environment results in greater improvements in aspects of functioning than traditional inpatient settings. Furthermore they provide greater privacy, freedom and autonomy for residents. Despite the differences between these units in, among other things, location and practices, the 'hostel–ward' remains the only new type of residential facility where the effectiveness has been evaluated empirically in a number of independent studies.

Falloon and Marshall (1983) studied the social interaction patterns of 28 residents in a large 'board-and-care' facility in Los Angeles. They concluded that some residents in this socially stimulating environment remained withdrawn, and were at times adversely affected by the stimulating environment. This, they believed, generated floridly psychotic symptoms and led some to escape to their rooms or to the nearby park. There was some evidence to suggest that, although the burden on family was eased by residential care, some individuals may have functioned better in a family milieu. This study, somewhat pessimistically, noted that relatively few of the people studied were able to take advantage of community facilities, without extensive staff assistance.

Falloon and Marshall found that the residents with patterns of high levels of social interaction tended to have very much larger social networks than the other 'withdrawn' group. Mulryan (1985) also looked at the network size of residents in group homes and hostels in England and Ireland. She found that while the English residents were more symptomatic and handicapped, with shorter psychiatric histories than the older deinstitutionalized Irish sample, the English group maintained a larger network. This was apparently accounted for by the greater degree of staff support and specialized daytime facilities available, in the context of which networks were generated and maintained.

Zipple and Elkind (1984) have considered the role of level of functioning in determining selection of 33 residents for a variety of residential facilities in the United States. While they found that those with the 'lowest' functioning were selected for the most structured environment, it was noteworthy that the degree of deviance, in terms of the resident's impact on the safety and comfort of both the community and residents, was the aspect of functioning given greatest weight.

Consumer evaluations have been an element in many studies, and in some it has formed the chief focus of the study. Lehman *et al.* (1982) asked 278 residents of Los Angeles board-and-care homes about their current life conditions and problems. The social problems of greatest concern to the subjects were their unemployment, poor finances and housing. The most commonly sought change in housing was to move to a flat of their own. In a British study (Kay and Legg, 1986) in which housing in London was reviewed for 100 people leaving psychiatric care, it was found that most patients had little involvement, choice or control over their discharge decisions and the arrangements for their rehousing. Eighty per cent of those interviewed were dissatisfied with their current housing, either because of hostel rules and regimes of 'enforced community' or because of the physical housing conditions. In future, three-quarters wanted their own independent housing, and to choose with whom they lived.

Kay and Legg found that many patients on discharge from hospital do not return to their most recent previous address. In a systematic study of this in New York city, Caton and Goldstein (1984) discovered that of 119 'chronic schizophrenics' discharged from hospital, 50 per cent changed their living arrangements at least once, and 21 per cent changed their living arrangements at least twice during one year. The principal reason given for the housing change reflected inter-personal problems, and 80 per cent of the changes involved going to or leaving family members. Pritlove (1983) also noted that a number of the younger residents did not settle success-fully in the group homes. The success of residential schemes should not be evaluated simply in terms of the status of current members, but should take account of the proportion and characteristics of those who are not accepted initially, or who leave after a brief period.

Some aspects of 'community care' have been fiercely criticized, in par-ticular the fast-growing use of seaside boarding houses, or other homes set up by private individuals to take in a number of discharged psychiatric patients. While these reports (Davidson, 1984; Fleming, 1984) are not formal evaluations, they raise concern about the quality of provision in such facilities. There may be a lack of access to day and other services, the physical and social environment may be impoverished and the independ-ence and autonomy of residents may be restricted. Many argue that the 1984 Registered Homes Act does not provide the powers needed to ensure good quality care.

## FUTURE SERVICES

'The juxtaposition of two major variables—a changing service system and a changing target population—has intensified problems in planning rel-evant services for the chronically ill psychiatric patient' (Bachrach, 1984, p. 976). This experience in the United States is highly relevant to Britain in this period of major change. In the United States Bachrach suggests that the new service structure has failed to meet the needs of the severely ill and highly dependent 'never institutionalized' patients, who have lacked access to services providing continuity and comprehensiveness of care.

There is no doubt that the large mental hospital has, for most of its residents, provided an impoverished, debilitating and dehumanizing environment and should be replaced with more effective and humane services. The responsibility of the service planners and providers now lies with ensuring that service users, especially those severely affected, are now at least as well, and preferably better, served than under the old order. Untested assumptions must be subject to close scrutiny. Is 'ordinary' housing always preferable to purpose-built housing? Is living in a group of two better for all than living in a group of four, and is four better than eight? Is it always undesirable to be visited at home by a psychiatrist, rather than go to a clinic? Indeed is it preferable not to see a psychiatrist at all, but to visit a GP? A real danger lies in proceeding apace with ordinary, exclusively small-scale, preferably unstaffed housing, in which the most disruptive cannot be accepted and for whom the hospitals will no longer provide long-term accommodation. Thus while ordinary housing may very well be suitable for, and preferred by, many, if not most, of the long-term mentally ill, and may provide for them the possibility of a greatly enhanced lifestyle, it may fail to provide at all for some, and empirical studies, including 'tracer' studies which follow up all those who come into contact with services must be set up.

Many new developments currently being planned in the UK are based upon the principles of 'ordinariness' and small scale. Brandon (1986) describes a plan for providing local and ordinary accommodation in three-bedroomed houses or maisonettes where two or three people live with varying degrees of support from full-time, part-time or visiting staff. The support would change as the needs of consumers change, and consumers would not be expected to move on as their need for support diminishes; support will be reduced. Brandon describes how consumers would look towards the use of existing community facilities such as local colleges, leisure centres and libraries, and they would not generally use 'a variety of facilities with the term "psychiatric" in front of it'. Schemes such as these have many real advantages; above all the opportunity for many who have lived in substandard, overcrowded and segregated accommodation to live in decent integrated housing with flexible support from the service providers.

The expressed aims of the new provision must, however, be evaluated in practice. Studies quoted above (Pritlove, 1983 and Falloon and Marshall, 1983) note the minimal integration of the residents into the 'community'. Furthermore a project which attempted to integrate psychiatric service users into an adult education centre (Wilson, 1984) had limited success.

Wing and Brown in 1970 demonstrated the value, in terms of reducing symptoms, of daytime activity. Wolfensberger in 1970 wrote of the normalizing nature of work, and in 1983 of the importance of valued social roles. Crucial to these is some form of day provision, without which users can become institutionalized at home. To write about community care is not to achieve it, and those who assume a golden age of integration, while failing to take account of the distressing experiences and disabilities of the long-term mentally ill, may in the long run do them a grave disservice.

In 1986 two plans for the development of mental hospital sites and services have been elaborated, which are in contrast to the model of dispersed ordinary housing. Wing and Furlong (1986) describe a plan for those with 'high-dependency needs' some of whom, they argue, require security, protection or shelter in two or more of the three major areas of life (housing, occupation and recreation). They believe that these individuals will require help from people and agencies familiar with the varied causes of social disablement, and may suffer a drop in quality of life if denied this specialized assistance. The term 'asylum' has had a bad press recently. They assert, however, the function it denotes remains a real need of some. Thus they propose a 'Haven Community' to be based on the grounds of Friern Hospital (a mental hospital in North-West London scheduled for closure). Here there will be four houses for those most needing care and shelter. Elsewhere on the site others will live in a range of houses and flats with a lower degree of supervision and, off the site but locally, will be 'peripheral group homes and supervised apartments'. Such a scheme, while drawing to some extent on the 'normalization' literature, is clearly at odds with its main thrust, providing as it does specialized staffed facilities, to some extent segregated from the local community, and for some in groups of as many as twelve people.

Wing and Furlong commend the use of part of the Friern Hospital site for facilities such as leisure and shopping centres which will, it is hoped, attract the local community to the site. Wallace (1986) reports in *The Times* (16 December) on a proposal for the redevelopment of Claybury Hospital, another large mental hospital on the outskirts of London, to create a town with shops, leisure centre, offices, flats and houses. However the architect proposes to retain within this new 'town' a 40-bed short-stay psychiatric unit, and flats and hostels for a further 300 people with psychiatric problems needing long-term accommodation. These schemes, which offer a different model of 'integration' from others hitherto, will also require evaluation.

In this chapter the central focus has been on long-term non-family accommodation. However, there may be new developments in the future for shorter-term accommodation. One special feature of mental illness is its fluctuating course, and while many good new schemes describe an inbuilt system of flexible support, at times more support may be needed than can be provided. Crisis residences, for the short-term relief of stress on an individual, or of burden on those caring for him/her, and as alternatives to inpatient admission (Lamb and Lamb, 1984; Weisman, 1985) are recognized as valuable in the United States. Some crisis residences may serve this function alone, while others may take the form of a spare room in a staffed hostel. Where a consumer is known to a certain group of staff, and/or does not require the special assessment or security that a hospital ward can provide, a brief stay in such a residence may prove more effective and less disruptive than an often over-long hospital admission.

## CONCLUSION

Community residential provision is entering a new phase. That the mental hospitals can be replaced with something better is not in doubt. Nor in doubt is the proposition that most people with long-term mental health problems prefer to live in 'ordinary housing', and currently there is a heartening concern to make this possible. However a civilization is evaluated by the care of its most vulnerable members. The needs of those with not only long-term but also severe mental health problems, resulting in 'social disablement', must be prominent in the minds of planners and providers. Specialized hospital hostels, small-scale staffed hostels, adult fostering and other special provision may well prove desirable and necessary for and to some. Unregistered lodgings, back wards, the streets and prisons should not be their lot.

## REFERENCES

Anstee, B H. (1985). An alternative form of community care for the mentally ill: supported lodging schemes . . . a personal view, *Health Trends*, **17**, 39–40.

Anthony, W., Cohen, M., and Cohen, B. (1984). Psychiatric rehabilitation. In J. Talbott (ed.) *The Chronic Mental Patient: five years later*, Grune & Stratton, New York, Chapter 10.

Apte, R. Z. (1968). Halfway houses: A new dilemma in institutional care, *Occasional Papers on Social Administration*. G. Bell & Sons Ltd, London.

Bachrach, L. L. (1978). A conceptual approach to deinstitutionalisation, *Hospital and Community Psychiatry*, **29**, 573–8.

Bachrach, L. L. (1984). Interpreting research on the homeless mentally ill: some caveats, *Hospital and Community Psychiatry*, **35**, 914–17.

Baxter, E., and Hopper, K. (1984). Troubled on the streets: the mentally disabled homeless poor. In J. Talbott (ed.) *The Chronic Mental Patient: Five Years Later*, Grune & Stratton, New York, Chapter 4.

Brandon, D. (1986). Pioneering heralds death of the hostel. *Social Work Today*, August.

Carling, P. J., and Ridgway, P. (1985). Community residential rehabilitation: an emerging approach to meeting housing needs. In P. Carling and P. Ridgway (eds) *Providing Housing and Supports for People with Psychiatric Disabilities*, NIMH, Rockville, MD, Chapter 1.

Caton, C. L. M., and Goldstein, J. (1984). Housing change of chronic schizophrenic patients: A consequence of the revolving door, *Social Science and Medicine*, **19**, 754–64.

Davidson, N. (1984). Hiving off mental health care, *Social Work Today*, **16**, 26.

DHSS (1975). *Better Services for the Mentally Ill*. Cmnd 6233, HMSO, London.

Falloon, I. R., and Marshall, G. N. (1983). Residential care and social behaviour: a study of rehabilitation needs, *Psychological Medicine*, **13**, 341–7.

Fleming, J. (1984). Psychiatric patients discharged without adequate support, *Senior Nurse*, **1**(15), 6.

Garety, P. A., and Morris, I. (1984). A new unit for long-stay psychiatric patients: organisation, attitudes and quality of care, *Psychological Medicine*, **14**, 183–92.

Goffman, E. (1961). *Asylums: essays on the social situation of mental patients and other inmates*, Doubleday, New York; Aldine, Chicago.

Goldberg, D. B., Bridges, K., Cooper, W., Hyde, C., Sterling, C., and Wyatt, R. (1985). Douglas House: a new type of hostel ward for chronic psychiatric patients, *British Journal of Psychiatry*, **147**, 383–8.

Good Practices in Mental Health (1985). *Housing Information Pack*, GPMH, London.

Gudeman, J. E., Dickey, B., Rood, L., Hellman, S., and Grinspoon, L. (1981). Alternative to the back ward: the quarterway house, *Hospital and Community Psychiatry*, **32**, 330–4.

Heginbotham, C. (1984). The myth of Sisyphus: turning mountains into molehills. In J. Reed and G. Lomas (eds) *Psychiatric Services in the Community*, Croom Helm, Beckenham, Chapter 20.

Heginbotham, C. (1985). Introduction. In *Good Practices in Mental Health Housing Information Pack*. GPMH, London.

House of Commons, Social Services Committee (1985). *Community Care with Special Reference to Adult Mentally Ill and Mentally Handicapped People*. Second Report from the Social Services Committee, HMSO, London.

Johnson, R. (1986). Opinions, *Ordinary Housing*, **1**, 2–3.

Kay, A., and Legg, C. (1986). *Discharged to the Community: a review of housing and support in London for people leaving psychiatric care*, City University, London.

King, R. D., Raynes, N. V., and Tizard, J. (1971). *Patterns of Residential Care*, Routledge & Kegan Paul, London.

Lamb, H. R., and Lamb, D. M. (1984). A non hospital alternative to acute hospitalization, *Hospital and Community Psychiatry*, **35**, 728–30.

Lehman, A. F., Reed, S. K., and Possidente, S. M. (1982). Priorities for long-term care: comments from board-and-care residents, *Psychiatric Quarterly*, **54**, 181–9.

Lovett, A. (1984). A house for all reasons: the role of housing in community care. In J. Reed and G. Lomas (eds) *Psychiatric Services in the Community*, Croom Helm, Beckenham, Chapter 8.

McAusland, T. (1985). Housing for people with long term psychiatric disabilities— beyond the 24 bedded unit? In *Good Practices in Mental Health: Housing Information Pack*, GPMH, London.

Mulryan, M. (1985). The social network of schizophrenic patients in varied settings. Unpublished M. Phil. thesis, University of London.

Pritlove, J. (1983). Accommodation without resident staff for ex-psychiatric patients. *British Journal of Social Work*, **13**, 75–92.

Raynes, N. V., Pratt, M. W., and Roses, S. (1979). *Organisational Structure and the Care of the Mentally Retarded*. Croom Helm, London.

Reed, J. (1984). The elements of an ideal service. In J. Reed and G. Lomas (eds) *Psychiatric Services in the Community*, Croom Helm, Beckenham, Chapter 7.

Ryan, P. (1979). Residential care for the mentally disabled. In J. K. Wing and R. Olsen (eds) *Community Care for the Mentally Disabled*, Oxford University Press, London.

Scott, H. J. (1986). Accommodation for mentally-ill people: the effects of the Housing (Homeless Persons) Act 1977, *Housing Review*, **35**, 10–13.

Shepherd, G. (1984). *Institutional Care and Rehabilitation*, Longman, London.

Wallace, M. (1986). Taking the people to the patients, *The Times*, 16 December.

Weisman, G. K. (1985). Crisis-orientated residential treatment as an alternative to hospitalization, *Hospital and Community Psychiatry*, **36**, 1302–5.

Wilkinson, G., and Freeman, H. (eds) (1986). *The Provision of Mental Health Services in Britain*, Gaskell, London.

Wilson, S. (1984). Chronic psychiatric patients in an adult education centre: socially integrated or isolated? Unpublished M.Phil. thesis, University of London.

Wing, J. K. (1986). The cycle of planning and evaluation. In G. Wilkinson and H. Freeman (eds) *The Provision of Mental Health Services in Britain*, Gaskell, London.

Wing, J. K. and Brown, ). (1970). *Institutionalisation and Schizophrenia: a comparative study of three mental hospitals, 1960–1968*, Cambridge University Press, London.

Wing, J. K. and Brown, G. W. (1970). *Institutionalisation and Schizophrenia: a comparative study of three mental hospitals, 1960–1968*, Cambridge University Press, London.

Wing, J. K., and Furlong, R. (1986). A haven for the severely disabled within the context of a comprehensive psychiatric community service, *British Journal of Psychiatry*, **149**, 449–57.

Wolfensberger, W. (1970). The principle of normalization and its implications to psychiatric services, *American Journal of Psychiatry*, **127**(3), 291–7.

Wolfensberger, W. (1983). Social role valorisation: A proposed new term for the principle of normalisation, *Mental Retardation*, **21**(6), 234–9.

Wykes, T. (1982). A hostel–ward for 'new' long-stay patients. In J. K. Wing (ed.) *Long-Term Community Care. Psychological Medicine*, Suppl. 2, pp. 41–55.

Zipple, A. M., and Elkind, M. (1984). The role of client level of functioning in residential placement decisions. *Psychosocial Rehabilitation Journal*, **7**, 56–65.

Community Care in Practice
Edited by A. Lavender and F. Holloway
© 1988 John Wiley & Sons Ltd

Chapter 9

# Day Care and Community Support

## FRANK HOLLOWAY

This chapter explores the provision of support to people with severe long-term mental illnesses who live in the community. Lack of adequate aftercare has been a major and continuing criticism of the deinstitutional-ization movement since its earliest days (Brown *et al.*, 1966). The widely canvassed failure of the American Community Mental Health Center movement to provide a truly comprehensive alternative to the state mental hospital has resulted in a further Federal initiative to promote the develop-ment of community support systems (Turner and Ten Hoor, 1978). These are specifically targeted at the chronically mentally ill, and should comprise a 'network of caring and responsible people committed to assisting a vulnerable population to meet their needs and develop their potential without being unnecessarily isolated or excluded from the community' (Turner and Shifren, 1979).

There has been no comparable initiative in Britain to the American community support programme, possibly because the process of deinstitu-tionalization has been less dramatic and its failures less publically acknow-ledged. The development of a coherent support system is vital to the success of community-based services. Day care is clearly an essential component of any system of support, and this chapter begins by reviewing the role of day care in contemporary psychiatric services. The focus is on the needs of the chronically mentally ill. This is followed by a broader discussion of community support, of which day care is but one element, and the chapter ends with some tentative suggestions for future service developments.

## DAY CARE FOR THE CHRONICALLY MENTALLY ILL

There is general agreement that day care forms a vital component of any good quality community-orientated psychiatric service. However, there is considerable confusion amongst both planners and practitioners about what day care actually is, what its legitimate functions are and how these functions are best carried out. One commentator has aptly described the development of day care as 'disordered' (Vaughan, 1983). There is no overall philosophy of care. Provision across the country is grossly uneven, and in many areas there is little evidence of coherent planning of services according to a rational assessment of need.

## The history of day care for the mentally ill

The first recorded psychiatric day hospital opened in Moscow in 1933 because of a shortage of inpatient beds. In 1946 Cameron opened the first day hospital in North America, at the Allan Memorial Institute in Montreal, and almost simultaneously Bierer opened the Paddington Social Psychotherapy Centre in London, which later became the Marlborough Day Hospital. Early proponents of the day hospital argued that, in comparison with traditional treatment, which at that time was almost entirely based in the mental hospital, a day hospital offered less risk of institutionalization, less stigma and allowed the patient to remain in contact with family and friends. At the same time it was hoped that day care would result in a saving in inpatient beds, and consequently money. Throughout the 1950s day care established itself in Britain, and by 1961 Farndale could write of a 'day hospital movement'.

Day care was slow to become established in the United States. However, the 1960s saw an explosion of interest in day care as a cheap and practical alternative to the state mental hospital. 'Partial hospitalization' was promoted as a key element in the plans of the Community Mental Health Movement.

Initially almost all psychiatric day care was provided by the hospital service. In the early years a number of distinct types of units were developed. The first day hospital in Moscow as a rehabilitative facility in which day care offered a half-way station in the transition between hospital and community. Some of the early day hospitals adopted the model pioneered by Bierer, in which the unit was run as a therapeutic community (Bierer, 1959). Bierer believed that faulty or inadequate relationships are a cause of mental illness. Consequently treatment should be of an 'experiential or situational nature' using the social group (although the day hospital would potentially offer the whole range of treatments, including drug therapy if necessary).

In this setting a major task of staff was, and still is, to create an appropriate therapeutic atmosphere. These principles have had a profound effect on the development of day care in this country (Blake *et al.*, 1984).

However, it was more common for early day hospitals to follow Cameron's 'medical' model. Harris described the Maudsley Day Hospital of the 1950s as functioning essentially as a hospital ward with the sole special characteristic that the patients went home at night. The unit would take patients who were so ill that admission to hospital would have been necessary had the day hospital not been available (Harris, 1957). Whether such patients would gain admission to a contemporary psychiatric unit serving an inner-city catchment area is another question.

Finally, some day hospitals, particularly those that developed in association with large mental hospitals, took on the role of providing long-term day care for the mainly psychotic population of patients who were discharged as these hospitals developed new patterns of care. Such day units often placed a heavy emphasis on work, having developed from an industrial therapy unit.

In some areas a two-tier service developed, with small well-staffed day units in the district general hospital providing a 'therapeutic' service for young, mainly neurotic patients while poorly staffed, low-status units in the mental hospital provided day care for an older, mainly psychotic and elderly population (Hassall et al., 1972). When the National Health Service came into being responsibility for the mentally ill was split. The Ministry of Health was, through the regional hospital boards, to run hospitals as treatment services. Local authorities were to provide preventive and after-care services, although this was never made a statutory obligation. In the event local authority day services for the mentally ill were non-existent before 1960, and were only developed on any scale after the establishment of social services departments in 1971.

Sadly there are few accounts in the literature of how a local day care service has developed over time in response to changing therapeutic fashion, the perceived needs of users or an increased understanding of what works in practice. Most accounts of projects or services are either uncritical descriptions of services that are quite new, or short-term evaluations. Descriptions of the social and demographic context within which a day care service operates are rare, despite abundant evidence that the use of all forms of health care is related to such factors as social deprivation. There is very little literature indeed on the development of day centre provision, reflecting the overall lack of research interest in local authority social services (Vaughan, 1983).

## The current pattern of day care

The government White Paper *Better Services for the Mentally Ill* (DHSS, 1975) envisaged a system of day care composed of two main elements. Local authority day centres would meet clients' immediate needs for shelter, occupation and support and provide families with relief from the strain of caring. The document described the functions of day centres in some detail. Day hospitals, however, were characterized only as places in which people would receive treatment under medical supervision: attenders would include inpatients in the new district general hospital psychiatric units as well as people living at home. Both would relate to sheltered employment and the voluntary sector. Long-term care would be the province of the day centre. The White Paper laid down norms for the number of places to be provided (30 places per 100,000 population for community attenders in day hospitals and 60 places per 100,000 in day centres).

After considerable expansion in provision throughout the 1960s and early 1970s, the rate of growth in day care has been more modest. In 1984 official statistics recorded 16,000 day hospital and 8000 day centre 'places' in England and Wales, which means that the planned figure for day hospital places has been reached, whilst local authorities are providing less than a quarter of the places expected of them. In the 1985, 32 out of the 108 social services departments in England provided no day centre places at all. Voluntary sector provision is even more unevenly distributed. Voluntary organizations provide some 1300 'day places' in 23 local authority areas but there is no voluntary day care in the other 85.

Even where there are local authority day centres it is very doubtful if the current pattern of day care reflects the neat distinction between treatment and long-term care envisaged in *Better Services* (Edwards and Carter, 1979). Many day hospitals provide long-term supportive care whilst some local authority facilities now offer short-term 'treatment'.

## Day care and the psychiatric services

The confusion that exists over the roles of day care is understandable when the many perspectives from which day care can be viewed are considered. From the viewpoint of the provider and planner of psychiatric services the major functions of day hospital care might fall into four main categories:

1. as an alternative to admission for people who are acutely ill and cannot be maintained as outpatients;
2. as a service of support, supervision and monitoring in the often difficult period of transition between a stay in an inpatient ward and life at home;
3. as a source of long-term structure and support for those with chronic handicaps, preferably in a friendly low-pressure environment; and
4. as a site for relatively brief intensive therapy for people with personality

difficulties, severe neurotic illnesses or in need of short-term focused rehabilitation.

In addition to these essentially clinical functions the day hospital might act as an information resource, a centre for training staff who provide community care and as a meeting place for people working in what might otherwise be a fragmented service.

A number of well-designed studies have shown that day care can provide a viable alternative to acute inpatient admission for selected patients (Wilder et al., 1966; Herz et al., 1971). However, it is not an effective alternative for patients who are elderly, suffering from dementia or are acutely confused due to the effects of physical illness or drug intoxication. Even when offered as an alternative to inpatient admission to patients suffering from neurotic conditions, day care may be clinically appropriate for only a minority of patients (Dick et al., 1985).

In current clinical practice the day hospital is frequently used as a stepping-stone into the community from the hospital ward, the rationale being that patients recovering from acute illnesses require support and monitoring, but to a less intense degree than inpatients. Transitional day care may be particularly useful when supplementing a policy of rapid discharge from inpatient care. Studies have shown that the adoption of an early discharge policy can result in massive savings in inpatient days, without any evidence of harm to patients or increased burden on relatives. Patients who had been readmitted many times before may do particularly badly with standard-length inpatient care (Endicott et al., 1979). This brief care approach has been extended by adding a low-key non-hospital residential setting to the inpatient/day hospital psychiatric unit (Gudeman et al., 1983). The availability of suitable alternative residential provision for patients who would otherwise have become long-stay is a crucial factor in determining the number of beds required to run a psychiatric service, and day care is no alternative for appropriate accommodation.

It may be that the real value of transitional care is to give the patient more confidence in returning to pre-existing social roles (and give family and therapists more confidence too!). Simple transitional care will be less appropriate for the patient who came into hospital with pre-existing social handicaps and for the 'revolving-door' patient, who will require long-term assertive community management.

Long-term day care is provided by NHS day hospitals and local authority and voluntary day centres. As we have seen, a number of the early day hospitals in Britain were established in the grounds of large mental hospitals. Where such facilities have been made available, former long-stay patients discharged from the mental hospital have continued to make use of supportive day care for long periods.

A number of surveys have been carried out looking at the clinical and social characteristics of long-term day patients. The average user of long-term day care has been described as suffering from schizophrenia, single, male, over 40 and living alone or with ageing parents (McCreadie *et al.*, 1984). This stereotype is less true in services where more day places are available in a greater variety of settings, and out of the large cities. Whatever the setting, the key characteristic of the long-term day attender is some form of impaired social competence, manifest either as a problem in making and maintaining satisfying social relationships or as an impairment of more basic aspects of social functioning such as self-care.

Controlled studies of the role of long-term day care are not plentiful (Herz, 1982) and tend not to take adequate account of the process of care. An exception is the multi-centre trial carried out by Linn and colleagues (1979). Schizophrenic patients discharged from ten Veterans Administration hospitals were randomly allocated to receive outpatient drug management alone or with additional supportive day care in a day treatment centre run by the hospital. All were considered suitable for long-term day care and as a group they suffered from chronic illnesses. The centres had common aims: to prevent admission to hospital, to improve social functioning and symptomatic disturbance and to contain the overall costs of care to the Veterans Administration. However, centres differed in the available resources and how these resources were used.

Although all centres improved social functioning, not all the centres reduced relapse rates compared with outpatient drug management alone. The 'good result' centres were characterized by a slower flow of patients, less professional staff hours and less group psychotherapy and family counselling. However, more recreational therapy, and more occupational therapy was provided. Successful centres showed a tendency to assign the patient to one worker for follow-up. In addition the 'good result' centres were considerably cheaper!

We know that people suffering from schizophrenia are sensitive to their environment: too much stress tends to precipitate a breakdown. An under-stimulating and impoverished social environment fosters the development of the so-called 'negative' symptoms of schizophrenia such as social withdrawal and lack of motivation (Wing, 1983). There is therefore a powerful rationale for the value of long-term day care in providing sustained non-threatening social support for patients suffering from chronic schizophrenia by means of a programme of activities individually tailored to provide the optimum degree of stimulation, together with practical help for the attenders' most pressing problems. We can be less clear about the needs of people suffering from other long-term psychiatric illnesses, although similar principles may apply.

The continuing care client will benefit from the availability of rather low-key long-term supportive day care, which may include the provision of sheltered work. This is not to deny that chronically mentally ill people have treatment needs. How are these needs to be met? Two strategies have been advocated. One is to ensure a regular review of patients' needs which is carried out within the long-term day setting, a review that includes the views of all involved professionals as well as day care staff (Wykes *et al.*, 1985). An alternative strategy is to admit patients to a rehabilitative day setting for assessment and the development of a long-term management plan.

Falloon and Talbot (1982) have demonstrated that the adoption of a goal-oriented approach to the short-term treatment of chronically disabled patients is feasible. They used detailed behavioural analysis to define goals for each attender at a day hospital and developed an individualized treatment plan to achieve these goals. The programme they initiated provided a range of treatments, including social skills groups, a work training programme and behavioural treatment packages for depression, anxiety, psychotic symptoms and family and marital conflict. Three accessory programmes were developed to be used after discharge, which took place within three months. These were a medication clinic, an outpatient counselling clinic and a recreational programme. In their report the authors demonstrated considerable success in attaining desired goals, particularly when the patient was involved in goal definition. Such a highly structured approach to day hospital care clearly demands a great deal of expertise and investment by staff, and the provision of appropriate resources for long-term care.

## Competing models of day care

Workers in local authority day centres might define their functions in very different ways from the four main functions described earlier. Whilst agreeing with their hospital colleagues that a primary task of day care is to break the cycle of readmission experienced by so many patients in contact with psychiatric services, day centre workers are likely to espouse a social model of psychiatric disorder. They may aim to provide social support, an opportunity to extend and develop social networks and an opportunity to achieve personal growth and integration. Centres may be attempting to encourage users to redevelop natural support systems, which for most of us come from a variety of sources: close relationships, family, friends, jobs, hobbies and membership of such social groups as clubs. The aim may be 'to build bridges to other sources of support' away from the day unit. Some centres may not expect users to be mentally ill at all, rejecting the use of such labels and allowing clients to define their own problems, which will be seen as problems of living. Clients may be encouraged to take a high degree of responsibility for themselves rather than receiving prescribed treatment.

Therapeutic community principles have had a significant impact on the development of local authority day care (Blake *et al.*, 1984). The London Borough of Kensington and Chelsea provides an integrated day care service based on these principles, with four centres catering for different client groups. Two activity-based therapeutic communities aim to improve the social skills and coping capacities of the most disabled, whilst two other centres have a strong psychotherapeutic orientation. The unit at the top of the hierarchy aims ambitiously at altering attenders' inner worlds. Not surprisingly the clientele at this centre are described as of above average intelligence, motivated and psychologically minded.

Selection of attenders for the appropriate setting in such a service is crucial. There is evidence that less articulate users, who are in general more chronically and severely handicapped, are discouraged from attending settings that are verbally oriented (Bender and Pilling, 1985). One great strength of the therapeutic community approach, at least in theory, is that it allows for the recognition of the feelings of staff, who may find working with a disabled client group demoralizing and distressing. Paradoxically, failure to resolve destructive dynamics within the community has been implicated in the dissolution of two leading psychotherapeutically oriented day hospitals (Roberts, 1980).

The system of day care in Kensington and Chelsea stands in sharp contrast to a number of other day care services that have been described, for example in the Scottish Day Care Survey (McCreadie *et al.*, 1984), in South Glamorgan (Pryce *et al.*, 1983) or in the old London Borough of Camberwell (Wing, 1982). In these services the focus of care is the person with long-term disabilities, and there is a heavy emphasis on the therapeutic role of industrial work. The Camberwell service has been evaluated by assessing the extent to which users' needs for treatment and care are met: this problem-orientated approach is reflected in the way the service has developed. It may be no accident that where interest is concentrated on the most handicapped patients the majority of users suffer from psychoses and have histories of multiple inpatient admissions.

Yet another approach to the development of a comprehensive day care service to the long-term mentally ill is provided by normalization, or social role valorization (Wolfensberger, 1983). This concept has had a powerful impact on mental handicap services in Britain and the United States, and now appears to be influencing policy-makers and practitioners in the field of mental illness. From this perspective a central aim of day care would be to provide users with a positive socially valued role. Preventing readmission to hospital and developing community support would be associated secondary aims. These aims would be carried out by developing and enhancing personal competence and social relationships, and by providing opportunities for the user to engage in appropriate leisure, educational and work-related activities. The normalization perspective does not necessarily deny the needs of long-term attenders at day units for specific therapeutic interventions based on problem-oriented or psychotherapeutic models of care, but makes the quality of life experience of users a central issue. It is, however, important to ensure that those adopting a normalization approach do not throw out the problem-oriented baby with the stigmatizing bathwater.

The difficulty of justifying a day care service divided between health authorities and local authorities, when in practice the distinctions are so blurred, has led to the development of a number of jointly run day units. An example of this is the Heatherwood Day Unit in Ascot, which has been open since 1977 (Vaughan, 1986). Cooperation appears to have been highly successful in this case, probably due to commitment by senior officers in both authorities. Clearly in these circumstances issues of control and inter-agency and inter-professional rivalry are likely to emerge.

## Day care and the user

Regular long-term users of day care must clearly value what they are offered. Indeed, they may value it so much that they do not want to be discharged, to the occasional discomfort of professionals who may mutter darkly about 'dependence'. People turn up to their day hospital or day centre either because they like what they get or because it is at least better than the alternatives. So what do users receive? At a minimum they get somewhere to go, away from wherever they live. Hopefully they are coming to a place that is physically comfortable and warm. Usually attenders are offered a cheap or free meal. There are other people around, and attenders may find the companionship of fellow-users to be very valuable. Some users find comfort in getting to know people who have had similar psychiatric problems to their own, and find that fellow-attenders are more supportive and understanding than the community at large. Others may value more especially the support and advice of staff, particularly at times of crisis. Most day settings offer some form of occupation or recreation, which in some units amounts to a highly structured programme of sheltered work. More specific services may be offered, such as psychiatric treatment (drugs, individual or group therapy aimed at specific problems), training in specific living skills and expert advice on, for example, welfare rights issues.

There have been few systematic attempts to discover what users find helpful about their day care. In a study of ex-attenders at Heatherwood Day Unit, where the typical attender is described as a middle-aged woman with neurotic symptoms living with her family (Vaughan and Prechner, 1985), patients rated the more traditional occupational therapy activities such as creative arts and crafts as being more beneficial than specific therapeutic activities such as group psychotherapy. There is some evidence that craft-based activities are more acceptable to women (Turner-Smith and Thompson, 1979), whilst men predominate in day services which mainly provide sheltered work (Pryce et al., 1983). The difficulty experienced by less articulate people in verbally oriented units has already been discussed.

Very little indeed has been written about the practices adopted in day settings, in other words what actually goes on. Certainly much time in many units is spent chatting to other attenders or simply doing nothing. Although staff often pay lip-service to the principle of developing individually tailored programmes matched to attenders' needs (however need is defined, itself a problematical issue) there must be some suspicion that the majority of settings purvey the block treatment typical of institutional care. Client-oriented management practices have been shown to be associated with a more personal approach to attenders' problems and a warmer quality of interaction between the staff and the users of day centres (Shepherd and Richardson, 1979). Client-oriented practices may be contrasted with the features of institutionally oriented care; clients being dealt with as a group rather than as individuals; lack of opportunity for clients to exercise autonomy; and social distance between staff and users. Attending a unit where your needs come first presumably improves your experience of the setting, although this has not been studied directly.

It is likely that in many day units the informal social networks that develop between attenders as they await or avoid the formal activities offered are of crucial subjective importance to users. The bulk of the social support available in day hospitals and day centres comes, of course, from other attenders.

If one analyses the place of day care in the lives of long-term attenders it appears to play a similar role to that of work. For these people day care may provide what Jahoda (1979) has called the 'latent' functions of work. Besides being a source of income (the 'manifest' function), work structures time, it enforces activity and provides a shared experience outside the confines of home, it links the individual to external goals and offers a sense of personal status and identity. If this analysis is accepted it follows that the treatment needs of day care users should not become the focus of their lives. It can be argued that these treatment needs are sessional in nature, and that the primary focus of day care should emphasize healthy functioning. The needs of the continuing care client for work as such are discussed more fully by Pilling in Chapter Ten.

A number of day care schemes aimed at the chronically handicapped specifically set out to emphasize healthy functioning—including, of course, those aimed at returning patients to work. Examples that have been described include the 'Unicentre' at Littlemore Hospital in Oxford (Gan and Pullen, 1984). This activity centre aims to meet some of the recreational and educational needs of clients in the Oxfordshire Rehabilitation Service by offering a very mixed programme of sessions covering communication, activities of daily living, creativity, use of community resources and use of general knowledge. Users have taken a large part in the development of the centre and there is emphasis on the exercise choice, a rare option for the chronically mentally ill. There is a weekly centre meeting for all users and staff. Community service volunteers are attached to the centre, which is complemented by a community day centre for the young chronically mentally ill run by the Oxford Mental Health Association (Hope and Pullen, 1985).

## The community mental health centre

A more radical approach to providing day care that is not illness oriented is presented by the North Derbyshire Mental Health Services project based at Tontine Road in Chesterfield (Milroy, 1985). This social work-based service is concerned with people who have had a history of 'psychiatric' disturbance but allows open access to all who perceive themselves to be in need. Sited in a former day centre for the physically handicapped, the project is described as a base for a therapeutic community, a social support club and a range of mental health groups including a local branch of the National Schizophrenia Fellowship. Therapeutic groups are run by outside workers, and the centre provides space for a day care service for the elderly run by a semi-independent voluntary organization. The project appears to be evolving rapidly, as accounts of its function vary from year to year: this may reflect responsiveness to needs or inherent instability in the organization.

Tontine Road is one particular form of community mental health centre. The CMHC movement is relatively new to Britain and, as a collection of papers recently published by the Kings Fund indicates, it is highly diverse in objectives and structures (McAusland, 1985). CMHCs may be based on day services, or may specifically exclude the provision of day activities in favour of a service providing assessment and therapy only. CMHCs may be run by the NHS or by the local authority, or may be a joint venture. Some are, in effect, small local psychiatric hospital units, with beds and 24-hour nursing cover as well as day care.

Accessibility to all those in need is a watchword of the CMHC movement. Who makes use of such services? In a large series of attenders at the walk-in clinic at the Mental Health Advice Centre in Lewisham the majority appeared to be suffering from transient distress reactions relating to adverse life circumstances or from long-term personality problems. Only 3 per cent were diagnosed as schizophrenic and a further 5 per cent as suffering from affective psychoses. Members of ethnic minority groups appear to have been under-represented amongst attenders (Bouras *et al.*, 1986). Although offering a useful service to a group of patients who would probably not otherwise receive specialist psychiatric help, such a centre may reflect a diversion of resources from the most severely ill. Furthermore it may be argued that CMHCs unnecessarily undercut the central role of primary care services, which are in this country the major source of help for psychiatric problems.

The delay in exporting CMHCs from the United States, where they have formed the backbone of the new pattern of psychiatric services for over 20 years, is an intriguing one. Ironically it occurs as the failure of the initial aims of the CMHC movement are being widely canvassed. Although set up with the intention of providing a fully comprehensive local service, CMHCs in fact predominantly treat young, single, mild to moderately disturbed patients in an outpatient setting (Mollica, 1980). The state mental hospital system remains the major source of inpatient care to the poor and the chronically disabled. Examples of highly successful CMHCs do exist, although some at least bear striking resemblances to the district general hospital psychiatric unit recommended in *Better Services* (Gudeman and Shore, 1984).

The original intellectual framework underpinning the movement has not stood the test of time. A social and highly politicized model of the causation of psychiatric disorder led some workers in CMHCs to abandon clinical care altogether, in favour of trying to reform society itself, although those now working in the CMHC movement appear to have lost their enthusiasm for political approaches that quite simply do not work (Mollica, 1980). Perhaps most disturbing of all from the viewpoint of public policy has been the well-documented flight of service providers from the care of the most disabled and disadvantaged patients, who may make little use of services that are not sufficiently assertive and fail to take their special disabilities into account.

Although CMHCs are currently fashionable there must be severe doubts about their relevance to the problems of the continuing care client. Unless planners and policy-makers can ensure that the needs of those with the most chronic and severe psychiatric disorders will be met by CMHCs, these facilities will not form an adequate substitute for the old, mental hospital-based, psychiatric services.

## PROVIDING COMMUNITY SUPPORT

The discussion so far has been confined to reviewing the history and utility of current day care provision. There have, however, been numerous attempts to synthesize this information and to identify the components of a comprehensive community-based system of support for the chronically mentally ill (Turner and Shifren, 1979; Stein and Test, 1980; Bachrach, 1982; Richmond Fellowship, 1983). Common themes emerge: the identification of persons in need; rapid intervention in crises; appropriate treatment to prevent relapse and minimize the disability and distress caused by illness; promotion of independent living skills and the fostering of satisfying and supportive social networks; support and education for relatives and carers; and attention to patients' basic needs for food, shelter and material possessions. There is also concern that the support system should ensure that the chronically mentally ill receive adequate general health care. Medical problems are frequent and may be presented in bizarre ways, or not be noticed at all by the patient and carers. It is vital that the support system itself is adequatley coordinated, and that users and their carers are guided through a fragmented and confusing array of helping agencies.

It is important to discuss a number of these elements of community support in more detail in order to demonstrate how interdependent and necessary they are for a satisfactory system of care to exist.

### Dealing with crisis

Crises often present as a request for admission to hospital. Indications for admission include unwillingness to comply with treatment, assaultive behaviour, severe suicidal intent and concurrent physical illness (Stein and Test, 1980). Sometimes patients and carers need a break from one another, although this need not necessarily require the use of a hospital bed.

Some health districts have set up specialized crisis intervention teams to respond to urgent calls for assistance (Waldron, 1983). The crisis intervention team owes much to Caplan's unified theory of crisis, in which a person's traditional pattern of coping breaks down. Caplan believed that the disequilibrium of the crisis provided an opportunity for the development of more adaptive coping skills (Caplan, 1964). Usually a crisis is seen as affecting more than the individual, and a family approach to assessment and management is often adopted.

The relevance of the crisis intervention model to the long-term mentally ill is not entirely clear. An alternative approach is the Training in Community Living Model developed by Stein and Test (1980). This form of community treatment, which has been favourably evaluated in the United

States and Australia (Hoult, 1986), is based on a clearly articulated model of the needs of the chronically mentally ill. The original programme used specially trained staff who were available on a 24-hour rota. Patients presenting for admission in psychosocial crisis were rapidly returned to the community. Symptoms were stabilized using medication, and an individualized programme prepared for each patient. Staff members assisted patients in the tasks of daily living, and in so doing provided practical training in social skills. The treatment team either worked in the patient's home, or, if the home setting was considered harmful, alternative accommodation such as a boarding house was found. The emphasis of the programme was on working with the patient in naturalistic community settings. Much time and effort was spent on educating the local community to respond to patients' needs. The community treatment team was assertive; actively maintaining contact with patients who defaulted from treatment.

Evaluations have shown the programme to be highly successful, in terms of improved social functioning, decreased symptomatology and increased satisfaction of both patients and carers (Stein and Test, 1980; Hoult, 1986). Significantly, the gains achieved are rapidly lost once the treatment team ceases its involvement. Although care must be taken in generalizing from small-scale research projects to clinical practice, the Stein and Test model offers an important pointer towards the future pattern of services for the chronically mentally ill. A three-year evaluation of the model in a British inner city area is currently under way (Marks et al., 1988). However, the community treatment approach can form only one component of a comprehensive psychiatric service. Crisis-oriented community treatment will founder if it is attempted without the backing of outpatient clinics, day care, sheltered workshops, social clubs, housing provision and inpatient facilities.

## Preventing relapse

Although many continuing care clients continue to suffer from disabling psychiatric symptoms, treatment of an acute episode of illness usually brings about a significant improvement in symptomatology. However, patients who have experienced an episode of psychiatric illness remain vulnerable to relapse or severe exacerbation of symptoms, and a key element of long-term psychiatric care is to prevent or minimize the possibility of relapse.

Most is known about strategies of relapse prevention in schizophrenia. A number of precipitating physical factors are known, including the use of drugs such as amphetamines and alcohol. The role of cannabis in precipitating psychiatric illnesses is less clear, although clinical experience points to a link between cannabis consumption and acute psychotic episodes in at least some vulnerable individuals. It is also known that the social environment may precipitate the recurrence of florid symptoms such as delusions and hallucinations (Wing, 1983). Stressful life events, which may not necessarily appear threatening or unfavourable, have been shown to precede the onset of acute illnesses in some patients (Birley and Brown, 1970). It is not known whether extra support can protect against the effects of stress, but clearly recognizing the perceived stress of a planned life event, such as a move into a hostel or starting work, may allow the client and therapist to explore ways of coping with stress.

For clients living with families, certain aspects of the emotional environment, notably relatives' criticism and over-involvement, may predispose to relapse. The role of 'expressed emotion' within families and possible strategies for intervention are discussed more fully in Chapter 11. There has to date been little work on the significance of 'expressed emotion' outside the family, and this is an important area for further research, since the majority of the long-term mentally ill do not live within a family.

Another form of stress is that provided by the therapist. It has repeatedly been shown that patients' psychiatric symptoms may get worse when they are put under pressure in over-enthusiastic rehabilitation programmes (Goldberg et al., 1977; Stevens, 1973). People working with the long-term mentally ill, especially with those suffering from schizophrenia, must be aware that patients are continually forced into a delicate balance between experiencing the stress of over-stimulation and the opposite danger of withdrawal into an under-active and isolated state.

There is a very considerable body of evidence that those patients who respond initially to treatment with antipsychotic drugs such as chlorpromazine and flupenthixol benefit from long-term maintenance medication (Hirsch, 1982). However antipsychotic drugs do produce potentially serious side-effects, notably various forms of movement disorder, and it has become an accepted part of psychiatric practice to treat patients on a minimum effective dose of antipsychotic drug (Manchanda and Hirsch, 1986). The role of long-term medication in patients who do not show clear-cut response to antipsychotic drugs is less clear, and can at present only be left to individual clinical judgment (Donaldson et al., 1983).

There has been much recent attention to the need actively to recruit patients and their carers to the drug treatment process by providing education and explanation in a structured format (Falloon et al., 1984). There is no doubt that optimal long-term management of psychotic disturbance requires a sensitive combination of drug treatment and attention to social factors (Falloon and Liberman, 1983).

There have been a number of exciting developments in the treatment of affective disorders using pharmacological, psychological and social interventions which may complement one another. A substantial body of evidence exists for the value of drug treatment in the prevention of relapse of severe affective disorders, including mania (Paykel, 1982). Although there is no doubt that social factors play a large role in the development of depressive disorders, and social functioning is frequently impaired in affective disturbances, the therapeutic effects of rehabilitative and social interventions have not been studied as systematically in affective disorders as in schizophrenia (Watts and Bennett, 1983a).

## Improving social competence

People with long-term mental illnesses tend to show poor levels of social competence. Social competence has a number of components: socialization skills (i.e. ability to relate to others); self-care skills (i.e. personal hygiene, care of clothing, care of personal apperance, concern with personal health); home management skills (i.e. cooking, shopping, cleaning, laundering, budgeting, etc.); ability to use community facilities (public transport, shops, financial services, statutory services, etc.); work skills; and literacy and numeracy skills. The starting point in enhancing an individual's social competence is an accurate assessment of their difficulties and abilities. It will be important to take account of the person's social circumstances (housing conditions, financial state and, most importantly, social network), since the social context will have a direct effect on what interventions are actually possible. Following the assessment an intervention programme may be developed that targets the particular needs of the client.

Surprisingly, there is very little empirical literature on skills training, with the notable exception of social skills training (Shepherd, 1986). However, a number of general points can be made about interventions aimed at improving social competence. Firstly, any skills training must take into account the problem of generalization. Training must help the individual to learn a particular skill in a way that will allow the skill to be put into practice in the appropriate setting. Shepherd (1977) has illustrated how particular social skills acquired in the special setting of a social skills group may fail to be transferred to outside 'ordinary' settings. The solution is to carry out the training in the setting in which the skills are to be used. If this is not possible it is necessary to simulate the conditions of the natural setting as closely as possible. Secondly, it is important to have clear goals that enable the client and therapist to direct their work and evaluate its success. The importance of clear goals to the success of any individualized programme has been demonstrated within the behaviour modification and social learning traditions (Paul and Lentz, 1977). Thirdly, a skills training programme will include a number of components: instruction, coaching, therapist/trainer modelling, role play, feedback on performance, social reinforcement contingent on appropriate behaviour, and the setting of practice or 'home work' tasks. Fourthly, in order to tackle the frequent problem of 'poor motivation', it is essential to work closely with the client to identify the skills to be addressed and the goals to be set. Finally, training programmes are unlikely to be effective unless the individual receives some emotional support during the intervention. This will require a member of the treatment team (e.g. the key worker) to offer regular counselling. Such regular meetings will enable staff to understand clients' inner worlds and relationship difficulties. This may not be the priority of skills-oriented training, but may well prove vital to the client's personal development.

Services must offer continuing care clients the opportunity to enhance their social competence. The extent to which a community care project aiming to integrate or reintegrate clients into the community provides such help will be an important area for the evaluation of the service. Day facilities clearly play a crucial role in the provision of this component of care.

## Fostering social networks

The long-term mentally ill tend to have very small social networks consisting mostly of family members (Mueller, 1980). Relationships are non-reciprocal: most of the aid flows from carer to patient. The causes of these impoverished social networks are complex: social contacts are lost during episodes of severe disturbance; patients are likely to be unemployed and poor and therefore to lack opportunities to develop and sustain relationships; many patients lack the self-confidence to mix with their more successful peers, and some have lost the skills of social interaction; many find social contact highly stressful and choose social withdrawal. Impoverished social environments encourage social withdrawal and promote the development of 'negative' symptoms (Wing and Brown, 1970).

There is a large and often contradictory literature on the relationship between social support and mental health (Henderson, 1984). Not all close relationships are experienced as supportive. Families characterized by high 'expressed emotion' predispose to relapse in both schizophrenia and depressive illnesses (Vaughan and Leff, 1976). Support from significant others and interpersonal stress are independent aspects of the social environment. Relapse after an episode of inpatient care is most likely in environments characterized by high levels of stress and lack of support (Goldstein and Caton, 1983).

A variety of approaches have been adopted to improve the quality and quantity of social networks. There is an extensive and optimistic literature on the family care of psychotic illness (Falloon *et al.*, 1984), which suggests that families containing a mentally ill member can be taught to adopt more positive styles of coping. Such treatment appears to have a direct benefit in reducing relapse rates, improving social functioning and decreasing vulnerability to adverse life events in the identified patient.

Families may become so depleted and depressed by the effects of chronic mental illness in a member that psychosocial treatment is ineffective. This has led to the development of 'network therapy' which uses the patient's social network to 'change dysfunctional patterns of interaction within the family, to re-energize the depressed nuclear family and to reconnect the nuclear family with its larger social system' (Schoenfeld *et al.*, 1986). Network therapy begins with an evaluation session involving the patient's nuclear family and several members of his or her social network. Family members are asked to formulate goals for treatment, and a series of meetings is convened to which relatives, friends, co-workers and significant others are invited. The meetings adopt a problem-solving approach. Resources within the family are mobilized, using a variety of experiential techniques, and an attempt is made to shift the burden of caring from the therapy team to the broader social network.

Many people with chronic mental illnesses come to lose their social network. It may then become necessary for the support system to develop a new social network. Day care and residential care can provide this artificial social network; many day care users are specifically motivated to attend by the social contact in their day unit (Holloway, 1988). It is important that any artificial network created encourages appropriate socially skilled behaviour. One of the ironies of psychiatric day care is that it may discourage people from relinquishing their symptoms for fear of losing the social support it offers.

It follows that the support system should, as far as possible, be encouraging the use of generic resources. Many people suffering from long-term mental illnesses are, despite their disabilities, quite skilled at using the pub, the library and the betting shop. Clearly, to encourage those patients who have become socially isolated to use community resources requires therapists to know what is available locally. Ideally professionals should be fostering the development of community support networks. However, limits to the tolerance of the community towards disturbed and deviant behaviour must be recognized. An alternative model of community support is the comprehensive psychosocial rehabilitation agency, run by and for users. The 'club house' model has had considerable success in the United States, Canada and Sweden. A major emphasis is on vocational rehabilitation, which underlines the importance of work and work-like activities in the support of the long-term mentally ill (Anthony *et al.*, 1984).

Yet another way of providing social support is the recruitment of befrienders, volunteers who develop personal relationships with mentally ill clients. At their best these contrived friendships are indistinguishable from natural friendships. The benefits of a befriending scheme are difficult to quantify, but proponents would point to an improvement in the ability of those being befriended to relate to others, to take initiative and to feel valued. Schemes dependent on volunteers are, of course, notoriously fragile.

## The coordination of care

The long-term mentally ill and their carers face a fragmented, confusing and ill-coordinated services system. This fragmentation has been exacerbated by the decline of the mental hospital and the development of locally based psychiatric services involving a multiplicity of caring agencies. How are we to ensure that patients and their supporters receive the help that they need when they need it? A number of principles can be stated with confidence. Firstly, those experiencing the most severe disabilities will only receive appropriate help from a service that is specifically targeted at their needs. Secondly, no single individual or profession has the breadth of skills required to meet all the needs of the continuing care client: a service system can only be effective if it relies on teamwork. Thirdly, patients or clients need a reference point, some person within the service system who takes individual responsibility for the coordination of care. Fourthly, the planning of care must take place within some coherent framework that allows for the formulation of aims and objectives, the planning of appropriate interventions and regular review of the outcome of care.

For all its faults, the mental hospital provided for those in society who were most vulnerable. Patients with long-term disabilities are not well catered for within district general hospital psychiatric units; indeed the necessary orientation towards treatment and rapid change may make their disabilities worse. Experience has shown that there is a continual tendency for care-givers working in community settings to offer their services to more immediately attractive 'deserving' or 'rewarding' client groups, who can be expected to respond to the 'therapy' that is offered to them. The solution is the development of a continuing care or rehabilitation team that is given the responsibility (and resources) to provide a service to the client group. Such a team will not provide all the necessary services, but will coordinate care and facilitate service development. Ideally the team should be the product of joint planning. An example of what can be achieved even within a short time scale is presented in Chapter 14.

The importance of team work in long-term psychiatric practice stems largely from the necessity of taking a comprehensive view of patients' problems (Watts and Bennett, 1983b). No single professional has the required range of skills and knowledge: good-quality care requires good inter-professional and inter-agency cooperation. However, barriers to effective teamwork abound. The varied professional and non-professional backgrounds of team members are both a source of strength and of potential conflict, since different groups have alternative conceptual frameworks in which patients' problems are seen. It is important that team members respect others' perspectives: no-one has the monopoly of wisdom in long-term psychiatry. Differences in status and pay may breed resentment on the one hand and defensiveness on the other. In our society direct care-givers have low status, and managers tend to avoid direct patient or client contact. This is unfortunate, since the modelling effect of senior staff is a powerful determinant of quality of care.

Some degree of conflict within a treatment team is inevitable, since long-term care presents inherent dilemmas, such as the necessity to balance demands for patients to adhere to a structured programme of rehabilitation and the importance of respecting autonomy and choice. These dilemmas may be acted out within the team. It is important that debate and dissent is encouraged within the team, since the very complex problems presented by patients demand innovation and flexibility in approach. Hierarchically organized teams, in which a single leader distributes tasks to other team members, tend to be inflexible. In contrast a decision-making process that involves all relevant members of the team results in more informed decisions that are more likely to be implemented. Staff teams that function well are often a source of support and motivation in the very demanding tasks of long-term care. Team meetings can, in addition, have an important supervisory function in monitoring the work of staff. Ideally teams should be cohesive, but not collusive.

Leadership is important to effective teamwork. Team meetings need to be chaired. When tasks are identified the chair of the meeting must specify what is to be done, allocate responsibility to team members for carrying out tasks, ensure that staff have the necessary skills to do what is required of them and feed back (in positive terms) on performance. In addition to providing structure to the tasks of the team, leaders must support the team in coping with the inevitable strains that the work produces, foster cohesiveness, communicate optimism about the potential of patients and demonstrate effective involvement with patients. Watts and Bennett (1983b) have argued that a distributed style of leadership, in which these functions are taken by a number of team members, is more likely to produce an integrated and effective team.

An important issue that the team must address is their relationship with the rest of the service system. Team members will have to orchestrate their responses to the wider system, both to obtain resources and to provide information on which management decisions will be based. It is also vital that the team is open to receiving information from the rest of the service. This will ensure that the team remains a healthy and open system. In turn managers must set clear aims for the team, whilst allowing a high level of autonomy in carrying out tasks. There is good evidence that autonomy motivates staff and encourages good practice (Raynes et al., 1979).

Despite the importance of teamwork, it is valuable to have a single team member take specific responsibility for the coordination of care to individual clients/patients. Various styles of 'key working' or case management have been adopted (Lamb, 1982; Pollock, 1986), from being given primary responsibility for particular therapeutic tasks to the role of a professional advocate who ensures that caring agencies meet their patients' needs. The key worker is perhaps best seen as that person who monitors the work of the team as a whole with a particular client, and is responsible for information-gathering, record-keeping, and ensuring that regular reassessment of progress is made. Effective key working requires the development of a close relationship with the patient or client, but this should never be exclusive.

The complexities of the problems presented to services by people suffering from long-term mental illnesses, and the resistance that these problems may show to change, make it vital that repeated systematic assessments are carried out. Interesting approaches to care planning have been developed in acute psychiatry (Parsons, 1986), continuing care for the elderly demented (Barraclough and Fleming, 1985), mental handicap services (Humphreys and Blunden, 1987) and psychiatric rehabilitation (Shepherd, 1983). Differing in detail, they share a desire to respect the person being planned for, and an active attempt to involve the patient/client in the planning process. Care planning owes much to the behavioural tradition, focusing on the identification of problems, the setting of clearly defined goals that are spelt out in terms of overt behaviour, the determination of a series of attainable steps to achieve these goals, and rigorous evaluation of the interventions provided. Authors emphasize the importance of capitalizing on the strengths of patients rather than focusing on weakness: the approach is 'constructionist', aiming to increase the range of appropriate client behaviours, in contrast to the traditional 'pathological' approach, which aims to reduce or eliminate negative behaviours. This style of care planning fits in well with the key worker system.

CONCLUSION

Unfortunately there is no blueprint available for the ideal system of community support for the chronically mentally ill that an average health district can dust off and put into practice. Support systems must evolve according to local conditions and local priorities. Inter-agency planning in the development of community care is crucial. Inevitably people suffering from long-term mental illnesses will make demands on a wide variety of agencies and professional groups. There is a need to have at the heart of any system of care a team whose specific task is the welfare of the continuing care client. The treatment team will aim to provide continuity of care, helping patient and carers through the service maze. Care to the individual is best coordinated by a key worker or case manager, who organizes a package of support, using a variety of agencies. This package will be based on an individualized assessment of need and a sensitive understanding of the person's inner world. Day care will be an important service element, offering an opportunity for social support and a setting for treatment programmes aimed at developing living skills and enhancing self-esteem. Ideally a range of day services will be available within a district, providing a variety of activities, social groups and therapeutic approaches.

There is a clear challenge to professionals to develop a flexible, accessible and informal community support service that assertively seeks to engage those in need.

REFERENCES

Anthony, W. A., Cohen, M. R., and Cohen, B. F. (1984). Psychiatric rehabilitation. In J. A. Talbott (ed.) *The Chronic Mental Patient*, Grune and Stratton, Orlando.
Bachrach, L. L. (1982). Assessment of outcomes in community support systems: results, problems and limitations, *Schizophrenia Bulletin*, **8**, 39–60.
Barraclough, C., and Fleming, I. (1985). *Goal Planning with Elderly People*, Churchill Livingstone, Edinburgh.
Bender, M. P., and Pilling, S. (1985). A study of variables associated with under-attendance at a psychiatric day hospital, *Psychological Medicine*, **15**, 395–402.
Bierer, J. (1959). Theory and practice of psychiatric day hospitals, *Lancet*, **ii**, 901–2.
Birley, J. L. T., and Brown, G. W. (1970). Crisis and life changes preceding the onset or relapse of acute schizophrenia: clinical aspects, *British Journal of Psychiatry*, **116**, 327–33.
Blake, R., Millard, D. W., and Roberts, J. P. (1984). Therapeutic community principles in an integrated local authority community mental health service, *International Journal of Therapeutic Communities*, **5**, 243–73.
Bouras, N., Tufnel, G., Brough, D. I., and Watson, J. P. (1986). Model for the integration of community psychiatry and primary care. *Journal of the Royal College of General Practitioners*, **283**, 62–6.

Brown, G. W., Bone, M., Dalison, B., and Wing, J. K. (1966). *Schizophrenia and Social Care*, Oxford University Press, London.

Caplan, G. (1964). *Principles of Preventative Psychiatry*, Basic Books, New York.

Creer, C., Sturt, E., and Wykes, T. (1982). The role of relatives. In J. K. Wing (ed.), *Long-term Community Care: experience in a London Borough. Psychological Medicine* Monograph, Supplement 2.

DHSS (1975). *Better Services for the Mentally Ill*, HMSO, London.

Dick, P., Cameron, L., Cohen, D., Barlow, M., and Ince, A. (1985). Day and full-time psychiatric treatment: a controlled comparison, *British Journal of Psychiatry*, **147**, 246–50.

Donaldson, S., Gelenberg, A. J., and Balderssarini, R. J. (1983). The pharmacologic treatment of schizophrenia: a progress report, *Schizophrenia Bulletin*, **9**, 504–27.

Edwards, C., and Carter, J. (1979). Day services and the mentally ill. In J. K. Wing and R. Olsen (eds) *Community Care and the Mentally Disabled*, Oxford University Press, London.

Endicott, J., Cohen, J., Nee, J., Fleiss, J. L., and Herz, M. I. (1979). Brief vs standard hospitalisation: for whom? *Archives of General Psychiatry*, **36**, 706–12.

Falloon, I. R. H., and Liberman, R. P. (1983). Interactions between drug and psychosocial therapy in schizophrenia. *Schizophrenia Bulletin*, **9**, 543–54.

Falloon, I. R. H., and Talbot, R. E. (1982). Achieving the goals of day treatment, *Journal of Nervous and Mental Disease*, **170**, 279–85.

Falloon, I. R. H., Boyd, J. L., and McGill, C. W. (1984). *Family Care of Schizophrenia*, Guildford, New York.

Farndale, W. A. J. (1961). *The Day Hospital Movement in Great Britain*, Pergamon Press, Oxford.

Gan, S., and Pullen, G. P. (1984). The Unicentre: an activity centre for the mentally ill, *Occupational Therapy*, **47**, 216–18.

Goldberg, S. C., Silvester, N. R., Hogarty, G. E., and Roper, N. (1977). Prediction of relapse in schizophrenic patients treated by drug and sociotherapy, *Archives of General Psychiatry*, **34**, 171–84.

Goldstein, J. M., and Caton, C. L. M. (1983). The effects of the community environment on chronic psychiatric patients, *Psychological Medicine*, **13**, 193–9.

Gudeman, J. E., and Shore, M. F. (1984). Beyond deinstitutionalisation: a new class of facilities for the mentally ill. *New England Journal of Medicine*, **311**, 832–6.

Gudeman, J. E., Shore, M. F., and Dickey, B. (1983). Day hospitalisation and an inn instead of inpatient care for psychiatric patients. *New England Journal of Medicine*, **308**, 749–53.

Harris, A. (1957). Day hospitals and night hospitals in psychiatry. *Lancet*, **i**, 729–30.

Hassall, C., Gath, D., and Cross, K. W. (1972). Psychiatric day care in Birmingham. *British Journal of Preventative and Social Medicine*, **26**, 112–20.

Henderson, A. S. (1984). Interpreting the evidence on social support, *Social Psychiatry*, **19**, 49–52.

Herz, M. I. (1982). Research overview in day treatment, *International Journal of Partial Hospitalization*, **1**, 33–44.

Herz, M. I., Endicott, J., Spitzer, R. L., and Mesnikoff, A. (1971). Day versus inpatient hospitalization: a controlled study. *American Journal of Psychiatry*, **127**, 1371–82.

Hirsch, S. R. (1982). Medication and physical treatment of schizophrenia. In J. K. Wing and L. Wing (eds) *Handbook of Psychiatry*, Volume 3: *Psychoses of Uncertain Origin*, Cambridge University Press, Cambridge.

Holloway, F. (1988). Users' views of their day care, *Health Trends* (in press).

Hope, J., and Pullen, G. P. (1985). 'The Mill': a community centre for the young chronically mentally ill—an experiment in partnership, *Occupational Therapy*, **48**, 142–4.

Hoult, J. (1986). Community care of the acutely mentally ill, *British Journal of Psychiatry*, **149**, 137–44.

Humphreys, S., and Blunden, R. (1987). A collaborative evaluation of an individual plan system, *British Journal of Mental Subnormality*, **3**, 19–30.

Jahoda, M. (1979). The impact of unemployment in the 1930's and 1970's, *Bulletin of the British Psychological Society*, **32**, 309–14.

Lamb, H. R. (1982). *Treating the Long-term Mentally Ill*, Josey Bass, San Francisco.

Linn, M. W., Caffey, E. M., Klett, J., Hogarty, G. E., and Lamb, H. R. (1979). Day treatment and psychotropic drugs in the aftercare of schizophrenic patients. *Archives of General Psychiatry*, **36**, 1055–66.

Manchanda, R., and Hirsch, S. R. (1986). Low dose maintainence medication for schizophrenia, *British Medical Journal*, **293**, 515–17.

McAusland, T. (ed.) (1985). *Planning and Monitoring Community Mental Health*, Kings Fund Centre, London.

McCreadie, R. G., Robinson, A. D., and Wilson, A. D. A. (1984). The Scottish survey of chronic day patients, *British Journal of Psychiatry*, **145**, 626–30.

Marks, I., Connolly, J., and Muijen, M. (1988). The Maudsley daily living programme, *Bulletin of the Royal College of Psychiatrists*, **12**, 22–4.

Milroy, A. (1985). Some reflections on the experience of the North Debyshire Mental Health Service Project—Tontine Road Centre, Derbyshire. In T. McAusland (ed.) *Planning and Monitoring Community Mental Health Centres*, Kings Fund Centre, London.

Mollica, R. F. (1980). Community mental health centres. An American response to Kathleen Jones. *Journal of the Royal Society of Medicine*, **73**, 863–70.

Mueller, D. P. (1980). Social networks: a promising direction for research on the relationships of the social environment to psychiatric disorder, *Social Sciences and Medicine*, **14A**, 147–61.

Parsons, P. J. (1986). Building better treatment plans, *Journal of Psychosocial Nursing*, **24**, 9–14.

Paul, G. L., and Lentz, R. J. (1977). *Psychosocial Treatment of Chronic Mental Patients: milieu vs social learning program*, Harvard University Press, Harvard.

Paykel, E. S. (1982). Medication and physical treatment of affective disorders. In J. K. Wing and L. Wing (eds) *Handbook of Psychiatry*, Volume 3: *Psychoses of Uncertain Origin*, Cambridge University Press, Cambridge.

Pollock, L. (1986). The multidisciplinary team. In C. Hume and I. Pullen (eds) *Rehabilitation in Psychiatry*, Churchill Livingstone, Edinburgh.

Pryce, I. G., Baughan, C. A., Jenkinson, T. D. O., and Venkatesan, A. (1983). A study of long-attending psychiatric day patients and the services provided for them, *Psychological Medicine*, **13**, 875–884.

Raynes, N. V., Pratt, M. W., and Roses, S. (1979) *Organizational Structure and the Care of the Mentally Retarded*, Croom Helm, London.

Richmond Fellowship (1983). *Mental Health and the Community*. Richmond Fellowship Press, London.

Roberts, J. P. (1980). Destructive processes in a therapeutic community, *International Journal of Therapeutic Communities*, **1**, 159–70.

Schoenfeld, D., Halevy, J., Hemley-van der Velden, E., and Ruhf, L. (1986). Long term outcome of network therapy, *Hospital and Community Psychiatry*, **37**, 373–76.

Shepherd, G. W. (1977). Social skills training and the generalisation problem, *Behaviour Therapy*, **8**, 100–9.

Shepherd, G. W. (1983). Planning the rehabilitation of the individual. In F. N. Watts and D. H. Bennett (eds), *Theory and Practice of Psychiatric Rehabilitation*. Wiley, Chichester.

Shepherd, G. W. (1986). Social skills training and schizophrenia. In C. B. Hollin and T. Trower (eds) *Handbook of Social Skills Training*, Pergamon Press, Oxford.

Shepherd, G., and Richardson, A. (1979). Organisation and interaction in psychiatric day centres. *Psychological Medicine*, **9**, 573–79.

Stein, L., and Test, M. (1980). Alternative to mental hospital treatment. I: Conceptual model, treatment programme and clinical evaluation, *Archives of General Psychiatry*, **37**, 392–7.

Stevens, B. C. (1973). Evaluation of rehabilitation for psychotic patients in the community, *Acta Psychiatrica Scandinavica*, **49**, 169–80.

Turner, J. E. C., and Shifren, I. (1979). Community support systems: how comprehensive? *New Directions for Mental Health Services*, **2**, 1–23.

Turner, J. E. C., and Ten Hoor, W. S. (1978). The NIMH Community support programme: pilot approach to a needed social reform, *Schizophrenia Bulletin*, **4**, 319–44.

Turner-Smith, A., and Thompson, I. G. (1979). Patients' opinions. A survey of effectiveness of a psychiatric day hospital, *Nursing Times*, 19 April, pp. 675–9.

Vaughan, C. E., and Leff, J. P. (1976). The influence of family and social factors on the course of schizophrenic and depressed neurotic patients, *British Journal of Psychiatry*, **129**, 123–37.

Vaughan, P. J. (1983). The disordered development of day care in psychiatry, *Health Trends*, **15**, 91–4.

Vaughan, P. J. (1986). A question of balance, *Health Service Journal*, **96**, 1260–1.

Vaughan, P. J., and Prechner, M. (1985). Occupation or therapy in psychiatric day care? *Occupational Therapy*, **48**, 169–71.

Waldron, G. (1983). Crisis intervention—is it effective? *British Journal of Hospital Medicine*, **308**, 367–73.

Watts, F. N., and Bennett, D. H. (1983a). Neurotic, affective and conduct disorders. In F. N. Watts and D. H. Bennett (eds) *Theory and Practice of Psychiatric Rehabilitation*, Wiley, Chichester.

Watts, F. N., and Bennett, D. H. (1983b). Management of the staff team. In F. N. Watts and D. H. Bennet (eds) *Theory and Practice of Psychiatric Rehabilitation*, Wiley, Chichester.

Wilder, J. F., Levin, G., and Zwerling, G. I. (1966). A two year follow-up evaluation of acute psychiatric patients treated in a day hospital, *American Journal of Psychiatry*, **122**, 1095–1101.

Wing, J. K., and Brown, G. W. (1970). *Institutionalism and Schizophrenia*, Cambridge University Press, Cambridge.

Wing, J. K. (1982). Long term community care: experience in a London Borough, *Psychological Medicine Monograph*, Supplement 2.

Wing, J. K. (1983). Schizophrenia. In F. N. Watts and D. H. Bennett (eds) *Theory and Practice of Psychiatric Rehabilitation*, Wiley, Chichester.

Wolfensberger, W. (1983). Social role valorisation: a proposed new term for the principle of normalisation. *Mental Retardation*, **21**, 234–9.

Wykes, T., Sturt, E., adn Creer, C. (1985). The assessment of patients' needs for community care, *Social Psychiatry*, **20**, 76–85.

Community Care in Practice
Edited by A. Lavender and F. Holloway
© 1988 John Wiley & Sons Ltd

Chapter 10

# Work and the Continuing Care Client

## STEPHEN PILLING

Work occupies a central position in the lives of most people. It can take many forms and have many different meanings; the *Oxford English Dictionary* offers 39 definitions. Its importance in maintaining an individual's psychological well-being has long been recognized. This is perhaps best expressed by Freud (1930), who wrote 'No other technique for the conduct of life so firmly attaches the individual to reality as laying of emphasis on work; for work at least gives him a secure place in a position of reality, in the human community.' This chapter is concerned with how work enables the continuing care client to develop the appropriate links with reality and the human community.

A distinction should be made between work and leisure especially as work and employment are often used synonymously. The definition of work used in this chapter is that of Jacques (1967), who states that work is 'the exercise of judgement or discretion within prescribed limits in order to reach a goal or objective'. Employment, however, is defined as the exchange relationship which exists between employer and employee, where the employee is rewarded, usually in financial terms, for the performance of work. In contrast, leisure is defined as the pursuit, in an individual's free time, of interests and hobbies which do not have goals or limits which are defined by external agencies. As can be seen from the above definitions these distinctions are not always clear-cut.

Although clearly concerned with the role work has in linking an individual to the social world, Freud and Jacques place a heavy emphasis on the intra-psychic or individualistic aspects of work. The social psychological aspects perhaps need greater stress, for it can be claimed that work provides a structure to individuals' lives that might otherwise not be obtainable. This is not to deny that work or employment can at times be harmful, physically or psychologically, or exploitative, but rather to emphasize that work offers individuals a way to develop their lives that few, if any, other activities do. If this view is accepted then it can readily be appreciated what a potentially powerful tool work can be in the development of services for the continuing care client group, whose lives are often characterized by a constant struggle against disintegration and social breakdown.

The social psychological significance of work is apparent, for example, in the effects of unemployment. Jahoda (1981) makes an important distinction between the latent and manifest functions of employment. The manifest functions she considers to be the payment for, and terms and conditions of, employment. The latent functions she describes as follows: (1) the imposition of a time structure (that is the temporal structuring of the waking day); (2) the provision of shared experiences and social contacts (in particular with people outside the primary social group); (3) the development of goals and purposes that transcend one's own; (4) the definition of personal status and identity; (5) the enforcement of activity. These functions provide a useful way to conceptualize the psychological value of work and have proved valuable in studying the psychological consequences of unemployment.

Empirical evidence (Warr, 1984) has demonstrated the impact of unemployment on psychological well-being. The increased apathy, indecision, loss of social contact, loss of self-esteem and inability to structure both leisure and daytime activity that occurs, provides support for Jahoda's conceptualization. Many studies of the continuing care client group also characterize them as apathetic, lacking in motivation, socially withdrawn, and unable to make use of their ample leisure time. Whilst it would be wrong to attribute all such problems to an absence of work, the similarities cannot be entirely ignored.

## THE HISTORY OF WORK IN THE MENTAL HEALTH SERVICES

Given the undeniable psychological importance of work, it is not surprising that it has played an important part in the development of mental health services. Its relative importance has waxed and waned; its role in treatment, rehabilitation and resettlement having been both the victim and beneficiary of changing fashions in psychiatric care and wider social and economic pressures.

John Conolly (1847), a pioneer in the development of modern psychiatric care, wrote in *The Construction and Government of Lunatic Asylums* that 'Among the means of relieving patients from the monotony of an asylum, and of preserving the bodily health, and, at the same time, of improving the conditions of the mind, and prompting recovery, employment of some kind or other ranks the highest.' Many country asylums followed Conolly's advice and gave work a central role in the treatment, rehabilitation and resettlement plans of their institutions. Many such institutions had their own farms, gardens and tailors, and became almost self-supporting communities. The days of chains and private madhouses were gone, and the Victorian work ethic, in combination with a growing humanitarian concern for the mentally ill, promised a brighter future in which self-improvement through work was possible.

However, the county asylums became overcrowded. The optimism about cure began to disappear and by the start of the First World War, when the mental hospital population was proportionally at its peak, the asylums had become custodial institutions where few of the residents engaged in any structured activity. The inter-war period saw little resurgence of interest, although by the mid-1930s records of visits to Dutch and German psychiatric services by British psychiatrists (Evans, 1929; 1933) commented on the success that had been achieved through the introduction of work therapy. The Second World War saw a major change in the attitude to, and the nature of, work in the mental hospitals. These were two major reasons for this: firstly, the shortage of labour resulting from the drain of personnel from industry into the armed services; secondly, a renewed optimism in psychiatry, characterized by the adoption of the 'open-door' and sociotherapeutic policies in many mental hospitals.

The impact of increased labour demand began to have an effect early in the war. The Disabled Persons (Employment) Act of 1944 arose from the deliberations of the Tomlinson Committee, which was concerned with the rehabilitation and resettlement of a wide range of disabled people into the workforce. It was not only concerned with the establishment of disabled people into employment, but also recognized that the provision of work-related activity in settings which simulated normal industrial conditions was the best way to achieve resettlement. A number of Industrial Rehabilitation Units (IRUs) (later to be renamed Employment Rehabilitation Centres (ERCs)) were established, initially to promote the development of 'work fitness'. The first unit opened in 1943 and today there are 27 ERCs. Although primarily concerned with the preparation of people for open employment, it was accepted that some people would require long-term sheltered work. To that end, a company, 'Remploy', was created in 1945. This company now has 80 factory sites and employs over 7000 disabled people, about 10 per cent of whom are registered disabled on psychiatric grounds.

These developments in government-led employment schemes were paralleled by a somewhat slower development of services within the National Health Service (NHS). In the 1950s a number of industrial workshops were established within the large mental hospitals (Bennett, 1970). These units had as their primary focus the resettlement of long-stay patients back into the community. By the end of the 1960s almost every large mental hospital in the country had its own industrial workshop. These workshops concentrated primarily on industrial subcontract work. Some units, such as that established by Donal Early at Glenside Hospital in Bristol, moved in part into the community to form locally based industrial therapy organisations. However, many units stayed within the large hospitals, and it could be argued that the resultant lack of change, either in the type of work activity or the setting, contributed to the declining interest in work in the mental health services in the 1970s and 1980s. The importance placed on work in the mental health services has also been influenced by the prevailing economic climate and the availability of employment.

## THE PRESENT POSITION OF WORK IN THE MENTAL HEALTH SERVICES

The move towards community-based care began to have a major impact on the mental hospital population in the 1950s and 1960s and work played an important part in the resettlement of many long-stay patients in the community. It is clear that much of the work-related activity presently carried out within the mental health services, particularly in the large mental hospitals, will not be able to make the contribution to rehabilitation and resettlement that it did in the 1950s and 1960s. The present population of the large hospitals is composed of an older and more disabled group of people, for many of whom work, although very important, is only part of an overall care programme. The possiblity of a return to open or sheltered employment, which offers a way to resettlement in the community, is unrealistic for the majority of this group, either by reason of age or disability. In addition, this older group of long-stay patients is being supplemented by a very disabled group of new long-stay patients for whom many of the present community-based services have proved inadequate. The challenge of providing a service for this group is very great, and it may be that some of the dissatisfaction with work-oriented services in both hospital and community settings stems from a perception that work has not helped these people.

The 1970s and 1980s have seen an economic recession in the advanced industrial nations unmatched since the 1930s. The consequent rise in unemployment, combined with advances in technology, is held to have permanently changed the nature of work and employment patterns. This has, in turn, led to a crisis of confidence amongst those providing work-related activities in the mental health services. This is illustrated in the title chosen by the British Institute of Industrial Therapy for their 1983 conference; 'Rehabilitation: the way ahead or the end of the road?' The industrial or manufacturing emphasis of many units appears misplaced when most of the employment opportunities for disabled people will be in service industries. Perhaps most importantly, the technological and economic changes of the past decade have led to serious questions being raised about the possibility of employment or work being a realistic option for many people. It is suggested that more effort should be focused on the development of leisure activities and the reduction of individuals' expectations that they will obtain work or employment. This is held to be the case particularly for disabled groups.

However, the problem is that work and employment meet a range of important psychological needs that few, if any, other activities can match. Indeed it could be said that the time we have for leisure is defined by the time we have free from work, and therefore that any attempts to develop people's leisure time without the benefit of work to help structure the day could be futile. That people still want to work—be they the long-term unemployed or the young school-leaver, whose expectations were formed in the 1980s—is a fact supported by empirical research (Warr, 1984). There is some reason to believe that many continuing care clients still want to work or to be employed. Community care faces major challenges over the next decade. If the needs of the continuing care client are to be met then the potentially powerful and wide-ranging psychological needs provided by work and employment must be acknowledged, and wherever possible harnessed to provide a more effective service.

The present position of work-related mental health services can appear bleak, particularly if it is combined with that of the Manpower Services Commission's (MSC) present services such as the ERCs and Remploy, which are themselves in something of a crisis. This crisis is exemplified by a decreasing ability on the part of the ERCs to place people in employment or further training (Cornes *et al.*, 1982). However, there are some sources of encouragement. The MSC has recognized the limits of ERCs as presently developed, and has begun to sponsor a number of innovatory schemes, often in partnership with other statutory or voluntary bodies. Some of these schemes, along with a number of other projects, will be described later in the chapter.

## EVALUATIVE STUDIES

Research studies have looked not only at work as an effective tool in treatment, rehabilitation and resettlement, but also as an outcome measure. For example, Anthony *et al.* (1972) reported that somewhere between 30 and 50 per cent of people were in employment within six months of leaving hospital. This dropped to around 20–30 per cent after one year. Other studies have demonstrated that hospital admission is often associated with loss of employment (Cole *et al.*, 1964).

The 1950s saw the development of the first rehabilitation units and the beginning of the first research programmes. Brown *et al.* (1958) demonstrated that people who found employment following discharge were less likely to be readmitted. In their study, of the 41 per cent of people who found employment, only 3 per cent were readmitted, whereas 54 per cent of those who did not find employement were readmitted. The study also demonstrated that there was no direct correlation between psychiatric symptomatology, severity of disability and ability to work (over a third of those in employment had psychotic symptoms and were rated at least moderately disabled). Later, Wing and Brown (1970), in their study of long-term patients in three psychiatric hospitals, were able to demonstrate that an increase in the level of occupation, including industrial therapy, was associated with an improvement in patients' clinical state. The studies emphasize the importance work and employment can have in promoting mental health in hospital and community settings.

Initial reports of work units within hospital services were largely descriptive. Early, who pioneered the development of industrial therapy at Glenside Hospital, produced a number of reports (e.g. Early, 1960) describing the establishment of the service. Early and Magnus (1968) noted that the marked impact industrial therapy initially had on hospital discharge rates tailed off after about two years. Such data caution against relying on work as the sole means of treatment or resettlement. This view is reinforced by the work of Wing *et al.* (1972), who conducted an evaluation of a newly established rehabilitation day hospital and associated workshop at the Maudsley Hospital. In this study fourteen people were placed in the day hospital and a matched control group of fourteen continued to receive standard community-based psychiatric care. At follow-up there was little difference between the two groups with regard to symptomatology, hospitalization and resettlement into work. Although some criticisms can be made of this study, including its small size and the even smaller number who had long-term experience of the industrial unit, the study raises an important note of caution about attempts to transfer the industrial workshop model from hospital to community settings.

The effectiveness of the services provided by ERCs (originally IRUs) for those with mental health problems has been the subject of extensive research. Wing and colleagues in a series of studies (Wing, 1966; Wing *et al.*, 1964) were able to demonstrate that both moderately and severely disabled clients could be helped by the services of an ERC. They showed that a positive attitude to work was an important predictor of success in an ERC. This was the case across all disability groups, and proved to be of more importance than psychiatric symptomatology. Wing and his colleagues felt that the more realistic settings, with non-mentally ill fellow-trainees, combined with the specific training that they offered, gave ERCs an advantage over similar units based in large mental hospitals. ERCs were also able to bring about a change to a more positive attitude towards work, and had the added advantage that their superior assessment techniques often enabled people to fit more easily into other sectors of the employment rehabilitation services.

Unfortunately the ERCs do not appear to have lived up to this early promise. The ERCs, like their hospital-based counterparts, have gone through a very difficult period in the past fifteen years. This process has been well documented by Cornes et al. (1982) in their report on employment rehabilitation services. It appears that policies developed in the 1940s and 1950s are proving increasingly ineffective. For example, in 1946, 84 per cent of ERC's clients were successfully placed (70 per cent in employment and 14 per cent in training). By 1977 this figure had fallen to 44 per cent with only 25 per cent moving to open employment. Although this decrease in successful placement was most marked from the early 1970s, comparative results from different ERCs suggest that it is not solely due to rising unemployment. This report challenges the commonly held view that the poorer performance of ERCs is a result of an increasing percentage of mentally ill clients. Their study shows that the number of people with mental illness using the services has remained around 20 per cent since the service's inception. There is also little evidence, in their study, to suggest that clients with mental health problems do worse than any other disability group. The report did, however, emphasize the importance for mentally ill people of both adequate preparation and orientation to work prior to joining an ERC. These clients also required a longer period of training than the standard ERC course offered.

The research reviewed so far does not provide very strong evidence for the effectiveness of work-related activity in the rehabilitation and resettlement of the continuing care client. Perhaps what can be said is that work has proved effective in certain settings and offers a promising starting point for the development of new and innovative community-based mental health services. Exactly what this promise is may be better understood from a review of the research which has sought to establish what, in particular, work has to contribute to the efficacy of mental health services.

Miles (1971, 1972) looked at the comparative effectiveness of industrial and occupational therapy with long-stay psychiatric patients. She demonstrated that industrial therapy produced more change than occupational therapy in patients' abilities and willingness to work. Perhaps more importantly, she demonstrated that social interaction increased more during the period of industrial therapy. Watts (1978) examined a number of aspects of work behaviour in a work rehabilitation unit and demonstrated that social relationship skills were most strongly associated with resettlement into employment. Wing and Freudenberg (1961) looked at the value of increased social stimulation, including such things as praise for improved performance, given to patients in a rehabilitation unit by their supervisors. They were able to demonstrate that social stimulation did improve overall productivity, which decreased again once the stimulation was withdrawn.

Wadsworth and colleagues (e.g. Wadsworth et al., 1962) examined a number of aspects of work performance of patients in the work unit of a mental hospital. Their studies emphasize the need for an appropriate level of supervision which can enable those with chronic schizophrenia to overcome their problems with fatigue and the organization of complex sequential tasks. Tasks should be organized in clear, easily achieved steps with opportunities for early success. It is important that the right level of supervision is maintained; supervision that is too intense can be over-stimulating. Walker (1979) looked at the effect of different methods of payment on work performance in an industrial workshop, and concluded that payment should be appropriate and contingent on performance and not, as is often the case, simply for tunring up or being on the books. Many workshops, particularly those run by the statutory services, are poorly funded and produce little of value that could be redistributed in a financial way amongst the workers. Even where this is possible the present restrictive Department of Health and Social Security rules on therapeutic earnings greatly limit what can be earned. This issue will be returned to at the end of the chapter.

The prediction of the successful return to employment has been the subject of much research and the area has recently been well reviewed by Anthony and Jansen (1984). They concluded that psychiatric diagnosis, psychiatric symptomatology and psychometric tests were poor predictors of successful return to employment. Ratings of individual performance in realistic work settings, social relationships skills and ego-strength were amongst the best predictors.

The final area of research to be reviewed is concerned with employment seeking and employment tenure. This can be summarized by the statement that for people with chronic mental health problems staying in employment is much more difficult than finding employment. This is not to deny that such people do not face prejudice from potential employers (Wansborough and Cooper, 1980); they clearly do. A number of recent studies have looked at the efficacy of the 'job club' method developed by Azrin et al. (1975) in the United States and recently adopted in this country by the MSC for use with the long-term unemployed. For example, Jacobs et al.

(1984) in California adapted the 'job club' model for the psychiatrically disabled. By concentrating on job-finding skills (locating jobs) they were able to place two-thirds of their clients in either work (50 per cent) or training (10 per cent). The average time spent with the club was just under 30 days, although a number stayed much longer. A job maintenance element was introduced into the project, offering long-term support to those individuals who had already been placed in employment.

Some indication of the difficulties individuals with chronic mental health problems face in maintaining employment comes from a study by Floyd (1984). He followed up over 150 people diagnosed as suffering from schizophrenia, and looked at their post-discharge experience of employment. He did not find employer prejudice to be a major problem; few people who lost jobs were dismissed; most gave them up voluntarily. Many had found the employment situation too stressful, and left their jobs to avoid the possible serious consequences of stress and over-stimulation. He found employment associated with job tenure was characterized by a high objective quality, including good clear feedback on performance and some freedom to organize work time, a good social climate (especially in small working groups) and a product that was perceived as being of interest and having high value. Roessler and Bolton (1985), in the United States, have conducted a similar study looking at clients discharged from a vocational rehabilitation unit. Their follow-up emphasized the need for specific counselling, good preparation work and support with matters as diverse as family relations, transportation and finance in order to secure job tenure.

The research described above has been conducted over the past 40 years in both hospital and community settings across a range of disability groups, although the focus has been primarily on the long-term mentally ill. Caution is required when drawing guidelines for future practice from this work because of the variable quality of the research, the changing nature of work opportunities available and the greater needs of the present-day continuing care client. However, some general points can be made. Firstly, work has a protective function. This can be in terms both of the prevention of readmission (Anthony et al., 1972) and in the development of symptomatology (Wing and Brown, 1970). For work to be effective in rehabilitiation and resettlement into employment it is apparent that preparation and training times may need to be extended beyond that provided to other disability groups (Cornes et al., 1982). The development of social relationship skills is also important for future resettlement (Watts, 1978) and it is encouraging to note that such skills do develop in work-related activity (Miles, 1972). The importance of clear structures, good supervision, and task specification has been highlighted (Wadsworth et al., 1962). The organizational structure of the workplace, with a proper stress on supervision, social relationships and feedback on performance, has implications for ensuring job tenure (Floyd, 1984). All work preparation should be conducted in as realistic a setting as possible, as this not only produces better results, but also allows for clearer prediction of future resettlement than do measures such as psychiatric diagnosis or psychometric tests (Anthony and Jansen, 1984). Job clubs have recently emerged as a successful means of securing employment, particularly if combined with measures to maintain job tenure (Jacobs *et al.*, 1984).

## MODEL SERVICES

This section provides a brief description of a number of work schemes. These schemes are not put forward as blueprints or ideals to be copied; rather they are used to illustrate how some of the important points referred to in the previous section can be put into practice.

At the Maudsley Hospital, the District Services Centre (DSC) provides part of the London Borough of Southwark with a largely community-based service. The daytime activities of the DSC are the primary source of rehabilitation and support for long-term mentally ill people resident in that part of the borough. The DSC has three workshops designed to meet differing levels of ability and provide different types of work. It maintains close links with the hospital-based vocational rehabilitation unit, which is a training workshop offering a range of work experiences with the specific aim of settling people in open and sheltered employment or in a place offering further training outside hospital. Both these services are provided by the NHS, but the final link in this chain is the independent Camberwell Rehabilitation Association (CRA). This is a small sheltered workshop located in industrial premises a mile or so away from the hospital, and which was established at the instigation of NHS staff and others to provide long-term work opportunities. The service demonstrates a clear recognition of the importance of work for the continuing care client and shows that the NHS can play a leading role in promoting this. The service thus offers to people of differing levels of disability a full assessment, a range of work activities and a system of preparing for those activities.

However, the service has its problems: its size (five separate workshops) seems daunting, and this clearly imposes restrictions on innovation, particularly in view of its close link to other NHS services. Its identification with the NHS and the location of the majority of the services on an NHS site presents problems for some in identifying the activities that take place there as work. The emphasis on a 'ladder' model of rehabilitation, with success being measured in terms of movement 'up the ladder' to more skilled or valued work, risks exposing clients and staff to the negative consequences of failure. Nevertheless there is much to be admired in the service's commitment to work. Of particular interest is the way in which the CRA was established. Instead of following the usual practice in mental health services of developing and then manufacturing an 'own product', the CRA bought out over a number of years a series of small manufacturing businesses. These now form the basis of a successful company which has sufficient work to be able to pay its workers approximately £80 a week.

Other hospital-based services have developed different approaches. For example Bec Enterprises, based at Tooting Bec Hospital in London, provides a range of work opportunities in such activities as catering and gardening. Fulbourne Hospital, Cambridge, has established an MSC work preparation unit on site, which assesses and prepares patients for future employment and training. It is staffed by the MSC and is an example of how links between statutory services can be developed to provide work opportunities.

The services described above are examples of some innovative developments within the NHS. However, the majority of NHS services are still industrial workshops on large mental hospital sites. With a few other exceptions it is the voluntary sector which has led the development of community-based work projects. This is because it is often only the voluntary bodies that have the flexibility of staffing and organization which work projects demand.

Lambeth Accord, established in 1984 with European Social Fund support and the backing of the local statutory services, has as its aim the integration of the disabled at all levels of society. A central part of Accord's work is Worklink, which is a 25-place unit for the assessment of employment suitability, general vocational training and specific training in office skills and catering. These last two were identified as areas where local job opportunities were greatest. There are a number of interesting aspects to Worklink. It is a mixed disability unit with approximately 40 per cent of its clients having mental health problems. Its assessment and preparation work is locally based and geared to identifying the skills necessary to work in something like a five-mile radius of the centre. (It is interesting to note that only 8 per cent of local jobs were in manufacturing industry.) The work preparation aspect of the centre involves placement for periods of around six weeks with local employers, so that this work experience can be used in both the assessment and preparation of individual's health, transport, housing and financial position can have on successful work placement, and although it explicitly does not offer services in these areas, it will pressurize other agencies to act on behalf of their workers. The training period offered is for six months, but can be extended up to twelve months if necessary. Many aspects of this scheme mirror the approach of the

American vocational rehabilitation units with their emphasis on individual work preparation programmes. Another similar scheme is the Vocational Rehabilitation Unit at Queen's Park Hospital in Blackburn, Lancashire. This scheme, which developed out of a traditional industrial therapy unit, uses a similar method of assessment (evaluation) and work preparation (work adjustment). Despite the limitations imposed by its NHS setting, it has developed an impressive preparation project for a mixed disability group, the majority of whom have mental health problems.

Both Worklink and Queen's Park are concerned with resettlement into employment, and are not concerned with the provision of long-term work opportunities. The Peter Bedford Trust (PBT), based in Islington, London, was established in 1969 and is concerned with the provision of long-term work. Central to PBT's philosophy is that individuals establish a sense of value in themselves and their relationships to others through work. There is also a recognition that not everyone would be able to, or wish to, return to open employment. Therefore the PBT has developed a number of workschemes, including a furniture collection, repair and retail service. This has the virtue of demanding and developing a range of skills and offering a range of experience to participants. The PBT draws participants from a variety of settings including mental handicap services, mental health services and the DHSS reception centres. In addition, through a separate company, John Bellars' Ltd (an office-cleaning business), the Trust offers an opportunity for full employment to its workscheme participants if they wish to move on. PBT has also developed a novel way of overcoming, to some extent, the limits imposed by the therapeutic earnings rule, through the development of a system of payment in kind which allows for a number of non-essential items (e.g. holidays, radios) to be earned through attendance at the workschemes.

The Many Hands project, developed by Kensington and Chelsea MIND, is a mental health scheme that aims to provide training or the chance to improve on existing skills in a number of areas that can lead to the establishment of some form of regular employment. The sceheme has concentrated so far on painting and decorating and carpentry courses. Initially training is for six months, largely in its own workshop. This is followed by a further six months where much of the training is 'on site'. After this one-year training period it is hoped that trainees establish themselves in teams that provide paid work for members at a level appropriate to the individual's work needs and abilities. The project will act as an employment agency for the teams; providing work as well as technical and management advice as appropriate. A particular attraction of this scheme is that it provides paid employment in a much more flexible way than many employers are prepared to do.

Another recent innovation is that of special needs worker cooperatives. A number of cooperatives have begun to include people with a range of disabilities as cooperative members (Sikking, 1986). The Gilleygate Food Cooperative in York, a wholefood bakery, is one such organization. This bakery, which wholesales and retails baked goods, offers places as cooperative members to people with a wide range of disabilities. Such people are effectively in open employment in a sympathetic but realistic environment. It also offers training and voluntary work opportunities for individuals who, for whatever reason, are unable to make the commitment that full membership of the cooperative requires.

All the schemes so far described have involved the establishment of a separate work unit, although the cooperative described above originally had no special brief and continues to operate as a commercial organization. This separate establishment of units inevitably limits the degree of integration into the local community. Such units, particularly in the voluntary sector, are vulnerable to change of policy, personnel and the uncertainty of funding. A number of schemes have developed in recent years which do not offer open employment but provide something similar. The Sheltered Placement Scheme (SPS) is an MSC-sponsored development. The SPS allows for a disabled person (as defined by section II of the Disabled Persons Act) to be placed in employment. It requires a sponsoring body, usually a local authority or voluntary organization, to locate and place an individual in full- or part-time employment and then negotiate with the employer what percentage of a non-disabled person's capacity the individual is able to work at. To qualify for the scheme an individual must perform at between 30 and 80 per cent of a non-disabled worker's capacity. When the percentage figure has been negotiated between the employer and the sponsoring body, the employer pays that percentage of the full wage, the balance being contributed by the MSC.

SPSs have expanded rapidly in recent times. The Shaw Trust, one of the more successful organizations in the field, have moved from having no placements in 1981 to over 700 in 1986. It is to be hoped that the MSC continues to support this innovative scheme. One difficulty with the SPSs is that it appears to be easier to place the mentally and physically handicapped than it does those with mental health problems. For example, only 2 per cent of the Shaw Trust's placements are for people with mental health problems. There are other ways in which work placements can be developed. The temporary employment placements, devised by the Fountain House Project in New York (Beard et al., 1982), offer individuals six months of work experience with a local employer, at the end of which the placement is made available to another member of the project.

The focus of this chapter is on mental health services, and so far mention of mental handicap services has been made only in relation to mixed-disability projects. However, it is the case that specialist employment services for mentally handicapped people are more advanced. A number of innovative projects are described by Porterfield and Gathercole (1985) in the King's Fund Project paper on the employment of mentally handicapped people.

## ESTABLISHING NEW WORK SCHEMES

The intention throughout this chapter has been to explore the relevance of work for the continuing care client. The evidence reviewed, and the model schemes presented, have shown that although work is an important element of the service, no clear or simple methods for providing it are available. Jahoda's (1981) 'latent' functions of employment provide a useful starting point for the development of a set of guiding principles to be considered when establishing any work scheme. The principles can be stated as follows: the clear structuring of time and day, the development of regular shared social contact, the enhancement of personal status and identity, the development of goals which transcend one's own, the enforcement of activity and the development and enhancement of individual skill. All newly developed work schemes should adhere to these principles, but some principles will become more or less important depending on the degree of disability of clients using the service. For example, with an SPS the principles of personal status and skill development may be paramount, but for a very disabled person who is withdrawn and disturbed the principle of a structure to time and day may be paramount.

If these principles are held in mind when establishing a new service they need to be considered along with the following factors.

### The setting

Non-hospital sites hold many advantages: status, identity and the range of social contracts can be enhanced more than on a hospital site. However, problems of access to, and use of, the service—particularly by more disabled clients—need to be borne in mind. Size is an important consideration. Few successful units go much above 30 people, and it is important to balance the flexibility offered by a small unit against the variety a large unit may be able to offer. The proper siting of work units near other manufacturing or service industries also provides a check against the drift away from work tasks into therapeutic activity that has been observed in some units.

## The funding

Siting services away from hospital sites tends to draw services away from statutory funding. Many organizations such as the Peter Bedford Trust or Lambeth Accord have become expert at attracting funding from a wide range of sources. However, attracting such funding is time-consuming and anxiety-provoking, and if this is combined with an entry into commercial activity this may involve almost unacceptable risks to the service users. It is also clear that statutory services cannot sponsor commercial ventures. The establishment of a charitable trust, in some form, is the usual solution chosen to overcome the difficulty statutory services encounter in commercial development. The proper development of such trusts depends on appropriate funding being channelled through the statutory services and bodies such as the MSC. In order for this to occur there needs to be a recognition on the part of such organizations of the importance of work-related activity in services for the continuing care client. If there is no such recognition then there is a danger that the healthy tension between service provision and financial management of the organization will degenerate into an exploitation of the service users.

## The mix of disabilities

A number of units, particularly those concerned with employment resettlement (e.g. ERCs; Lambeth Accord), serve a mix of disability groups. There is some evidence to support this kind of mix, but against it is the enhancement of stigma that may well occur when a number of disadvantaged groups are brought together under one roof. The different speed of preparation time needed by the long-term mentally ill could lead to the creation of a disadvantaged or stigmatized group within the resettlement units; witness the prejudice against the mentally ill within the ERCs. Possibly the best solution is for there to be a mixture of non-disabled people and people with mental health problems in work preparation units. In providing long-term sheltered work it is probable that the most disabled would be best catered for in specialist units where the problem of integration is addressed through the fullest possible integration of the unit into the locality, rather than through the mixing of disability groups on one site.

## The payment of clients

This remains a major problem. Schemes such as the SPS pay the full rate as in open employment, whilst others such as the CRA offer payment at rates approaching that of open employment. However, such schemes are few in number. Over 20 years ago Freudenberg (1966) stated four principles to be followed when determining payment done for work as part of psychiatric rehabilitation. These were that an individual should receive proper payment for the job, that there should be an agreed minimum wage, that service work should be given equal weighting with industrial work and that payment should not exceed that obtainable in open employment. These principles represent a reasonable starting point for the development of a policy for the payment of clients engaged in work-related activity. The implementation of such principles has to start with changes in the policy governing long-term sheltered work and work rehabilitation for the disabled. This requires a review of the present levels set for therapeutic earnings (unchanged for over ten years) and greater flexibility in the rules governing qualification for various disability allowances, so that long-term eligibility is not compromised by short-term rehabilitation courses. Pending any changes in the therapeutic earnings rules, then methods such as the payment-in-kind policy of the Peter Bedford Trust should be considered.

## The nature of the work

The type of work a unit takes on and develops will need to reflect both the needs of the clients and the needs of the local area. Many hospital-based units are still engaged in subcontract packing and similar tasks. Although this has a number of elements, including its simple structure and identifiable end-product, which are important for the more disabled client, it remains dull and repetitive for many people and a real disincentive for some to work.

For those interested in employment rehabilitation the methods developed in this country by units such as Worklink at Lambeth Accord or the vocational rehabilitation unit at Queen's Park, Blackburn, offer a useful model. When developing long-term sheltered work there are a wide range of options to be considered, such as the marketing of an 'own product', as has been done by Portugal Prints (the MIND workshop in London) with greetings cards or through the buying out of existing businesses as the CRA have done. Other schemes such as Bec Enterprises or the Peter Bedford Trust Furniture Workscheme have sought to provide a service to a local area.

Whatever the task chosen, two points need to be borne in mind. Firstly, wherever possible long-term work units should choose activities which demand a range of skills and activities so that people with different ranges of disabilities can be involved. For example, the wholesaling and retailing of wholefoods could create a variety of demands, including the simple and repetitive filling of one-pound bags of beans, the design and manufacture of appropriate packaging, and approaching and dealing with potential customers. Secondly, most of the ventures described in this chapter, such as retailing of goods or the baking of bread, require skills for their successful execution that are not usually found in the statutory services, so careful consideration has to be given as to how these skills can be obtained.

## The staffing of work units

Recruiting the staff with both the technical and commercial skills that a work unit requires will never be easy. Although unfavourable salary comparisons make it difficult to recruit from manufacturing or service industries it is desirable that people with such backgrounds form the bulk of the staff of the units. Some staff, particularly those with a proper 'entrepreneurial' spirit, from the statutory services can make a successful transition to work units. Otherwise, whilst an understanding of any sympathy for those with mental health problems is a necessity, the role of NHS and social service staff is best restricted to the provision of advice and consultancy services. Such a staffing policy would also help to guard against the drift to therapy, referred to previously.

## CONCLUDING COMMENTS

The provision of work-related activity is a potentially powerful tool in community care. It can be as beneficial, albeit in different ways, to the most disabled client, who will always remain in sheltered employment, as to the least disabled client seeking a return to open employment. In a world of limited resources and restricted vision this potential must be forcefully asserted.

## REFERENCES

Anthony, W. A., and Jansen, M. A. (1984). Predicting the vocational capacity of the chornically mentally ill, *American Psychologist*, **39**, 537–44.
Anthony, W. A., Buell, G. J., Sharratt, S., and Althoff, M. E. (1972). Efficacy of psychiatric rehabilitation, *Psychological Bulletin*, **78**, 447–56.
Azrin, N. H., Flores, T., and Kaplan, S. J. (1975). Job finding club: a group assisted program for finding employment, *Behaviour Research and Therapy*, **13**, 17–27.

Beard, J. H., Probst, R. N., and Malamud, T. J. (1982). The Fountain House model of psychiatric rehabilitation, *Psychosocial Rehabilitation Journal*, **5**, 47–53.

Bennett, D. H. (1970). The value of work in psychiatric rehabilitation, *Social Psychiatry*, **5**, 224–30.

Brown, G. W., Carstairs, G. M., and Topping, G. G. (1958). Post-hospital adjustment of chronic mental patients, *Lancet*, **ii**, 685–9.

Cole, N. J., Brewer, D. L., Allison, R. B., and Branch, C. H. H. (1964). Employment characteristics of discharged schizophrenics, *Archives of General Psychiatry*, **10**, 314–19.

Conolly, J. (1847; republished 1968). *The Construction and Government of Lunatic Asylums and Hospitals for the Insane*, Dawsons of Pall Mall, London.

Cornes, P., Alderman, J., Cumella, S., Harradence, J., Hutton, D., and Tebbutt, A. G. (1982). *Employment rehabilitation: the aims and achievements of a service for disabled people*, Manpower Services Commission, HMSO, Sheffield.

Early, D. F. (1960). The Industrial Therapy Organization (Bristol), *Lancet*, **ii**, 754–7.

Early, D. F., and Magnus, R. V. (1968). The Industrial Therapy Organization (Bristol) 1960–1965, *British Journal of Psychiatry*, **114**, 335–6.

Evans, A. E. (1933). Tour of Dutch mental hospitals and clinics, *Journal of Mental Science*, **75**, 192–202.

Evans, A. E. (1933). A tour of some mental hospitals in Western Germany, *Journal of Mental Science*, **79**, 150–66.

Floyd, M. (1984). The employment problems of people disabled by schizophrenia, *Journal of Social and Occupational Medicine*, **34**, 93–5.

Freud, S. (1930; republished 1985). *Civilization and its Discontents*, Pelican Freud Library, Volume 12, Penguin, London.

Freudenberg, R. K. (1966). 'Work therapy in psychiatric hospitals', Maudsley Bequest Lecture, 7 February 1966.

Jacobs, H. E., Kardashian, S., Keel Kreinberg, R., Ponder, R., and Simpson, A. R. (1984). A skills-orientated model for facilitating employment among psychiatrically disabled persons, *Rehabilitation Counselling Bulletin*, December, pp. 87–96.

Jacques, E. (1967). *Equitable Payment*, Penguin, London.

Jahoda, M. (1981). Work, employment and unemployment: values, theories and approaches in social research, *American Psychologist*, **36**, 184–91.

Miles, A. (1971). Long-stay schizophrenic patients in hospital workshops, *British Journal of Psychiatry*, **119**, 611–20.

Miles, A. (1972). The development of interpersonal relationships among long-stay patients in two hospital workshops, *British Journal of Medical Psychology*, **45**, 105–14.

Porterfeild, J., and Gathercole, C. (1985). *The Employment of People with Mental Handicap*, Kings Fund Project Paper, King Edwards Hospital Fund, London.

Roessler, R., and Bolton, B. (1985). Employment patterns of former vocational rehabilitation clients and implications for rehabilitation practice, *Rehabilitation Counselling Bulletin*, March, pp. 179–87.

Sikking, M. (1986) *Co-ops with a Difference: worker co-ops for people with special needs*, ICOM Co-Publications, London.

Wadsworth, W. V., Wells, B. W. P., and Scott, R. F. (1962). The organisation of a sheltered workshop, *Journal of Mental Science*, **108**, 780–5.

Walker, L. G. (1979). The effects of some incentives on the work performance of psychiatric patients at a rehabilitation workshop, *British Journal of Psychiatry*, **134**, 427–35.

Wansborough, N., and Cooper, P. (1980). *Open Employment After Mental Illness*, Tavistock Publications, London.

Warr, P. (1984). Job loss, unemployment and psychological well-being. In V. L. Allen and E. van der Vliert, (eds) *Role Transitions*, Plenum Publications, New York.

Watts, F. N. (1978). A study of work behaviour in a psychiatric rehabilitation unit, *British Journal of Social and Clinical Psychology*, **17**, 85–92.

Wing, J. K. (1966). Social and psychological changes in a rehabilitation unit, *Social Psychiatry*, **1**, 21–8.

Wing, J. K., and Brown, G. W. (1970). *Institutionalism and Schizophrenia*, Cambridge University Press, Cambridge.

Wing, J. K., and Freudenberg, R. K. (1961). The response of severely ill chronic schizophrenic patients to social stimulation, *American Journal of Psychiatry*, **118**, 311–22.

Wing, J. K., Bennett, D. H., and Denham, J. (1964). Industrial rehabilitation of long-stay schizophrenic patients. Medical Research Council Memo No. 42, HMSO, London.

Wing, L., Wing, J. K., Stevens, B., and Griffiths, R. D. (1972). An epidemiological and experimental evaluation of the industrial rehabilitation of chronic psychotic patients in the community. In J. K. Wing and A. M. Hailey (eds) *Evaluating a Community Psychiatric Service*, Oxford University Press, London.

Community Care in Practice
Edited by A. Lavender and F. Holloway
© 1988 John Wiley & Sons Ltd

Chapter 11

# The Role of Relatives

## BRIGID MACCARTHY

This chapter is written from the perspective of family members who are supporting people receiving continuing care in the community. The effect that families and clients have on each others' level of functioning and mental health is explored, and the role of services in providing professional interventions is described.

Since the late 1950s the policy of maintaining people with long-term psychiatric disturbances in the community has led to large numbers of relatives or close friends replacing the state as the main providers of daily care. In some households families are reintegrating someone who has lived for years in a large institution. More often, relatives are accommodating to an increasingly supportive role, as the full extent and long-term nature of the disturbed family member's social handicaps gradually become apparent.

People in need of continuing care who live with family or friends rather than alone or in hostels seem to represent the success stories of community care. However, these people rarely live a 'normal' life in the community. More often they remain confined within the boundaries of their homes. High unemployment, housing shortages and a scarcity of long-term state-funded residential placements partly account for this. Neither patient nor family are likely to be offered alternatives, whatever their qualify of life.

Stages in the process of adjustment to providing long-term support for a family member have been largely ignored (Kreisman and Joy, 1974). The family's caretaking career begins before their first contact with services, the point at which the psychological problems of the disturbed member receive official recognition. Families may need support from services not only at times of crisis, but also when they are undergoing transitions which occur in the life cycles of all families. Although the problems and needs of supporters have been acknowledged for two decades, there is a dearth of research on their specifically long-term requirements (Atkinson, 1986).

However, studies of the process by which families adapt to chronic physical illness and to organic disorders can usefully provide an indication of what these stresses are likely to be (Shapiro, 1983; Gilleard, 1984; Livingstone et al., 1985). In planning both services and specific interventions account needs to be taken of the wide range of problems of this group in order to provide appropriate and comprehensive support.


## BEFORE THE FIRST CONTACT WITH SERVICES

Events preceding the first contact with professional help—and immediately surrounding admission, diagnosis and the initiation of treatment—may have a profound effect on relatives' subsequent relationship with the patient and with services. Fear, resentment and faulty expectations dating from this early stage may continue to cause difficulties years later. The social failures and disturbed behaviour of the patient, the preliminary meanings attached to unusual behaviour by the family, the supportive capacities of their social network and the quality of their contact with service personnel all contribute to the effectiveness of the relatives' efforts to support the patient and provide a positive atmosphere in the home.

The quality of the relatives' relationship with the patient before the onset of the illness has a significant influence on how they respond to the role of supporter. Relatives tend to be more critical of disturbed family members if previously relationships were strained (Leff and Vaughn, 1985). Similarly, supporters of the elderly mentally infirm are likely to ask for inpatient care earlier in the process of deterioration (Gilhooley, 1986). However, poor premorbid relations do not consistently result in reluctance to assume a supportive role. Increasing dependency may reveal previously untapped resources of confidence, self-sufficiency or affection in the supporter that had been stifled by the dynamics of the premorbid relationship (Gilleard, 1984; Fadden et al., 1987).

The period before difficult or unusual behaviour is identified as psychiatric disturbance—and thus is, to some extent, contained by being recognized and labelled by services—can be peculiarly taxing for relatives. Among people who develop psychotic disorders, those who show poor premorbid social adjustment and a slow onset of disturbance often have parents who have over-protective, intrusive or negative attitudes (Goldstein, 1985). A prolonged gap between the onset of symptoms and contact with services may be associated with more critical or rejecting attitudes among relatives (MacMillan et al., 1986). During this phase, when formal or informal support is often lacking, relatives have to deal with their own confusion and anxiety while trying to minimize the patient's distress and loss of social functioning. Even many years later, relatives vividly recall incidents before services became involved. They particularly remember bewildering and unpredictable swings from normality to disturbance. Attempts to seek help frequently fail. The disturbed family member can often conceal their problems from outsiders. Hard-pressed GPs and social workers may offer reassurance or referral to other services, rather than the immediate and practical help the relative seeks (Creer and Wing, 1974). Such initial experiences can create distrust between relatives and service personnel for many years.

The relatives' early attempts to reframe difficult behaviour as psychiatric illness requiring treatment can earn the patient's long-lasting resentment and distrust. It may serve to confirm the sufferer's sense of personal failure and rejection or reinforce delusional beliefs. Relatives are forced to choose between colluding with pathological beliefs and behaviour or defining the problems as requiring medical attention. Indeed, their early support for hospital admission, medication or rehabilitation regimes often becomes the focus of antagonism, particularly at times of relapse. The most painful expression of these dilemmas comes when relatives are directly involved in applications for compulsory admission to hospital under the Mental Health Act. It seems prefereable to avoid this, where possible, by asking social workers to make the application instead.

How family members understand the patient's behaviour has a profound effect on their practical and emotional response. The speed and manner of seeking help are influenced by whether the family view the behaviour as a medical or psychological, rather than a legal or social, problem (Harrison *et al.*, 1984). When symptoms are seen as enduring features of the patient's character, rather than as psychological disturbance, they may be seen as untreatable and deserving of criticism and blame. Such issues of definition can create continuing management problems (Meyerstein and Dell, 1985). Conflicting models held by different family members can cause distress to all concerned, delay contacts with services and increase the chance of the family developing ineffective day-by-day management strategies (Birchwood and Smith, 1986). These attitudes form early in the process of adjustment, and are difficult to change, even with an intensive educational programme (Berkowitz *et al.*, 1984). In part, differing models of illness appear to be linked to pervasive cultural and class values. Non-Western societies tend to endorse a more impersonal model, where disturbed behaviour is construed as an illness and the individual is absolved of blame. Families in such societies typically display less criticism and a greater commitment to continuing to support the disturbed member within the family (Jenkins *et al.*, 1986), while the patient's disturbance shows a more rapid recovery and a less chronic course (Cooper and Sartorius, 1977).

The patient's social and economic role in the family, and the size and characteristics of the family's social network, are important determinants of the manner and speed with which disturbed behaviour comes to the attention of psychiatric services. Patients who occupy key economic roles in the family reach treatment sooner, as do those who have closely interwoven networks, who choose friends rather than kin as intimates and who know other people with a history of psychiatric treatment (Perrugi and Targ, 1982). People who are poorly integrated socially also tend to be more disturbed when they finally seek treatment. Thus those who are slow to reach psychiatric services are more likely to be living with relatives with negative attitudes, in a dependant role, and to have little social contact apart from kin for whom mental illness is an unfamiliar or stigmatized condition. Such factors isolate the patient and the family from formal and informal support throughout their career in community care.

## DIAGNOSIS AND EARLY MANAGEMENT PLANNING

The time of the family's first contact with mental health services is formative. Relatives often recall receiving strong support from GPs and from other relatives who are less emotionally involved, and so can deal matter-of-factly with distressing practical issues. However, poor and insensitive service, procrastination and long and frustrating waits in emergency clinics are also common. The first admission is the time when relatives are most extensively interviewed by clinical staff, yet this is frequently a one-way process: information is extracted but not provided. Sometimes relatives are given no choice about whether they want the patient to be present when they are interviewed. They occasionally report that their first opportunity to speak with senior clinicians took place in front of dozens of strangers during a busy ward round.

The way that people describe disturbance to clinicians is strongly influenced by cultural norms and models of illness. Doctors, and particularly psychiatrists, however, also hold a range of beliefs about the significance of particular factors in specific illnesses, which influence the way in which they conduct interviews. If the doctors' beliefs do not mesh with those of the family, both parties are likely to emerge from the interview dissatisfied and with a sense of not having being listened to (Gaines, 1982).

The belief that parents are largely to blame for their child's psychosis is now treated with scepticism, yet much recent research has focused on the influence of the family on the patient, and rarely vice-versa (Kreisman and Joy, 1974). Consequently the psychiatrist's initial questioning may inadvertently serve to enhance the guilt and self-blame already present in the family. A family who prefer to hold a physical explanation for their sick member's behaviour may feel threatened by questions about how they all get along together. Another family might feel ignored by questioning about symptoms and signs, which passes over their descriptions of their efforts to cope. Early miscommunications of this sort are often remarked upon by relatives who remain dissatisfied with the services they receive. While continuing to act as the major caretakers, their relationships with staff are strained: they may later be reluctant to cooperate with management plans which in turn may evoke negative feelings in staff (Birley and Hudson, 1983).

A persistent concern of relatives is the need for more information about diagnosis and prognosis (Creer and Wing, 1974; Creer et al., 1982). Prognosis is a particularly pertinent issue for those providing long-term continuing care. Recently, efforts have been made to supply relatives with this kind of information (Berkowitz et al., 1984; Anderson, 1986). However, relatives do not seem simply to lack vital information. The search for causal and moral explanations is more urgent in conditions of uncertainty (Folkman, 1984). Later, the apportioning of blame seems to evolve into critical or over-involved attitudes which are progressively less easily modified. An educational approach seems to alleviate some distress, but does little to alter beliefs about the causes of problems and about how much responsibility the sufferer should carry. A direct attempt to hand over information will fail if the proffered model conflicts too markedly with relatives' existing attitudes or coping style: not everyone copes better with painful experiences when they know what to expect (Miller and Mangen, 1983).

Educational programmes have usually been part of a larger intervention package, and as yet the value of supplying clear and detailed information alone has not been assessed. Some relatives derive considerable relief and sense of support from receiving information alone, while it seems to help others to engage with subsequent treatment (Anderson, 1986). Many clinicians, however, are still hesitant to discuss such issues directly— caution which is perhaps often justified. They may be uncertain of the precise diagnosis, fear the adverse effects of labelling, or want to protect families from a pessimistic outlook. Moreover, psychiatrists have proved to be very poor predictors of functional outcome in individual cases (Greenley, 1979), and much of the 'information' they would pass on is still a matter for debate and may even change as conditions in society or psychiatric practice change (Bleuler, 1978). The problem of balancing the benefits of providing clear information at an early stage against these real uncertainties should not deter clinicians. It suggests that supplying accurate and meaningful information cannot always be achieved at once and in a standardized way with all families. Providing relatives with information needs to be conducted as a process of negotiation, not as a correction of an educational deficit (Tarrier and Barrowclough, 1986) and seems most likely to achieve its desired effects when it is conducted as part of a continually developing partnership between clinician and supporter.


PLACEMENT

Professionals may have their own set of prejudices about the appropriate place for an adult with long-term psychological problems to live. In Britain, at least among the middle classes, adult children are expected to live away from home before marriage. This convention is reinforced by the fear that family living can exacerbate or maintain disturbance. Clinicians are more reluctant to encourage spouses to separate, even though living with a psychiatrically disturbed spouse can damage mental health (Fadden *et al.*, 1987).

Paradoxically, there is another prevailing belief that community care should be privatized, non-statutory care, provided by the family where possible, since the family is seen as the place where genuine care is dispensed. This idealized model of society has meant that care is given in the community, but not by the community. The state hands the caring role over to one or two adults, usually female, at an enormous economic saving. This ideology, together with the propensity of many women to follow an ethic of caring, persuades the clinician to advocate, and potential carers to assume, demanding supportive roles as a duty. Neither party can readily question whether the patient continuing to live with the family is really the best option. Group homes and other alternatives are seen as a poor substitute for the family model, rather than as a positive option (Dalley, 1988).

In the end, practical considerations often resolve these ideological conflicts. The Italian experience affords an instructive example of how contradictory beliefs and practices can be. Despite the conviction, partly enshrined in the legal reforms of 1978, that both families and asylums are damaging and repressive institutions (Jones and Poletti, 1986), the great majority of Italian patients live with their families or remain in psychiatric hospitals. In Italy it is customary for unmarried adults to continue to live with their parents, and in many places the severity of the housing shortage makes alternative arrangements impossible. Yet therapists are reluctant to work with families, so contact between professionals and the family is often restricted to rather hostile interactions which focus on separating or rescuing the patient from the family.

Researchers have given little attention to the patient's desire to live with relatives. However, Scott and Alwyn (1978) found that patients' views on the tenability of the family unit predicted the outcome of a home placement better than those of the relatives. Similarly, Hooley and Hahlweg (1986) report a close association between depressed patients' marital dissatisfaction and their spouses' levels of criticism. While patients may often be the best informant about their ability to survive in the family, their clinical state may temporarily affect their sense of security and acceptability in the family. Clinicians have to balance these conflicting considerations.

In Britain now, families rarely fail to accept the patient back into the home after a first hospital admission (MacMillan *et al.*, 1986). Once established, these arrangements usually continue, even when the patient has remained severely disturbed for many years and are only terminated by the death or severe disability of the chief supporters. Relatives are notoriously reluctant to complain, despite experiencing severe stress. Indeed, some are adept at foiling professional efforts to separate them (Meyerstein and Dell, 1985).

Many factors influence relatives' willingness to take on and maintain their supportive role. Initial reluctance to accept a discharged patient back into the home is greater after longer spells of inpatient care unless relatives continue to visit (Rawnsley *et al.*, 1962). Fear of the stigma of mental illness and disliking the patient before the onset of disturbance all increase the chance of early clinical deterioration and rapid readmittance to hospital (Greenley, 1979; Gilleard, 1984). Patients occupying a key role in the household are more likely to be encouraged to return home as quickly as possible, although they seem to cope better with living in households where low levels of role-performance are tolerated. Supporters become less motivated to continue to provide care when they can no longer maintain a mutual relationship with the sufferer. Both reported burden and critical attitudes appear to increase the longer the patient is disturbed (Hoenig and Hamilton, 1969; Gibbons *et al.*, 1984; Hogarty, 1985). Supporters of the elderly who are younger, employed, have a wider social life and other dependents are more ready to opt for institutional placement (Gilhooley, 1986).

Families who do continue to support their disturbed relatives seem to be a rather unusual group (Gillis and Keet, 1965). They often present a picture of chronic adjustment, in which the personal needs and expectations of individual family members, both supporters and sufferers, have been sacrificed to accommodate the continuing presence of the disabled member. Whether this situation maximizes the disturbed member's level of functioning, or is an unacceptable infringement of the quality of life of the rest of the family, should be constantly under review. As Brown and his co-workers remarked as long ago as 1966, 'the fact that parents do not complain is not a valid reason for the clinician to reject alternative disposals without deep consideration' (Brown *et al.*, 1966).

## LONG-TERM ADAPTATION

The reactions of families learning to accept long-term disturbance often pass through recognized stages. Denial, guilt and blaming often characterize early stages of adjustment, and anticipatory mourning may follow the realization of the implications of a pessimistic prognosis. Relatives report feeling sorrow for the loss of the disturbed person's expected future and the loss of the future they had planned together (Creer and Wing, 1974). Over-protectiveness, temporary rejection and 'doctor-shopping' can also occur, and are particularly disruptive to the formulation of long-term management plans which rely on collaboration with relatives. The situation is further complicated by the uncertain prognosis of most psychiatric disorders. The process of adjustment is constantly challenged by changes in the patient's level of disturbance. An episodic pattern, with repeated cycles of hope and distress, is peculiarly stressful for relatives (Hatfield, 1978). Coping strategies which are adaptive for acute illnesses may be counterproductive in chronically disabling conditions (Folkman, 1984). It may be some years before relatives or staff can know for certain that the sufferer will need long-term, even if intermittent, care.

Adaptive attitudes towards the long-term disabled are a matter of balance: high expectations encourage high levels of social functioning (Greenley, 1979), yet resignation and the adoption of a disability model reduces stress in both relatives and patients (Gilleard, 1984). Some relatives seem to cope better if they can retain even an illusory belief that a return to previous levels of functioning will be possible. Others seem less critical in dealing with day-to-day problems and more able to facilitate an optimal, albeit reduced, level of functioning when they have fully accepted a disability model. Clinicians must be sensitive to the strengths of each family's appraisal of their situation; otherwise they may contradict attitudes which seem maladaptive, but in practice protect both supporter and sufferer and enable the family unit to remain intact (Birchwood and Smith, 1986).

## THE EFFECT OF SUFFERERS ON THEIR RELATIVES

Having a mentally ill person living in the household can have a negative impact on the rest of the family. Researchers have developed the concept of 'family burden' to explore the stress families experience as a consequence of their supportive role. Two types of stress have been distinguished, and need to be assessed independently as far as possible: objective stresses such as economic hardship, loss of autonomy and exposure to disruptive or frightening behaviour, and the subjective distress which relatives report or attribute to their role. A comprehensive review of conceptual and methodological issues in the measurement of burden can be found in Platt (1986).

In the past, assessment of burden has tended to confound the measurement of external stress with the relatives' reactions to their difficulties. Thus only those things which relatives are prepared to admit to finding a burden have been counted as burdensome. This methodological confusion tended to minimize the amount of stress that can be quantified, particularly as these relatives are notoriously uncomplaining. Policy-makers may thus have been encouraged to overlook some very substantial distress that has resulted from the wholesale implementation of community care.

Research results give an inconsistent picture of levels of burden. In some studies, supportive relatives have been included who have considerable contact with a patient, but do not live with them (e.g. Gibbons et al., 1984; Creer et al., 1982). As even a short break from continuous care seems to reduce subjective burden, such over-inclusive sampling may underestimate the general level of distress of full-time supporters. The consensus is that at least 60 per cent of households have had to contain at least moderate levels of disturbed behaviour, a similar proportion suffer some hardship, often severe, and only 10 per cent or less completely escape hardship because of their supporting role. Moreover, Grad and Sainsbury (1968) found that 20 per cent of their initial sample remained heavily burdened two years later.

Assessment of the relatives' own mental health by means of psychiatric interview or self-report checklist is an important adjunct to the investigation of burden. Behavioural disturbance that relatives are not annoyed by, or cope with to their own satisfaction, may still take a toll on their health and well-being. An accurate understanding of the relationship between these different aspects of 'family burden' is needed to inform the everyday practice of clinicians who are involved in making judgments about appropriate placements.

Few studies report on psychological difficulties in relatives. When these have been adequately assessed, perhaps a third of relatives have been found to need help with serious psychiatric symptoms incurred by their supportive role (Creer et al., 1982; Fadden et al., 1987) but many more report frequent feelings of anxiety, anger, guilt and a great sense of loss. Adolescent children living with chronically depressed parents also show increased levels of psychiatric morbidity (Hammen et al., 1987). Disturbances are more marked when the children have to cope with life-events, even positive ones (Hirsch et al., 1985). Living with disability appears to reduce children's capacity to respond adaptively to change.

People with long-standing psychological difficulties are more likely to find spouses with similar problems, and some of this disturbance is likely to be passed on to children through the influence of genetics or environment. These factors will account for some of the disturbance shown by relatives, estimated at three times the rate for an equivalent population (Fadden *et al.*, 1987). However, longitudinal studies suggest that much of the psychiatric disturbance may be attributed specifically to the supporters' burdens. Calculating the costs of maintaining a patient in need of continual care in the community should include that of providing psychiatric treatment for up to one-third of the main dispensers of this care.

Which behavioural problems cause most distress? Actively disturbed behaviour appears to be acutely distressing to relatives, but negative symptoms such as apathy, self-neglect and social withdrawal seem more likely to cause conflict and disrupt the relationships between the family and the sufferer (Birchwood and Smith, 1986). They can lead to the reversal of roles or the loss of reciprocity in relationships. Parents find they have to cajole adult children to get out of bed and remind them to wash each day; wives may have to assume entire responsibility for organizing household affairs. Although relatives do adapt to such specific changes in daily routine, these role changes are deeply felt and may be expressed indirectly in anxiety about what will happen when they die, or in resentment about the loss of a companion.

Restrictions on social life are frequently mentioned as particularly burdensome. Living with long-term psychological disturbance seems to severely limit relatives' social contacts (Anderson *et al.*, 1984). In early studies in the 1950s (Clausen and Yarrow, 1955) it was assumed that relatives withdrew because they were afraid of the stigma attached to mental illness. However, possibly only those relatives who can tolerate a very restricted social life persist in providing long-term care. Brown *et al.* (1972) found that isolated parents had a more negative attitude to the patient, but isolated spouses were less negative. Relatives of people suffering a first episode of schizophrenia spend less time with the patient, if they have a critical attitude towards them (MacMillan *et al.*, 1986). This may reflect a process of withdrawal, which will end in separation. In contrast, relatives of chronically ill psychotic patients spend more time in their company than those living with acutely ill patients, and they are more likely to be over-involved (MacCarthy *et al.*, 1986). Spouses with chronically depressed partners may spend much of their waking day in their company (Fadden *et al.*, 1987). Relatives of long-term day-care attenders have very few social contacts other than the patient. Few are employed, and many are isolated within their homes.

Thus, social isolation may in some cases help relatives tolerate their supportive role, and may not necessarily be experienced as stressful; but for those who are unhappy with the limitations imposed on their lives by the patient's disabilities, the virtual solitary confinement experienced by some is peculiarly stressful. Such isolation may also be disabling for patients. There is a risk that it leads to institutionalization outside the hospital gates, which does little to enhance independence or the patient's quality of life. Relatives report that social isolation is more distressing than financial or employment difficulties. The former seems to be a more pervasive problem, which impairs the relationship between patient and supporter, and reduces coping resources more fundamentally than material hardship.

Financial and employment difficulties do also occur. They are likely to be greatest when the patient is married, particularly if the spouse cannot take on the role of main breadwinner. Although early onset might be expected to cause more economic burden because the illness has greater power to interfere with long-term earning power, in practice, higher levels of pre-morbid functioning seem to be associated with greater burden. Many patients in continuous care have never become financially independent. Parents who have always supported their child seem to find their child's transition to patient status less difficult to adapt to materially. When onset occurs later, many older patients have debts to settle or possessions to dispose of. These practical matters often have to be sorted out by the supporter, and are the focus for much conflict and distress. The effect on relatives' employment status is also variable. Often supporters are retired or cannot work. The few who do hold jobs often negotiate flexible arrangements with employers so that time-off does not lead to loss of earnings, but frequently loses them the chance of promotion or more interesting work. Unemployability may therefore help to select-in relatives prepared to offer long-term support (Gilleard, 1984).

It is not clear how the various types of stress are related. How much stress relatives feel may determine how much disruption patients' problems cause in the household: relatives who are highly stressed will be less able to cope adequately. If this is the case, interventions could most usefully focus on reducing relatives' stress levels in order to enhance their coping skills. Alternatively, relatives' distress may be more closely linked to how disrupted their own social functioning has been by their supportive role. If this is the case, social work support which attempted to alleviate social isolation, financial hardship and employment difficulties would be a more appropriate intervention. Studies in which families are followed throughout the process of adjustment are needed to clarify which are the important links between these variables in order to plan effective interventions.

Although the objective hardships for families increase the longer the illness lasts (Hoenig and Hamilton, 1969; Grad and Sainsbury, 1968), resignation, which seems to alleviate subjective stress, becomes more common (Gibbons *et al.*, 1984). Those relatives who cannot adopt an attitude of resignation, or find other ways of decreasing the distress caused by persistent behaviour problems and mounting hardship, eventually separate from the patient (Gilhooley, 1986).

In the past, services which responded to severe behaviour disturbance by admitting patients for protracted inpatient care were significantly more effective at reducing burden than those which tried to avoid admission whenever possible. Community-oriented services, however, indirectly helped to keep the patient out of hospital by increasing relatives' tolerance of difficulties (Hoenig and Hamilton, 1969). Now, less and less use is made of hospital-based facilities in the care of long-term patients, but relatives complain that care teams are not responsive to their needs or opinions, particularly when they ask for short-term admission during periods of disturbed behaviour (Birley and Hudson, 1983). Even in a progressive day care service, staff often do not consult relatives (Creer *et al.*, 1982).

Day care is very much welcomed by supporters of patients needing continuous care. Most relatives, even those elderly or disabled supporters who have no particular plans for the time they gain, feel more able to get on with their own lives during the time that the patient is attending the day centre. High levels of day care reduce distress and household disruption among supporters of the dementing elderly (Gilleard, 1984), but its effect on burden among supporters of the long-term mentally ill has still to be tested. Since there has been little consistency in how family burdens have been defined and assessed over the past two decades, the opportunity to evaluate the effect on the family of these global changes in policy about how care is provided has been lost.

## THE EFFECT OF THE FAMILY ON SYMPTOMS

Families, particularly parents, were long suspected of contributing to the onset of psychotic disorders. Although carefully conducted studies have not supported this radical version of the argument (Goldstein, 1985), family life does appear to have some influence on the course of most psychiatric disorders, through factors which affect the occurrence of core symptoms.

Brown and his colleagues (1958) discovered that patients discharged to live with close relatives survived in the community less successfully than those who went to live in more emotionally neutral circumstances, such as lodgings and hostels. A highly reliable technique of measurement, known as 'expressed emotion' (EE) was developed to assess the emotional atmosphere in families (Vaughn and Leff, 1976a). Markedly critical or over-involved, intrusive attitudes voiced in interviews by key relatives of patients suffering from schizophrenia were strongly associated with a later increase in acute psychotic symptoms. Chances of this occurring were further increased if the patient spent long hours in the company of high-EE relatives, or failed to take the medication prescribed. If all these factors were working against the patient there was a 92 per cent chance of a worsening of symptoms, within nine months after discharge. In contrast, a patient living in a low-EE family with low levels of face-to-face contact and taking adequate medication had only a 12 per cent chance of deteriorating (Vaughn and Leff, 1976b). A similar pattern of protective factors was found two years after the key admission, although the importance of main-tainance medication for patients living in low-EE homes emerged more strongly (Leff and Vaughn, 1981). Since these basic findings were estab-lished, further studies have explored their significance for other disorders and in other cultures (Jenkins et al., 1986; Wig et al., 1987). With minor variations, remarkably similar results have been found in these different contexts.

The EE measure itself, although highly reliable, is only a summary index of relatives' feelings, and can do no more than suggest what might be happening in interactions between patients and relatives. Close similarities have been found between relatives' attitudes expressed during interviews and their behaviour during live encounters (Miklowitz et al., 1984). Rela-tives' attitudes to the patients' illness and to particular behavioural prob-lems are also systematically related to EE variables: those relatives who refuse to recognize the legitimacy of the illness and attribute difficult behaviour to wilfulness or long-standing personality traits are more likely to express critical or over-involved attitudes (Leff and Vaughn, 1985). Coping styles also reflect emotional attitudes. Low-EE relatives are charac-teristically tolerant of abnormal behaviour and have worked out consistent reponses so that they can set limits without conflict, while remaining empathic and supportive. Highly critical relatives tend to nag or argue with the patient about unacceptable or disturbed behaviour and struggle to gain control over phenomena which are essentially beyond their control (Hooley, 1985). They are also more likely to respond variably or unpredict-ably, particularly when the patient is chronically disabled, thus providing a confusing and stressful environment (MacCarthy et al., 1986). Instead, a flexible but consistent coping style appears to be associated with good family adjustment a couple of years after admission (Birchwood and Smith, 1986).

Concentrating particularly on safeguarding those suffering from long-term disabling conditions from experiencing a return of acutely distressing symptoms or readmission to hospital may be inappropriate. Factors which affect social functioning, such as lack of motivation, apathy and social withdrawal—negative symptoms which are common to many disorders—were assumed to be a response to long-term institutionalization. Now it is clear that they also occur in patients treated entirely in the community, and are frequently particular sources of burden and conflict in the family. Consequently there is a need to discover what exacerbates such phenomena, and what kinds of home environment minimize their disabling effects.

An interesting series of studies, begun in the early stages of deinstitutionalization in the 1960s, showed that although the return or intensification of positive symptoms often leads to readmission, such symptomatic changes are not closely related to levels of social functioning. Patients' level of functioning some years after hospitalization does not seem to be closely related to how disturbed they were previously. Instead, when relatives were optimistic during the period of acute disturbance, about the level of disability to be expected years later, the patient achieved higher levels of social functioning (Freeman and Simmons, 1963; Greenley, 1979). Thus, family attitudes seem to have a significant influence on these aspects of the sufferer's well-being as well as on the probability of relapse. An issue of considerable practical importance is whether there is a trade-off between high levels of functioning and the risk of relapse: efforts to minimize that risk may inadvertently encourage deterioration in functioning.

So far the results of research on family burden have not been clearly integrated with those of research on family atmosphere. Investigations have tended to focus on one or other direction of effect, so that the relationship between aspects of family burden and the emotional attitudes and expectations of supporters have not been explored. For example, the effect on patients' well-being and level of functioning of continuing to live with a severely burdened relative has not been assessed. Similarly, the effects of high-EE attitudes on relatives' experience of burden, or the power of a very positive attitude to alleviate the negative effects of severe objective burden, is unknown.

## FOCUS OF INTERVENTIONS

A clear understanding of the relationships between family burden, adverse attitudes and behaviours in relatives and the course of the patients' disorder should provide a basis for planning effective interventions. Research findings have indicated which patterns of disturbed behaviour disrupt family functioning, which aspects of supporters' behaviour are potentially detrimental to the well-being of the sufferer and which families are most in need of help.

There has been a remarkable convergence of views among therapists working with families containing long-term psychotic members who come from very different traditions of family therapy. The consensus is that family work with this population should focus on maintaining the patient at an optimum level of functioning in the community rather than searching for a cure. In this model, blame for the onset of the patients' disturbance is explicitly or implicitly lifted from the shoulders of the relatives, who are enlisted as therapeutic agents, working alongside professionals, and sharing their aims.

Family work, however, needs to address the supporter's concerns as well as attempting to enhance the patient's adjustment. This does not necessarily entail intensive interventions. The majority of relatives supporting people with long-term disabilities have made a permanent adjustment to their role, and will not need continual intensive input. However, a substantial proportion of these relatives are heavily burdened, and dissatisfied with their contacts with professionals, which, in traditional services, are very limited (Leff *et al.*, 1982).

Few services have the resources to provide elaborate and labour-intensive intervention packages. The revival of interest in intensive family work with this population should not distract staff from making the low-key changes in their priorities and routine management practices that research indicates is badly needed. Rapid, practical and non-judgmental responses to early appeals for help at onset, careful and sensitive interviewing during the admission phase, respect for the relatives' own explanatory models, and detailed education about diagnosis and prognosis should become a matter of course. Tolerance for the stages of grieving and adjustment reached by relatives and persistent support which can be easily mobilized during acute crises should characterize the basic relationship between care staff and supporters. If a relationship of trust has been established at non-crisis times the professional system can be responsive to the needs of the relatives in their own right, without appearing to imply that they require treatment themselves. For example, it might enable relatives to look critically at the level of burden they experience, so that separation, should it be in the interests of either the patient or the relatives, would be achieved appropriately, and without resistance.

Acute symptoms can be managed, in all but a small percentage of the long-term mentally ill, by effective medication and a flexible and responsive use of inpatient care when disturbed behaviour reaches an intolerable pitch and the family can no longer cope. Burden can be substantially relieved by the same strategies. Relatives need to be able to identify behavioural problems which are beyond their ability to manage without support, and to know how to ask for this support as quickly and unambiguously as possible, without feeling a sense of guilt or failure. 'Family' work might at times appropriatley include the entire professional support system involved in the patient's day-to-day treatment, to ensure that the lines of communication between family and staff work efficiently. If relatives could gain confidence that they will be reliably backed up in times of crisis, this would enhance their tolerance of disturbed behaviour, a major factor in keeping people out of hospital, and increase their willingness to cooperate with management and medication regimes (Anderson, 1986).

A series of intervention trials (Leff *et al.*, 1982; Falloon *et al.*, 1985; Hogarty *et al.*, 1986) have attempted to modify negative or high-EE attitudes and behaviours in relatives in an effort to reduce the rate of relapse. The outcomes of these trials have been most encouraging about the efficacy of family interventions as an adjunct to pharmacological therapy, in improving the adjustment of recently discharged patients in the community.

The success of the interventions suggests that EE and equivalent factors in the relative are causally related to relapse, and are not simply responses to difficult behaviour. Indirectly, therefore, high levels of EE seem to be a stable trait in the relative, albeit one that is specific to the relationship with the patient. However, EE does appear to be systematically related to aspects of the patient's behaviour, and families can shift spontaneously from high to low levels of EE as acute episodes resolve (Brown *et al.*, 1972; Hogarty *et al.*, 1986). Further, the patient's behaviour has usually been assessed in terms of variations in core symptoms, whereas high levels of EE seem to be generated more by negative symptoms and poor role performance than by these acute symptoms. Therefore, EE levels in the family may be the result of a complex and long-term interaction between the patient's behaviour, premorbid relationships and family burden. Taking more variables into account in assessing family responses to long-term disability, may suggest that interventions in some families could profitably focus less on relatives' behaviour and more on such interactive issues.

There is a danger that concentrating therapeutic efforts on lowering relatives' EE in order to minimize the possibility of an exacerbation of core symptoms may ignore the problem of how the best possible levels of independent functioning and social role performance can be maintained. Efforts to turn a critical or over-involved household into a typically low-EE one may inadvertently provide an unchallenging environment where high levels of social withdrawal are tolerated and deficits in self-help and social skills are coped with rather than confronted. Interventions which facilitate attitudes and coping strategies which minimize behavioural deficits and enhance independence and self-help skills, may be the most cost-effective use of resources, leaving the management of severe disturbance largely in the hands of professional services.

The EE findings have encouraged therapists to work with high-EE relatives. This may be premature while the mechanisms linking family attitudes and the patient's functioning are still not clear. The 'scattershot' nature of the earlier intervention trials has not helped to clarify this, or to pinpoint which aspects of such families' interactions are particularly harmful (Barrowclough and Tarrier, 1984). Nor do we know whether the atmosphere in high-EE homes increase stress, or if low-EE families offer protection against external stresses. The independent effect of warm or positive attitudes is also unclear. High-EE relatives supporting a patient in continuing care, who display warmth, may be good at maintaining high levels of functioning, despite recurring episodes of acute disturbance. Low-EE families that lack warmth may be providing a disabling environment, by using disengagement as a strategy of chronic adjustment, in order to cope with long-term burdens arising from providing continuous care. Hogarty (1985) has questioned whether low-EE relatives can offer the support necessary to help patients cope with life-event stresses which are known to precipitate relapse in some psychotic and depressed patients. Explorations of interactions between separate measures of family attitudes and patients' symptoms and social functioning are needed to help clinicians identify families which have most to gain from intensive interventions.

Although specific therapeutic ingredients have not yet been isolated from packages of intervention both the trials conducted in Los Angeles (Falloon et al., 1985) and Pittsburgh (Hogarty et al., 1986) have carefully assessed changes in a range of functioning, and are a fertile source of ideas. Particularly helpful are their detailed accounts of strategies designed to improve patients' tolerance for stress, including family arguments, and to increase their social functioning. In the Pittsburgh trial the process of individuation has been given a central place. Both patients and relatives are encouraged to enhance their level of contact outside the family, in preparation for eventual separation.

Such projects are extremely taxing on resources and are unfeasible for most clinical teams to implement. Research is needed to examine the efficacy of less intensive and extensive family work, which can be easily integrated into ordinary clinical practise. A low-cost group counselling project for relatives has produced some positive results (Atwood, 1983). One minimal intervention with a group of relatives providing continuous support for long-term severely disturbed people in day care effectively relieved the supporters' sense of isolation and shame, and they became less critical of the patient. In addition, the patients' self-help skills improved significantly (Kuipers et al., 1987). Attempts to integrate clinical practice by following a vulnerability model for long-term psychotic and neurotic disturbances has led to a demand that treatment approaches should recognize phases in the course of the disturbance and the family's response to it. Treatment packages are likely to be most cost-effective and acceptable to consumers if components are used to meet the specific needs of individual families as they arise during the family's life cycle (Heinrichs and Carpenter, 1983).

Supporting people with long-term psychiatric disabilities is challenging and stressful for all concerned. Relatives have to carry an extra burden of personal distress as well as provide 24-hour care. They deserve every possible support from professionals, including help in identifying the toll their caring role takes and the full right to terminate it when they choose. Family work should focus on relatives' independent needs as much as on factors which facilitate the patient's adjustment if they are not to be an exploited resource in the network of community care.

## REFERENCES

Anderson, C. M. (1986). Psychoeducational family therapy. In M. J. Goldstein, I. Hand and K. Hahlweg (eds) *Treatment of Schizophrenia: family assessment and intervention*, Springer-Verlag, Berlin.

Anderson, C. M., Hogarty, G., Bayer, T., and Needleman, R. (1984). Expressed emotion and social networks of parents of schizophrenic patients. *British Journal of Psychiatry*, **144**, 247–55.

Atkinson, J. M. (1986). *Schizophrenia at Home: a guide to helping the family*, Croom Helm, London.

Atwood, N. (1983). Supportive group counseling for the relatives of schizophrenic patients, in *Family Therapy in Schizophrenia*, W. R. McFarlane (ed.), Guilford Press, New York.

Barrowclough, C., and Tarrier, T. (1984). Psychosocial interventions with families and their effects on the course of schizophrenia: a review. *Psychological Medicine*, **14**, 629–42.

Berkowitz, R., Eberlein-Vries, R., Kuipers, L., and Leff, J. (1984). Educating relatives about schizophrenia. *Schizophrenia Bulletin*, **10**, 418–29.

Birchwood, M., and Smith, J. (1986). Schizophrenia. In J. Orford (ed.) *Coping with Disorder in the Family*, Croom Helm, London.

Birley, J., and Hudson, B. (1983). The family, the social network and rehabilitation. In F. N. Watts and D. H. Bennett (eds) *Theory and Practice of Psychiatric Rehabilitation*, Wiley, Chichester.

Bleuler, M. (1978). The long-term course of schizophrenic psychosis. In L. Wynne, R. L. Cromwell and S. Mattysse (eds) *The Nature of Schizophrenia*, Wiley, New York.

Brown, G. W., Carstairs, G. M., and Topping, G. G. (1958). Post-hospital adjustment of chronic mental patients, *Lancet*, **ii**, 685.

Brown, G. W., Bone, M., Dalison, B., and Wing, J. K. (1966). *Schizophrenia and Social Care*. Maudsley Monograph No. 17, Oxford University Press, Oxford.

Brown, G. W., Birley, J. L. T., and Wing, J. K. (1972). Influence of family life on the course of schizophrenic disorders: a replication, *British Journal of Psychiatry*, **121**, 241–58.

Clausen, J. A., and Yarrow, M. R. (1955). The impact of mental illness on the family, *Journal of Social Issues*, **11**, 3–64.

Cooper, J., and Sartorius, N. (1977). Cultural and temporal variations in schizophrenia: a speculation on the importance of industrialisation, *British Journal of Psychiatry*, **30**, 50–4.

Creer, C., and Wing, J. (1974). *Schizophrenia at Home*, National Schizophrenia Fellowship, Surbiton, Surrey.

Creer, C., Sturt, E., and Wykes, T. (1982). The role of relatives. In J. K. Wing (ed.) *Long Term Community Care: Experience in a London Borough. Psychological Medicine* Monograph, Supplement 2.

Dalley, G. (1988). *Ideology of Caring, Rethinking Community and Collectivism*, Macmillan, Basingstoke.

Fadden, G., Bebbington, P., and Kuipers, L. (1987). Caring and its burdens: a study of the spouses of depressed patients, *British Journal of Psychiatry*, **151**, 660–7.

Falloon, I. Boyd, J. L., McGill, C. W., Williamson, M., Razani, J., Moss, H. B., Gilderman, A. M., and Simpson, G. M. (1985). Family management in the prevention of morbidity of schizophrenia. Clinical outcome of a two-year longitudinal study, *Archives of General Psychiatry*, **42**, 887–96.

Folkman, S. (1984). Personal control and stress and coping processes: a theoretical analysis, *Journal of Personal and Social Psychology*, **46**, 839–52.

Freeman, H., and Simmons, O. (1963). *The Mental Patient Comes Home*, Wiley, New York.

Gaines, A. D. (1982). Cultural definitions, behaviour and the person in American psychiatry. In A. J. Marsella and G. M. White (eds), *Cultural conceptions of Mental Health and Theory*, Reidel, The Hague.

Gibbons, J. S., Horn, S. H., Powell, J. M., and Gibbons, J. L. (1984). Schizophrenic patients and their families. A survey in a psychiatric service based on a DGH unit, *British Journal of Psychiatry*, **144**, 70–7.

Gilhooley, M. L. M. (1986). Senile dementia: factors associated with caregivers' preferences for institutional care, *British Journal of Medical Psychology*, **59**, 165–71.

Gilleard, C. J. (1984). *Living with Dementia: community care of the elderly mentally infirm*, Croom Helm, London.

Gillis, L. S., and Keet, M. (1965). Factors underlying the retention in the community of chronic unhospitalised schizophrenics, *British Journal of Psychiatry*, **111**, 1057–67.

Goldstein, M. J. (1985). Family factors that antedate the onset of schizophrenia and related disorders: the results of a fifteen year prospective longitudinal study. *Acta Psychiatrica Scandinavica*, **71** (Suppl. 319), 7–18.

Grad, J., and Sainsbury, P. (1968). The effects that patients have on their families in a community care and a control psychiatric service—a two year follow-up, *British Journal of Psychiatry*, **114**, 265–78.

Greenley, J. R. (1979). Family symptom tolerance and rehospitalisation experiences of psychiatric patients. In R. Simmons (ed.), *Research in Community and Mental Health*, Vol. 1, pp. 357–86.

Hammen, C., Adrian, C., Gordon, D., Burge, D., Jaenicke, C., and Hiroto, D. (1987). Children of depressed mothers: maternal strain and symptoms as predictors of dysfunction. *Journal of Abnormal Psychology*, **96**, 190–8.

Harrison, G., Ineichen, B., Smith, J., and Morgan, H. G. (1984). Psychiatric hospital admissions in Bristol, II. Social and clinical aspects of compulsory admission. *British Journal of Psychiatry*, **45**, 605–11.

Hatfield, A. (1978). Psychological costs to the family of living with schizophrenia, *Social Work*, **23**, 355–9.

Heinrichs, D. W., and Carpenter, W. T. (1983). The coordination of family therapy with other treatment modalities for schizophrenia. In W. R. McFarlane (ed.), *Family Therapy in Schizophrenia*, Guilford, New York.

Hirsch, B. J., Moos, R. H., and Reischl, T. M. (1985). Psychosocial adjustment of adolescent children of a depressed, arthritic or normal parent, *Journal of Abnormal Psychology*, **94**, 154–64.

Hoenig, J., and Hamilton, M. W. (1969. *The Desegregation of the Mentally Ill*, Routledge & Kegan Paul, London.

Hogarty, G. E. (1985). Expressed emotion and schizophrenic relapse: implications from the Pittsburgh study. In M. Alpert (ed.) *Controversies in Schizophrenia*, Guilford, New York.

Hogarty, G. E., Anderson, C. M., Reiss, D. J., Kornblith, S. J., Greenwald, D. P., Javna, C. D., and Madonia, M. J. (1986). Family psychoeducation, social skills training and maintenance chemotherpy in the aftercare treatment of schizophrenia, *Archives of General Psychiatry*, **43**, 633–42.

Hooley, J. M. (1985). Expressed emotion: a review of the critical literature, *Clinical Psychology Review*, **5**, 119–39.

Hooley, J. M., and Hahlweg, K. (1986). The marriages and interaction patterns of depressed patients and their spouses: comparison of high and low EE dyads. In M. J. Goldstein, I. Hand and K. Hahlweg (eds) *Treatment of Schizophrenia: family assessment and intervention*, Springer-Verlag, Berlin.

Jenkins, J. H., Karno, M. de la Selva, and Santana, F. (1986). Expressed emotion in cross-cultural context: familial response to schizophrenic illness among Mexican–Americans. In M. J. Goldstein, I. Hand and K. Hahlweg (eds) *Treatment of Schizophrenia: family assessment and intervention*, Springer-Verlag, Berlin.

Jones, K., and Poletti, A. (1986). The 'Italian experience' reconsidered, *British Journal of Psychiatry*, **148**, 144–50.

Kreisman, D. E., and Joy, V. D. (1974). Family response to the mental illness of a relative: a review of the literature, *Schizophrenia Bulletin*, **10**, 34–57.

Kuipers, L., MacCarthy, B., Hurry, J., and Lesage, A. (1987). Counselling for relatives of the long-term mentally ill. Paper read at World Psychiatric Association meeting, Reykjavic.

Leff, J. P., and Vaughn, C. E. (1981). The role of maintenance therapy and relatives' expressed emotion in relapse of schizophrenia: a two-year follow-up, *British Journal of Psychiatry*, **139**, 102–4.

Leff, J. P., and Vaughn, C. E. (1985). Patterns of response in high EE and low EE relatives of psychiatric patients. In C. E. Vaughn and J. P. Leff (eds) *Expressed Emotion in Families: its significance for mental illness*, Guilford, New York.

Leff, J. P., Kuipers, L., Berkowitz, R., Eberlein-Vries, R., and Sturgeon, D. (1982). A controlled trial of social intervention in the families of schizophrenic patients, *British Journal of Psychiatry*, **141**, 121–34.

Livingstone, M. G., Brooks, D. N., and Bond, M. (1985). Patient outcome in the year following severe head injury and relatives' psychiatric and social functioning, *Journal of Neurology, Neurosurgery and Psychiatry*, **48**, 876–81.

MacCarthy, B., Hemsley, D. J., Shrank-Fernandez, C., Kuipers, L., and Katz, R. (1986). Unpredictability as a correlate of expressed emotion in the relatives of schizophrenics, *British Journal of Psychiatry*, **148**, 727–31.

MacMillan, J. F., Gold, A., Crow, T. J., Johnson, A. L., and Johnstone, E. C. (1986). Expressed emotion and relapse, *British Journal of Psychiatry*, **148**, 128–33.

Meyerstein, I., and Dell, P. F. (1985). Family therapy versus schizophrenia and the psychiatric–legal establishment. In S. B. Coleman (ed.) *Failures in Family Therapy*, Guilford, New York.

Miklowitz, D. J., Goldstein, M. J., Falloon, I. R. H., and Doane, J. A. (1984). Interactional correlates of expressed emotion in the families of schizophrenics, *British Journal of Psychiatry*, **144**, 482–7.

Miller, S. M., and Mangan, C. E. (1983). Interacting effects of information and coping style in adapting to gynecologic stress: should the doctor tell all? *Journal of Personality and Social Psychology*, **45**, 223–36.

Perrugi, R., and Targ, D. B. (1982). Network structure and reactions to primary deviance of mental patients. *Journal of Health and Social Behaviour*, **23**, 2–17.

Platt, S. (1986). Measuring the burden of psychiatric illness on the family: an evaluation of some rating scales, *Psychological Medicine*, **15**, 383–93.

Rawnsley, K., Loudon, J., and Miles, H. (1962). The attitudes of relatives of patients in mental hospital, *British Journal of Preventive Social Medicine*, **16**, 1.

Scott, R. D., and Alwyn, S. (1978). Patient–parent relationships and the course and outcome of schizophrenia, *British Journal of Medical Psychology*, **51**, 343–56.

Shapiro, J. (1983). Family reactions and coping strategies in response to the physically ill or handicapped child: a review, *Social Science and Medicine*, **17**, 913–931.

Tarrier, N., and Barrowclough, C. (1986). Providing information to relatives about schizophrenia: some comments. *British Journal of Psychiatry*, **149**, 458–63.

Vaughn, C. E., and Leff, J. P. (1976a). The measurement of expressed emotion in families of psychiatric patients. *British Journal of Social and Clinical Psychology*, **15**, 157–65.

Vaughn, C. E., and Leff, J. P. (1976b). The influence of family and social factors on the course of psychiatric illness, *British Journal of Psychiatry*, **129**, 125–37.

Wig, N. N., Menon, D. K., Bedi, H., Leff, J., Kuipers, L., Ghosh, A., Day, R., Korten, A., Ernberg, G., Sartorius, N., and Jablensky, A. (1987). Expressed emotion and schizophrenia in North India. *British Journal of Psychiatry*, **151**, 156–73.

*Section D*

# The Evaluation of Community Care in Action

Chapter 12

# Day Care in an Inner City

TONY WAINWRIGHT, FRANK HOLLOWAY, and
TRAOLACH BRUGHA

This chapter is both an evaluation of day care and an attempt by three writers to debate their disparate views on evaluation methods. Inevitably the disputes that exist are more philosophical than practical, but they do have important implications for the way human services are evaluated.

The chapter begins with a description of the day services for people with long-term mental illnesses who live in East Lambeth using contemporary epidemiological methods of health services research (HSR). Wing (1986) has described how HSR methods may be incorporated in a cycle of evaluation, planning, implementation and re-evaluation as a logical aid to the development of a comprehensive psychiatric service. This presentation is followed by an explanatory introduction to, and evaluation of, one of the day units from the perspective of normalization theory (Wolfensberger, 1983). An attempt is then made to compare and contrast the conclusions from the two evaluations.

THE CATCHMENT AREA

Together East Lambeth and South Southwark form the Camberwell Health District in South London. Its population was, in 1981, 213,000, of whom 40 per cent lived in the East Lambeth sector. Camberwell is one of the most socially deprived health districts in the country. There are high proportions of pensioners living alone, unemployed people, one-parent families, un-skilled workers and residents over 85 years of age. Within the district poor housing and overcrowding is common, and residents frequently change address. There is a large ethnic minority population, comprising mainly first-, second- and third-generation immigrants from the West Indies.

There are, however, areas of considerable affluence to the south of the district.

## THE PSYCHIATRIC SERVICES

In common with many inner urban areas the pattern of psychiatric services is highly complex. The district contains two teaching hospitals. The Maudsley Hospital provides services to the South Southwark sector and is administered by a special health authority (SHA). Psychiatric services to East Lambeth are the responsibility of the Department of Psychological Medicine based at Kings College Hospital, which is managed by the Camberwell Health Authority. Some long-stay patients remain in Cane Hill Hospital, the mental hospital in Surrey that historically served the area (Wing and Hailey, 1972). Confusingly, the Camberwell Health Authority retains statutory responsibility for planning services for the whole district, although in practice the extensive and innovative developments that have taken place in South Southwark have stemmed from the work of enthusiastic professionals working within the Maudsley (Birley, 1974; Bennett, 1981; Wykes, 1982). The District Services Centre, the focus of long-term community care within South Southwark, is a national demonstration centre for psychiatric rehabilitation.

Many of the factors identified by the Audit Commission in their report on community care as inhibiting the development of new patterns of services are at work in the area (Audit Commission, 1986). The health district is not coterminous with local authorities boundaries, and straddles two London boroughs. Traditionally cooperation between agencies has been poor. However, both local authorities have stood out against central government policy and attempted to provide a wide range of social and other services to their local communities, although neither has paid particular attention to the needs of the metally ill.

The district's social deprivation is reflected in a heavy utilization of all forms of medical care (Golding et al., 1986). Psychiatric services are particularly heavily used and admission rates for South Southwark and the Borough of Lambeth as a whole are well in excess of the national average (Wing and Der, 1984, GLC, 1985). An unpublished census identified twice the national average of beds occupied by 'acute' psychiatric patients from East Lambeth. An even higher rate of bed usage is reported in South Southwark (Wing and Der, 1984). This introduction has described the context of the services in Camberwell Health District as a whole. The rest of the chapter is concerned with the day services in the East Lambeth sector of the district.

## DAY SERVICES IN EAST LAMBETH

### St Giles day hospital

A psychiatric day hospital was opened in the grounds of St Giles Hospital in 1974. Initially it was intended that it would provide short-term and transitional day care for patients living in the community and offer day activities for the adjacent district general hospital inpatient unit, which has subsequently closed. In the event longer-term users accumulated. Although planned as a '110-place' day hospital (with 30 of these places taken up by inpatients) daily attendances currently average 55, which represents the number that can comfortably be accommodated in the building. There are 110 patients 'on the books', with most patients attending either two or three days a week. Only a handful of current inpatients make the taxi journey to the day hospital, although the majority of referrals are discharged inpatients.

The unit is staffed by a multidisciplinary team with medical input provided by eight doctors on a sessional basis. There is also a technical instructor who runs a woodwork shop. The Inner London Education Authority (ILEA) provides a number of teachers. The operational policy states that two main streams of care are provided: a 'rehabilitation' stream for users who have active programmes aimed at a return to independent living, and a 'support' stream for users who have long-term needs. 'Support' and 'rehabilitation' patients attend on different days, although a number of very disabled 'support' patients come up every weekday. In addition there is a steady trickle of referrals for 'acute' day care, usually when the inpatient unit is full. All patients have an allocated key nurse and junior psychiatrist, whilst some have an additional key worker from another discipline. A varied programme is offered by the unit, including recreational and diversional activities such as needlework, a sports group and an exercise group, life skills training and a range of therapeutic groups. The operational policy states that patients should receive an individual programme which reflects their individual needs. The patient day revolves around lunch, which is provided free of charge: morning coffee and afternoon tea provide other substantial landmarks to the day. There is a limited ambulance service.

### Local authority day centres

Three local authority day centres were opened in Lambeth between 1970 and 1975. Initially two centres provided light industrial work, but as a result of council policy this was abandoned. Each day centre has a catch-ment area and must relate to the two health districts serving Lambeth. The centres each have a distinct character, although all have a common level of resources and utilize a key worker system. They are open to all people from the borough with mental health problems, including those who refer themselves. Some clients are referred on: the under-20s to ILEA youth provision (which is not limited to the psychiatrically ill) and the over-65s to provision for the elderly, for example luncheon clubs. Those identified as mentally handicapped will be referred on to a local social education centre.

One centre provides a relatively structured seven-hour day, with lunch separating a morning 'therapeutic' session during which users attend individually programmed group activities and an afternoon 'drop-in' ses-sion in which clients engage in recreational activities which they them-selves initiate. The centre was purpose-built to high standards, although it is not well adapted to its present use because of a lack of suitable small rooms for the group work and counselling offered by the staff. A second centre offers a similar range of activities in a large converted house, which has recently been refurbished.

In contrast a third day centre, a 'community mental health centre', operates quite differently. Three 'levels of work' are described. Firstly there is a 'drop-in' open three days a week for a total of fourteen hours a week. This is freely available to any Lambeth resident, and offers a friendly unstructured environment where food can be purchased cheaply, and cooked. A limited range of recreational activities is also available within the very cramped premises. The aim is to provide a 'flexible and responsive environment' to 'anyone in the community who considers themselves to have a mental health problem'. The 'drop-in' has the feel of a club, and there is a very non-psychiatric atmosphere about the centre. Secondly, individual sessions with a centre worker are offered to clients from the catchment area. An approach is adopted in which the client defines what help and advice is needed from the workers. Thirdly, centre workers provide input to various community and mental health projects in the surrounding area.

## The voluntary sector

Within the voluntary sector there is an innovative day centre that aims to attract young Afro-Caribbean people living in the area who have had mental health problems and who may be suspicious of the statutory services (Moodley, 1987). The only sheltered work available to East Lam-beth residents, apart from places at the local Remploy factory (a light industrial company specializing in the provision of sheltered work) and services provided to the occasional patient taken in by the Maudsley Hospital, lies within the voluntary sector in a small work-oriented day centre. The work centre aims to resettle attenders in open employment, although in practice attenders rarely progress to paid employment.


## EVALUATING THE DAY SERVICES

One of the authors (F.H.) has recently completed an evaluation of day care for long-term mentally ill people in East Lambeth. Population-based epidemiological methods were used. This study evaluated the effectiveness of the services by assessing the needs for clinical and social care of each user. Health service evaluation by means of the assessment of met and unmet needs for clinical interventions is a well-established technique in the field of epidemiology (Alderson, 1983). This form of evaluation attempts to assess whether those who have particular problems (physical, psychological, social) for which there are known, potentially helpful remedies (i.e. interventions, treatments or supports) have been given full access to adequate amounts of these remedies (Brugha, 1984). The principle has been applied in studies of 'new' long-stay psychiatric inpatients (Mann and Cree, 1976), day psychiatric service attenders (Wykes *et al.*, 1982) and casual non-compliant users of day services (Compton and Brugha, 1988).

The study first identified the psychiatric day units used by people from East Lambeth. Local authority day care services for the elderly and the mentally handicapped were excluded, although undoubtedly some people suffering from mental illnesses do use these facilities. The small amount of specialist provision for dementia within the district was also excluded.

Patients were found in six units: St Giles day hospital, the three local authority day centres, the work centre run by a voluntary organization and the local Remploy (sheltered work) factory. The Afro-Caribbean Centre described above had not opened when the study began. In addition a small number of patients attended the district services centre at the Maudsley. A census of these units identified 133 users from the catchment area, of whom 115 were defined as 'long-term mentally ill'; that is they had been in continuous contact with mental health services for a year or more.

Only 9 per cent of the users went to one of the three units offering sheltered work. The paucity of work opportunities for users of all levels of disability stands in striking contrast to the situation in the South Southwark sector. In South Southwark there are three sheltered workshops catering for differing levels of disability within the district services centre (DSC), the rehabilitation day hospital. Adjacent to the DSC is a vocational resettlement unit. A voluntary organization, the Camberwell Rehabilitation Association, runs a workshop providing paid employment for fourteen people. In addition one of the two local authority day centres provides some sheltered work. Over half of the long-term mentally ill users of psychiatric day care in South Southwark receive sheltered work or industrial rehabilitation (Brugha *et al.*, 1988). This disparity within a health district underlines the extent to which the services available to the mentally ill depend on accidents of geography and planning rather than any systematic assessment of what people need.

### Characteristics of the service users

When the census had been completed, attenders at each unit were approached to take part in an evaluation of their care. All but five of the 115 long-term mentally ill users were prepared to be included in the study. Information was collected about their personal and clinical characteristics from an interview with the users. This included a structured psychiatric interview, the Present State Examination. Day care staff completed a complementary questionnaire designed to assess the patients' clinical and social problems. Where available the case notes were reviewed. The study used techniques developed by the MRC Social Psychiatry Unit in a complementary survey of day care for the long-term mentally ill in South Southwark (Brewin *et al.*, 1987, 1988; Brugha *et al.*, 1988).

Some of the sociodemographic and clinical findings are summarised in Table 12.1. The overall sex ratio was nearly equal, although of the ten attenders at work-oriented units eight were male. Users were predominantly middle-aged. Less than a fifth currently lived with a partner, although in all half lived with a relative. Just under half of the users were diagnosed as suffering from schizophrenia. This was the commonest diagnosis amongst attenders at all the units except the community mental health centre (CMHC), where less than a quarter of users received this diagnosis. The majority of CMHC attenders suffered from neurotic problems or alcohol abuse.

The proportion of long-term mentally ill users in the service as a whole who were Afro-Caribbeans or ethnic Asians, 24 per cent, was identical to the proportion of 'black' people living in the catchment area. 'Black' people were under-represented amongst CMHC attenders, despite attempts by the staff to cater for ethnic minorities. Most attenders had substantial past psychiatric histories: the mean time since first contact with psychiatric services was fifteen years and the average number of previous psychiatric admissions for all users was 3.7. The CMHC attenders had had on average only 1.7 admissions. Comparison on these crude characteristics between

Table 12.1 Sociodemographic and clinical characteristics of long-term mentally ill day care users (percentages).

| | |
|---|---|
| Percentage male | 48 |
| Proportion aged | |
| 20–39 years | 36 |
| 40–59 years | 47 |
| 60+ years | 17 |
| Diagnosis | |
| Schizophrenia | 48 |
| Manic depressive psychosis | 14 |
| Neurosis | 20 |
| Personality disorder | 6 |
| Other | 12 |
| Marital status | |
| Married/cohabiting | 18 |
| Single | 50 |
| Separated/widowed/divorced | 32 |
| Usual accommodation | |
| Living with relative | 48 |
| Living independently | 35 |
| Living in hostel/group home | 17 |

units showed that the users of the CMHC, which operated as a drop-in service, were quite different from users of the services as a whole.

## Clinical assessment of users

The study investigated in more depth the clinical and social problems presented by users. Physical illness, psychiatric symptoms, behavioural disturbance and social functioning were assessed. Twenty-two problem areas were rated. These problems represent the psychiatric morbidity experienced by attenders (Wing, 1972). When someone experiences a problem, for example delusions and hallucinations, he or she may be said to have a potential need for treatment and care (Brewin et al., 1987). Table 12.2 shows the frequency with which the 22 problems were identified amongst long-term mentally ill users of the day services: these are the sorts of problems that will have to be tackled by staff in any day service for the chronically mentally ill.

A high proportion of users in all diagnostic categories, including schizophrenia, were found to experience depression and/or neurotic symptoms such as anxiety. Categorical diagnosis appeared to be of limited relevance. Nearly two-thirds of the sample received antipsychotic medication,

Table 12.2   Clinical and social problems of day care users
in the East Lambeth Psychiatric service.

| Problem | Percentage of users showing problem |
|---|---|
| Delusions/hallucinations | 26 |
| Depression | 38 |
| Anxiety/obsessions | 34 |
| Poor concentration | 52 |
| Drug/alcohol abuse | 14 |
| Physical illness | 36 |
| Side-effects of medication | 30 |
| Slowness/underactivity | 18 |
| Socially embarrassing behaviour | 23 |
| Aggression | 7 |
| Psychosocial distress | 75 |
| Personal hygiene | 12 |
| Shopping | 24 |
| Cooking | 25 |
| Household chores | 32 |
| Managing money | 21 |
| Use of public transport | 18 |
| Use of public amenities | 27 |
| Social interaction skills | 30 |
| Literacy/numeracy | 15 |
| Decision-making | 20 |
| Material welfare | 18 |

and amongst these patients side-effects (Parkinsonian symptoms, akathi-
sia and tardive dyskinesia) were noted in 48 per cent. Severe behavioural
problems were uncommon: apparently aggressive attenders were rapidly
discharged or transferred to other services.

Much of the morbidity found was accounted for by impaired social
functioning, either a lack of daily living skills or very poor interpersonal
skills. Problems with shopping, cooking and managing money were not
infrequently due to lack of opportunity to perform the skill rather than
inability.

## Comparisons between units

Comparison of the frequency of individual problems between the day
centre and day hospital attenders revealed few differences. Day hospital

Table 12.3 Resources, problems and unmet needs in day units in the East Lambeth services for the long-term mentally ill.

| Unit | Number of attenders in sample | Attendances per staff member | Mean problem score | Percentage unmet need |
|---|---|---|---|---|
| St Giles day hospital | 66 | 3.3 | 6.4 | 30 |
| Day centre A | 17 | 5.0 | 7.2 | 32 |
| Day centre B | 6 | 4.3 | 5.2 | 70 |
| Community Mental health centre | 13 | 4.0 | 4.1 | 40 |
| Work centre | 3 | 6.0 | 5.0 | 7 |
| Remploy | 3 | N/A | 3.0 | 50 |

attenders were significantly more commonly depressed, a finding that has been reported previously (Edwards and Carter, 1979; Wykes *et al.*, 1982). The number of clinically significant problems rated for each patient provides an index of psychiatric morbidity: a total problem score. Overall the range and distribution of problem scores of the users of NHS and local authority day care was identical. The highest average morbidity was encountered in one of the day centres, whilst attenders at the community mental health centre had a significantly lower average morbidity score than attenders at this day centre and St Giles Day Hospital (Table 12.3). This confirms the impression gained from the other measures, and is consistent with the finding of Bender and Pilling (1985) that a verbally oriented day centre retained the more intelligent and articulate of its referrals.

The similarity of long-term mentally ill users of NHS and local authority day care found in this survey has been noted in other studies (Carter, 1981; Wykes *et al.*, 1982). The logic of a jointly managed, integrated day service appears overwhelming.

**Needs assessment**

After identifying the clinical and social problems of the users, the study assessed the extent to which these problems were being adequately managed by the services, using the 'needs assessment' technique (Brewin *et al.*, 1987) discussed by Shepherd in Chapter 6. Needs may be said to be met when services provide the appropriate treatment and care for a given problem. For example treatment of clinical depression by an adequate dose of an antidepressant drug would be meeting a need, whilst failure to provide skills training to a patient who has problems in cooking or using public transport would result in a need being unmet. It has already been noted that this is, quite intentionally, a precise and narrow definition of need. The relevance of a broader definition is discussed more fully below.

For each patient a profile was made of his or her clinically significant problems. Day care staff were then asked what response the services had made to these problems. Standard criteria were prepared to define what represented an appropriate and adequate response for each problem area: if the response was inadequate the existence of an unmet need was rated. It must be emphasized that although these judgments of need were carried out in a reliable fashion, according to standard criteria that reflect current good rehabilitation practice, the study was not designed to present evidence that attenders would benefit were the recommended interventions to be provided. Longitudinal experimental studies are the appropriate method for achieving such an aim.

The unmet needs that were identified often required simple interventions that were well within the means of the service to provide, such as alterations in medication or counselling patients who were distressed by intractable symptoms. (The drug treatment practices in the service were assessed in a separate exercise reported elsewhere (Holloway, 1988).) Staff were at times unaware of problematic symptoms, and some lacked skills or confidence to provide coping advice to patients and relatives. One of the commonest specific interventions that was not provided was behavioural assessment and/or treatment. Unmet need for care for problems of social functioning almost invariably meant a requirement for some form of skills training. Skills training was not available at some settings, and facilities were everywhere limited. A number of the unmet needs that were identified required the development of a structured programme to monitor and modify an attender's deviant behaviour, to provide a carefully graded set of activities to improve concentration or to help a severely disorganized individual through the day. There was a pervasive lack of structure throughout the East Lambeth day care service.

There was no evidence that overall unmet need was commoner amongst attenders at the less well-resourced local authority units than at the NHS units. However, the ratio of unmet needs to problems varied significantly between units (Table 12.3). These differences cannot be explained by the available staffing within units or by the levels of disability of attenders. The least effective unit, one of the local authority day centres, was in considerable organizational turmoil at the time of the assessment, and shortly thereafter closed for redecoration and a complete change in staff.

In addition to assessing users' needs for treatment and care, an attempt was made to rate their needs for particular kinds of day or residential care. Needs for services are conceptually quite different from needs for care (Brewin et al., 1987). Fourteen of the 110 users did not appear to require any form of day care. A quarter of the users were rated as needing some form of sheltered work, either in a relatively open setting such as the Remploy factory or, more commonly, in a highly sheltered setting without expectations of a degree of commercial productivity. A third of the sample were felt to require an occupational therapy-based day unit such as St Giles day hospital or one of the more traditional day centres. The remainder required some less structured kind of day care such as a social club, or were not compliant with a structured day regime.

## Users' views of their care

Since the study was initiated a new managerial climate within the NHS has encouraged interest in the views of the consumer of services, who has hitherto largely been considered to be a passive recipient of treatment and care. As part of the study an attempt was made to find out what users from East Lambeth thought about their day care. There was a considerable degree of satisfaction: 65 per cent were rated as satisfied or having no criticism, whilst only 6 per cent were entirely critical of the service. Two-thirds wished to continue attending their day unit for the foreseeable future. Such high degrees of satisfaction are common in studies of consumer views of health care (Slater *et al.*, 1982), and are not particularly revealing.

In an attempt to dig deeper attenders were then asked 'In what way does this unit help you?' A content analysis of the responses was made. The commonest reply was that the unit offered a chance to meet people: 'It helps me mix with people', 'It helps loneliness to meet people here.' The activities offered were important: 'Activities keep your mind occupied', 'The activities the craft and the dressmaking.' For some just getting out of the house is important: 'It breaks the monotony of the house.'

Some users mentioned the support that they received from staff or fellow-attenders: 'If you feel rotten you can tell someone', 'It's helpful to share problems.' Others mentioned the practical benefits of attending, such as a free meal or welfare rights advice. One man who lived in a common lodging house noted that his alternative to day care would be to sit in the park or the public library. There were other positive comments: 'It helps to improve my concentration', 'It's a relaxing place to come', 'It makes me more confident.' One young man suffering from schizophrenia that had not responded to treatment stated that the day hospital 'evens me out . . . proves me wrong about things and gives me a feeling of reality'. Few users made comments relating specifically to the therapies available at the settings, possibly because of the way the question was asked.

## Implications of the research

The evaluation of the day service as a whole revealed a paradoxical situation. There was considerable unmet need for treatment and care within day settings where significant numbers of users also required less treatment and care of the kind that they were receiving. With the exception of the work-oriented units, each day setting appeared to be carrying out a multiplicity of roles for different clients: occupational therapy unit for some, workplace for others and social club for many. Clearly the way resources such as skilled staff are used is crucial to effective functioning, and resources were not being deployed effectively. It was also notable that the successful work centre had good links with the local psychiatric services: staff at the centre acted as effective advocates with the psychiatric service to ensure that medical aspects of management were optimal. In contrast workers at the other non-NHS units reported considerable difficulty in gaining access to, or recognition from, the psychiatric services. One major cause for the high level of unmet need recorded in this study was general difficulty in carrying out regular, systematic review of the progress of clients. Adequate systems of review are an essential component of successful services for chronically disabled clients (Wykes *et al.*, 1985; Compton and Brugha, 1988).

Although there are clear methodological limitations to the assessment of users' views of their day care, the results indicate that attenders felt that they benefited from the service. This perception of benefit did not appear to come primarily from the 'therapies' that were available, but came instead from the opportunity to meet people, the (often very skilled) support from staff and the practical activities that were provided.

There is an apparent tension between what the users report they receive from their day care (social contact, activity, support) and the 'needs assessment' which focuses on the treatment provided for the clinical and social problems of attenders. It is, however, known that chronically handicapped day care attenders can with some accuracy define their key problems (MacCarthy *et al.*, 1986). When attenders have been actively involved in problem identification they are more likely to show improvement (Falloon and Talbot, 1982).

## THE DAY HOSPITAL FROM A NORMALIZATION PERSPECTIVE

## Normalization principles

The ideas of Wolf Wolfensberger and his colleagues have become increasingly influential in the development of 'human services' (Wolfensberger, 1972; Wolfensberger and Thomas, 1983). It is clear that Wolfensberger is intensely committed to the cause of the disabled, the downtrodden and the marginal in society. He came to believe that it was vital to combat the social devaluation that he viewed as playing a pivotal role in the lives of people with disabilities, developing a set of ideas initially subsumed under the rubric of normalization (Wolfensberger, 1972) and more recently social role valorization or SRV (Wolfensberger, 1983).

The central contention of what is essentially an ideological system is that all human services (and particularly those serving people who are subjected to discrimination, are marginalized or devalued) should aim to enable users to reach as valued a social position as possible. Human services should achieve this through the use of methods that are highly valued by society. (A discussion of the profound implications of this statement can be found elsewhere (Wolfensberger, 1975).) An effective but culturally despised method of management might therefore have to be rejected in favour of a less effective but culturally valued one. For example the development of a highly structured residential facility run on token economy lines might have to be rejected in favour of a less structured and more homely facility even if the latter was known to be less effective in modifying people's behaviour.

Wolfensberger states that many characteristics of human service systems are determined by very negative beliefs about disability that are unconsciously held by service planners and providers. These beliefs reflect stereotypes that are common to society at large, and are extremely powerful. They must be recognized and challenged if high-quality services that enhance the devalued status of disabled people are to be developed.

Wolfensberger (1980) has strongly asserted that evidence in favour of normalization principles may be found in studies carried out in disciplines as widely separated as behavioural theory and political science. An analogy can be drawn with the science of ecology, which draws its inspiration from many sources, and has developed an ideological framework (Felce *et al.*, 1985). Although some normalization principles are open to empirical investigation, SRV may best be seen as a paradigm: that is a set of assumptions which reflect a way of viewing the world. The ethical components of normalization, such as the assertion that services that promote the personal rights of clients are better than those that do not, are not testable.

## The concept of need

The concept of social need is inherent in the idea of social service (Bradshaw, 1972). However, human need may be approached from a variety of perspectives (Maslow, 1954; Brewin *et al.*, 1987), and discussions about meeting needs often lack clarity in the definition of terms (Baldwin, 1986).

Normalization theory addresses this area by making the following assumption:

Everyone shares the same needs but people differ in the ease with which they are able to meet their needs.

No matter how disabled someone is, he or she must be afforded the same opportunities and rights as any other citizen. Ensuring that ordinary human needs such as those identified by Maslow (1954) are met is the central task for any human service system.

Within this framework the function of any treatment or care provided to service users is to enable them to meet their ordinary human needs. Treatment needs such as those described in the 'needs assessment' above are therefore not denied in normalization theory, but the focus of the services is shifted to the more general notion of the life experience of users. Normalization theory asserts that for services to be effective they must be non-stigmatizing. This is based on the proposition that stigma is a central problem faced by people with disabilities. Unless services address this issue users will remain disadvantaged, however successful it is in other ways.

## PASS and PASSING

PASS (program analysis of service systems: Wolfensberger and Glen, 1973) and PASSING (programme analysis of service systems implementation of normalization goals: Wolfensberger and Thomas, 1983) are instruments that have been developed to evaluate human services from the normalization perpsective. Like all standardized instruments they have been designed to be used in a particular way. One essential ingredient is the use of a team of people (rather than a single rater working alone) to make the evaluation, so that the choices made by the service can be measured against the ideas of a group of people. Teams receive intensive training in normalization theory and the practice of PASSING before carrying out an evaluation.

There are 42 ratings in PASSING. These cover two broad categories: elements of the programme related primarily to 'client social image enhancement' and elements related primarily to 'client competency enhancement'. (Texts in the normalization tradition are noted for precise but rarely elegant language.) Ratings made in PASS and PASSING are governed by a set of rules. Strict criteria have been set out to determine whether, and in what ways, a service follows or fails to follow normalization principles. The evaluating team is instructed to concentrate on what the situation actually is, rather on why things are as they are.

## Image enhancement ratings

PASSING assumes that services unwittingly convey messages about the people who use them. Users of the services are likely to be particularly sensitive to these messages because of their impact on their own personal self-evaluation. Messages of particular importance concern: clients social status, roles, similarity to valued members of society, competencies, and miscellaneous other attributes, in order to make life conditions of such (devalued) people more valued' (Wolfensberger and Thomas, 1983). A service is evaluated by the extent to which the messages it conveys are positive, and the extent to which the service 'refrain[s] from unnecessarily conveying negative images about the people it serves' (*ibid.*). Four main areas are considered: the physical setting: the way people are grouped by the service: the activities provided to clients: and the language and labels used to describe clients.

## Competency enhancement ratings

Services often describe their aims in terms of 'improving users' functioning' or 'social skills training'. From a normalization perspective it is important to enhance users' competence because it is a seriously devaluing characteristic to be incompetent. Incompetence will also impede the person from interacting in socially valued settings and adopting socially valued roles. Furthermore, if a person does have a disability they may be able to compensate for it if they possess some socially valued characteristic.

Three areas are assessed: (1) the capacity of the service to enhance competence, (2) the provision by the service of high quality environments within which competency may be enhanced and (3) the use of effective, valued and relevant methods. PASSING assumes that modelling is a powerful phenomenon and that consequently grouping disabled people together will impede competency enhancement.

## Evaluating St Giles day hospital

In this chapter an evaluation will be presented of the St Giles Day Hospital based on the PASSING method. This account of the day hospital is not definitive and it differs from a proper PASSING practice evaluation. The evaluation was not carried out by a group of people trained in the PASSING method but reflects the views of a single observer (T.W.). However this observer has worked at the day hospital for six years, is familiar with the ideas of SRV and has participated and team-led in PASS and PASSING practice evaluations. For ease of presentation the image enhancement and competency enhancement ratings will be presented under the same headings.

## Who are the people and what are their needs?

In a full-scale practice evaluation the team begins by describing the people who use the service. Each team member gets to know one of the users and tries to produce a vivid and rich picture of the life of the person he or she has met. From these accounts (together with any available statistical data on demography, diagnosis, etc.) a summary of the characteristics of the users is made. This exercise has not been carried out for day hospital attenders, but a flavour may be conveyed by the following description made by one of the authors (T.W.):

> Some of the people who attend the day hospital were: Proud, tough, very disabled, brilliant, caring, talented, resourceful, have a good sense of humour, clever, poor, fearful, colourful, have symptoms, young black and beautiful, on benefits, gentle, questioning, religious, political, have families, completely alone, tolerant, bewildered, responsible, live in rough areas, angry, friendly.

Once the users have been described, an attempt is made to identify their needs in terms of the needs we all share. These needs would include the following:

> friends, a good job, a decent income, company, understanding, good food, a home in a safe area, intimate relationships, the opportunity to contribute, a quiet mind . . .

In order to ensure, in the case of the day hospital users, that their needs are met, the service may have to provide specific forms of treatment and care. It will be important for the service to be clear about what falls within its province. Outside the total institution many needs will be met away from the service. This is entirely appropriate, since valued people receive different things in different places.

## The culturally valued analogue

The next task for the PASSING team is to define what the 'culturally valued analogue' of the service would be. Looking at St Giles day hospital what would socially valued citizens call something with a similar function in their lives? The day hospital was a place that the majority of users went to during/on weekdays between the hours of 9 am and 5 pm. Often users attended for several years. One obvious equivalent is work, a term actually employed by some users for their attendance. However, attendance at the day hospital is unpaid, and only in the woodwork department are the activities carried out remotely like work in the ordinary sense. The day hospital is very unlike its 'culturally valued analogue'.

## Separation of programme activities

The PASSING team investigates the extent to which functions provided by the service are separated in the way that they are for the rest of us: this is termed 'culturally appropriate separation of programme functions'. This concern derives from the sociological critique of the 'total institution'. The existence of such an institution, catering for all needs, implies that its users should not meet other people and are not entitled to use ordinary services. The day hospital provides a plethora of activities including therapy, medical care, work, education, leisure and the occasional holiday. In addition it functions as a social club and a free luncheon club. In fact the only thing it does not provide is a place to sleep. It would appear that the day hospital, rather surprisingly, provides little separation of programme activities: this makes it likely that it presents seriously negative images to the outside world about the capabilities and entitlements of users. Furthermore one might suspect that this multiplicity of roles would make it difficult for the unit to carry out any one task successfully.

## The physical setting

The importance of high-quality physical settings is taken very seriously by large companies, which tend to pay great attention to their corporate image. The physical setting is an obvious source of positive and negative images about service users. The day hospital building is new and rather unattractive. It blends poorly with the surrounding area. It is sited within the grounds of a decaying and largely disused old hospital. Part of the site is closed off by security fencing to prevent further vandalism. The interior is dirty, despite recent wall-washing and some painting. The efforts of the domestic staff have been unable to prevent the floors and toilets remaining dirty, and the furniture is now very worn out. Lighting is by strip lights. The building is poorly insulated and ventilated: too hot in the summer and too cold in the winter. Overall the setting is uncomfortable.

Applying the same evaluation technique produced the following judgments:

> It projects an image of users (and staff!) who lack any aesthetic sense, and who do not deserve a setting of high quality or beauty. It in no way resembles

its culturally valued equivalent, a high-quality place of work. It has elements that resemble a hospital outpatients department, a benefits office or housing office: these images are potentially damaging. It is not culturally valued to be sick or be in need of welfare handouts. Moreover the building is judged to convey inappropriate messages about the age of the people who use it. Internally it resembles a school or playschool rather than a place for adults. One room, used for music appreciation, is painted in nursery style with lambs and rainbows. The walls are covered with pictures and collages. The exterior of the building is reminiscent of a school, and the overall effect is to project a child-like image of the users.

The day hospital site was formerly a workhouse for the old and indolent (St Giles is the patron saint of cripples and mendicants). On the campus are a venereal diseases clinic, a drug dependency clinic, an assessment centre for children with developmental delay and the base for a community assessment and treatment team for people with learning difficulties (a non-stigmatizing term for mental handicap. The St Giles centre for home-less people and a social services area office are nearby. There would seem to be a heavy concentration of services that carry a negative stereotype, reinforcing damaging images of the day hospital users.

The PASSING method also requires consideration of the capacity of a locality within which the service is set to absorb the disabled population without them becoming an obvious feature of the neighbourhood. Where service users do not stand out in the area they are more likely to be considered as individuals rather than as examples of one type of disability or another. The day hospital is set in a busy neighbourhood with a good variety of local amenities, and if it were the only such local service it would have little impact on the area and social integration could be carried out with little difficulty. However Camberwell contains a concentration of psychiatric facilities and numerous hostels for homeless and vulnerable people. The area contains a high proportion of people with serious social problems.

Accessibility of the service to potential users and their friends and relatives is another important area for evaluation. The day hospital lies outside its catchment area, and many users face a complicated bus journey to reach it. This may prevent people from making use of a facility from which they might gain benefit, and may discourage the involvement of carers.

### Interactions between staff and users

The nature and quality of the interaction between staff and users is a crucial component of service evaluation. One PASSING rating in this area often causes dismay to helping professionals. The evaluators ask whether the staff, defined in terms of identity and skills, enhance or demean the image of users? The image associated with nurses is one of sickness. Therapists are associated with an image of psychological problems, social workers deprivation and psychiatrists madness. Paradoxically the therapeutic skills that the staff at the day hospital have developed in their formal training, helpful and relevant though they may be, are judged not to promote a positive image of the users. From a PASSING perspective this can only be negative. Similarly the activities promoted by the therapists, such as painting in groups during the day, taking part in psychodrama and having individual sessions with the psychologist, are all likely to create quite negative images.

The PASSING team questions whether the service promotes 'life-enriching' interactions between the various people who take part in the service: the rating addresses the social distance between users and providers. At the day hospital this social distance is large and actively promoted by the use of technical (psychotherapeutic) languages leading to the maintenance of appropriate boundaries between staff and patients. Staff are discouraged from having social contacts with users out of hours, even though some close friendships between staff and users occur. There are separate staff toilets. Some areas are out of bounds to users. Staff and users eat together only infrequently.

The language used to address people will have an important bearing on individuals' perceived competence and status. Attenders are described as 'rehab' and 'support' 'patients'. Medical jargon is employed. People are addressed largely by their first names, except the doctors who are referred by their professional title. Little attention appears to be made to the preferred ways in which users wish to be addressed. This may be seen as a failure by the service to consider an important area of dignity. Furthermore, the use of medical language and labels provokes negative images of the users and reinforces their perceived incompetence.

## Autonomy and rights of users

A service may also violate users' autonomy and rights, a risk always facing those who by virtue of disability become users of human services. There is an inevitable tension between the needs of the consumer and the needs of the organization and its representatives. If one accepts that the culturally valued equivalent of the day hospital is paid employment, certain rights that would be accepted within the workplace simply are not considered within this day hospital (or the rest of the local day service). Users do not have a choice of employer: you accept the day placement you are offered or passively withdraw from the system. A wage, career prospects and union representation would not be felt appropriate to users' status as patients.

## Involvement with socially valued citizens

A further concern of PASSING is the extent to which the service promotes relationships between users and socially valued citizens outside itself. Considerable effort is made in this day hospital, particularly by the occupational therapists, to find non-segregated activities for users and hence to foster social relationships outside the service. However, the service as a whole tends to organize itself on segregated lines, for example by providing a regular social evening that is restricted to users. One annual highlight is the coach trip to the seaside, an event that is enjoyed by all. Enjoyable as it is, normalization principles would suggest that this segregated outing loses any value for potential social integration.

## Meeting users' needs

PASSING considers the extent to which users' needs are met in a number of ways. Does the service provide opportunities for the development of greater independence and hence access to more socially valued roles? Does it use the most effective methods of skills development? Does it use the most modern technology? Failure to monitor the progress of attenders in any systematic way, a failure identified in the HSR evaluation of the East Lambeth service as a whole, makes it difficult to say whether the methods of skill development used within the day hospital are effective. The service has not been seen to be committed to evaluating its performance.

## Expectations of users

One important feature that structures the day hospital week is the distinction between days for 'resettlement' or 'rehabilitation' patients, about whom there are some positive expectations, and 'support' patients, who are not judged capable of significant change. In practice the distinction is not one of need but of age: young people are allocated to 'rehab' days whilst older people attend the 'support' days. Pressure of numbers makes meaningful skills training difficult. Low expectations of all users are reflected in the times at which patients are asked to attend. People arrive later than a normal working day, between 9.30 and 10 am, and leave much earlier. They are thus marked out as different from workers, which has devaluing consequences. The way time is structured is significant: bad rehabilitation practice results in users spending large parts of the day doing nothing at all (Wing and Brown, 1970).

## Development of individuality

PASSING stresses the importance of the service enhancing the individuality of its users, for example whether the service provides places for people to keep their personal belongings. None of the day hospital users has a secure place to keep personal possessions. Users may hang their hats and coats at the front entrance, which in view of the many posters prominently displayed announcing the presence of thieves in the building, may not be a very useful facility. Another example is the pervasive use within the day hospital of group activities. There is little scope for people to be treated as individuals within some of the groups, which are not closely targeted on problems of specific relevance to group members. (This observation of the indiscriminate use of group therapy within rehabilitation settings has been made before (Stevens, 1973).) However, the service is aware of the importance of supporting people's individuality and uniqueness, as is demonstrated by the framing and display of two of the users' paintings.

## Programme address of client need

The PASSING evaluators ask a final question: does the service, taken as a whole and considering what it should properly be doing, meet the needs of the people who depend on it? This rating should ideally be made in a dialogue with the service providers. At the day hospital the bulk of the available activities are of a therapeutic nature (counselling, medical treatment, skills training, group psychotherapy). For the majority of users the major need might well be for paid employment or training related to employment, although specific data concerning this were not collected. The users of the service also have a pressing need to be seen as valued by society at large: the day hospital is not conscious of this issue and sends out messages about the users that are seriously devaluing. Moreover, the service fails to demonstrate that the therapeutic methods it does employ are effective. It is difficult from this analysis to argue that the day hospital meets the needs of its users within the PASSING framework.

## Feedback

Feedback to the service is an important element of a PASSING evaluation. The feedback given to the service providers might focus on three levels of functioning of the system, and could take in the following form, although of course considerably expanded. At an individual level the day hospital might review its policy on how people may relate to each other after 'work'. At the service level it could review the potentially stigmatizing messages being sent out about users by the interior and exterior of the building. At a system level the likely closure of the unit in 1991 offers the current team an opportunity to become involved in planning a service that can more effectively meet the needs of its users.

This chapter has been discussed with the day hospital team. Space precludes a full presentation of their views. The team believed that evaluation, in promoting critical self-examination, can be helpful. However, the PASSING evaluation was perceived as failing to take account of the good aspects of the service and as wilfully ignoring the constraints under which the staff operated. The team felt that the very real needs of attenders and the nature of their problems were ignored, and especially took issue with the failure of the PASSING evaluation to take account of the internal experiences of the clients.  The PASSING evaluation also produced personal distress in the staff, which inhibited them from accepting the valid criticisms that were made. The proposition that working on a group basis detracted from individuality was dismissed: it was argued that therapeutic groups would help attenders learn about their individuality. Finally, the team took issue with the assumption, central to social role valorization, that it was possible to identify what is and what is not socially valued.


## HOW DO THE EVALUATIONS COMPARE?

Despite the employment of contrasting techniques both evaluations produced apparently quite similar results. It should be noted that these findings do not necessarily imply that all psychiatric day care facilities within the NHS are likely to be found similarly wanting in performance— indeed the methodologically similar HSR evaluations carried out in the neighbouring area of South Southwark (Wing, 1982; Brewin et al., 1987) provide an important counterbalance. However, the two evaluations were different in ways that follow quite logically from their contrasting perspectives.

The sharpest difference between the evaluations is seen in the way the service users were described. In the evaluation of the East Lambeth service as a whole users were described in essentially negative terms as people who suffer from particular kinds of problems, have a particular psychiatric diagnosis and fall into particular ethnic and age groups. In the PASSING evaluation of the day hospital very different terms were employed of users, and their strengths as well as weaknesses as individuals were identified. The PASSING evaluation employed a broad (universal) concept of 'basic human need', whilst in the evaluation of the East Lambeth service need was defined much more specifically in terms of the delivery of effective treatment and care for particular clinical and social problems. The imagery associated with the service, and the means by which treatment and care is delivered, ignored in the first evaluation, was seen to be of critical importance within the SRV framework. (The apparent absence of a concern with the quality of physical surroundings and the personal rights of service attenders is not, of course, necessarily a characteristic of all epidemiologically based HSR evaluations (see for example Wing and Brown, 1970; Wykes, 1982).) There were broad areas of agreement. Both evaluations concluded that 'work' most closely describes the activity of the service from the users' perspective. Both noted that the wide variety of tasks undertaken by the day hospital appeared to give rise to difficulties, and that a more focused approach might be more appropriate and effective. In neither evaluation did the day hospital appear effective in meeting the needs of its users, be these needs narrowly or broadly defined.

There is a final paradox to these evaluative studies, which may be seen as highly critical of the services. Users appeared to express satisfaction with the services they receive. One might view this satisfaction as reflecting their institutionalized attitudes. However, it may reflect the considerable success of staff in the units studied in promoting an accepting atmosphere in which staff and users felt a sense of belongingness. There is, for example, a long tradition of cohesiveness amongst the staff team at the day hospital which has been transmitted to the users.

Normalization theory owes much to the sociology of deviance. Within this framework certain kinds of behaviour, for example those traditionally associated with mental illness, become labelled as deviant. This social definition of an individual as having a devalued identity is seen as the central problem faced by people with disabilities. How a person is perceived and treated by others will, according to Wolfensberger (1983), strongly determine how that person subsequently behaves. The power of social circumstances to influence behaviour explains the great attention paid by normalization to the physical and social context in which services are located. The PASSING framework encourages us to take seriously important issues about the way services are provided, such as the imagery surrounding a service, that might otherwise be ignored. However, PASSING addresses other issues, such as the efficacy of the help provided to individuals, only weakly.

The traditional psychiatric way of looking at problems has tended to locate pathology within the individual, and to view the social difficulties that afflict the mentally ill as secondary phenomena. The appropriate management of mental illness, according to such a model, lies in physical or psychological manipulations addressed at the (internal) problems of the individual. During the past 20 years theory and research on the psychology of learning (i.e. social learning theory: Hodgson, 1984) and of personality (i.e. situationism versus trait theory: Mischel, 1973) have made necessary a radical modification of such a viewpoint. The needs assessment technique and the evaluation of a human service based on normalization principles are perhaps best seen as contrasting but complementary ways of trying to bring about a measure of improvement in the overall quality of services for some of the most disadvantaged members of society.

## ACKNOWLEDGMENTS

The study of day care in East Lambeth was carried out whilst F.H. was in receipt of an MRC Training Fellowship. We would like to thank staff and users of all the day units in the area for their generous cooperation.

## REFERENCES

Alderson, M. (1983). *An Introduction To Epidemiology*, Macmillan Press, London.

Audit Commission (1986). *Making a Reality of Community Care*, HMSO, London.

Baldwin, S. (1986). Problems with needs—where theory meets practice. *Disability, Handicap and Society*, 1, 139–45.

Bennett, D. (1981). Camberwell District rehabilitation service. In J. K. Wing and B. Morris (eds) *Handbook of Psychiatric Rehabilitation Practice*, Oxford University Press, London.

Bender, M. S., and Pilling, S. (1985). A study of variables associated with under-attendance at a psychiatric day care centre. *Psychological Medicine*, 15, 395–402.

Birley, J. L. T. (1974). A housing association for psychiatric patients, *Psychiatric Quarterly*, 48, 568–71.

Bradshaw, J. (1972). A taxonomy of social need. In G. McLachlan (ed.) *Problems and Progress in Medical Care: essays on current research*, 7th series, Oxford University Press, London.

Brewin, C. R., Wing, J. K., Mangen, S. P., Brugha, T. S., and MacCarthy, B. (1987). Principles and practice of measuring needs in the long-term mentally ill: the MRC needs for care assessment. *Psychological Medicine*, 17, 943–8.

Brewin, C. R., Wing, J. K., Mangen, S. P., Brugha, T. S., MacCarthy, B., and Lesage, A. (1988). Needs for care among the long-term mentally ill: a report from the Camberwell High Contact Survey, *Psychological Medicine* (in press).

Brugha, T. (1984). Needs for care: developing and evaluating services for the chronically mentally ill. *Irish Journal of Psychiatry*, Spring, pp. 10–13.

Brugha, T. S., Wing, J. K., Brewin, C. R., MacCarthy, B., Mangen, S., Lesage, A., and Mumford, J. (1988). The problems of people in long-term psychiatric day care: an introduction to the Camberwell High Contact Survey. *Psychological Medicine* (in press).

Carter, J. (1981). *Day Services for Adults*, George Allen & Unwin, London.

Compton, S., and Brugha, T. (1988). Problems in monitoring needs for care of long-term psychiatric patients: a study of casual attenders. *Social Psychiatry* (in press).

Cumella, S., and Bennett, C. (1985). The content of long-term psychiatric day care. Unpublished manuscript.

Edwards, C., and Carter, J. (1979). Day services and the mentally ill. In J. K. Wing and R. Olsen (eds) *Community Care and the Mentally Disabled*, Oxford University Press, London.

Falloon, I. R. H., and Talbot, R. E. (1982). Achieving the goals of day treatment. *Journal of Nervous and Mental Diseases*, **170**, 279–85.

Felce, D., Thomas, M., De Kock, U., Saxby, H., and Repp, A. (1985). An ecological comparison of small community-based houses and traditional institutions for severaly and profoundly mentally handicapped individuals. *Behaviour Research and Therapy*, **23**, 67–73.

Golding, A. M. B., Hunt, S., and McEwen, J. (1986). Health needs in a London District. *Health Policy*, **6**, 175–84.

Greater London Council (1985). *Mental Health Services in London*, GLC, London.

Hodgson, R. J. (1984). Social learning theory. In P. McGriffin, M. F. Shanks, and R. J. Hodgson (eds) *The Scientific Principles of Psychopathology*, Grune & Stratton, London.

Holloway, F. (1988). Prescribing for the long-term mentally ill: a study of treatment practices. *British Journal of Psychiatry* (in press).

Mac Carthy, B., Benson, J., and Brewin, C. R. (1986). Task motivation and problem appraisal in long-term psychiatric patients. *Psychological Medicine*, **16**, 431–8.

Mann, S., and Cree, W. (1976). 'New' long stay psychiatric patients. A national sample survey of fifteen mental hospitals in England and Wales 1972/3, *Psychological Medicine*, **6**, 603–16.

Maslow, A. (1954). *Motivation and Personality*, Harper, New York.

Mischel, W. (1973). Towards a cognitive social learning reconceptualization of personality. *Psychological Review*, **80**, 252–28).

Moodley, P. (1987). The Fanon Project, *Bulletin of the Royal College of Psychiatrists*, **11**, 417–418.

Slater, V., Linn, M. W., and Harris, R. (1982). A satisfaction with mental health scale. *Comprehensive Psychiatry*, **23**, 68–74.

Stevens, B. C. (1973). Evaluation of rehabilitation for psychotic patients in the community, *Acta Psychiatrica Scandinavica*, **49**, 169–80.

Wing, J. K. (1972). Principles of evaluation. In J. K. Wing, and A. M. Hailey (eds) *Evaluating a Community Psychiatric Service*, Oxford University Press, London.

Wing, J. K. (1982). (ed.) Long term community care in a London borough, *Psychological Medicine Monograph, Supplement 2*, Cambridge University Press, Cambridge.

Wing, J. K. (1986). The cycle of planning and evaluation. In G. Wilkinson and H. L. Freeman (eds), *The provision of Mental Health Services in Britain: The Way Ahead*. Gaskell, London.

Wing, J. K., and Brown, G. W. (1970). *Institutionalism and Schizophrenia*, Cambridge University Press, Cambridge.

Wing, J. K., and Der, G. (1984). *Report of the Camberwell Psychiatric Register 1964–1984*, MRC Social Psychiatry Research Unit.

Wing, J. K., and Hailey, A. M. (1972). *Evaluating a Community Psychiatric Service*, Oxford University Press, London.

Wing, J. K., Wing, L., and Hailey, A. (1970). The use of case registers in evaluating and planning psychiatric services. In *Psychiatric Case Registers*. DHSS Statistical Report Series No. 8, HMSO, London.

Wolfensberger, W. (1965). Embarrassments in the diagnostic process, *Mental Retardation*, **3**, 29–31 (National Institute of Mental Retardation, Toronto).

Wolfensberger, W. (1972). *The Principle of Normalization in Human Services*, National Institute of Mental Retardation, Toronto.

Wolfensberger, W. (1975). Values in the field of mental health as they bear on policies of research and inhibit adaptive human service strategies. In J. C. Schoolar, and C. M. Gaitz (eds) *Research and the Psychiatric Patient*, Brunner/Mazel, New York.

Wolfensberger, W. (1980). Research, empiricism and the principle of normalisation. In R. Flynn, and K. Nitsch (eds) *Normalisation, Social Integration and Community Services*, University Press, Baltimore.

Wolfensberger, W. (1983). Social role valorization: a proposed new term for the principle of normalisation, *Mental Retardation*, **21**, 234–9.

Wolfensberger, W., and Glen, L. (1973). Programme analysis of service systems (PASS): a method for the quantitative analysis of human services. *Handbook of the National Institute on Mental Retardation*, Toronto.

Wolfensberger, W., and Thomas, S. (1983). *Program Analysis of Service Systems' Implementations of Normalisation Goals (PASSING). Normalization Criteria and Rating Manual*, 2nd edition, Canadian Institute of Mental Retardation.

Wykes, T. (1982). A hostel ward for 'new' long stay patients: an evaluative study of 'a ward in a house'. In J. K. Wing (ed.) *Long-term Community Care: experience in a London Borough. Psychological Medicine* Monograph, Supplement 2.

Wykes, T., Sturt, E., and Creer, C. (1982). Practices of day and residential units in relation to the social behaviour of attenders. In J. K. Wing (ed.) *Long-term Community Care: experience in a London Borough. Psychological Medicine* Monograph, Supplement 2.

Wykes, T., Sturt, E., and Creer, C. (1985). The assessment of patients' needs for community care, *Social Psychiatry*, **20**, 76–85.

Community Care in Practice
Edited by A. Lavender and F. Holloway
© 1988 John Wiley & Sons Ltd

Chapter 13

# Out of the Cuckoo's Nest:
# the Move of T2 Ward
# from Bexley Hospital to 215
# Sydenham Road

PAUL CLIFFORD

This chapter is about the move of a small rehabilitation ward from a large psychiatric hospital to an ordinary street some ten miles away. At the time of writing the move had only just taken place so it is far too early to evaluate the project's success or failure. Instead, what follows will concentrate on the process of the project's development, trying to bring out issues of relevance to others embarking upon similar ventures.

T2's development and style of work is considered in Part 1, and some issues arising during the planning of the move to Sydenham Road described in Part 2. Two recurrent themes are the importance of history to the process of change and the need to understand the relationship between institutional structures or practices and the emotional life of the institution. These are old ideas but can be easily forgotten in the drive to create new services.

The development of a community-based care for the long-term mentally ill is an enormous task. This has to do with both the organizational complexities of re-siting and delivering services and the inherent difficulties in dealing with people with severe psychological disturbance. Such basic problems may underlie local conflicts, conflicts which at the time often appear to be the sole product of personality clashes, management failure or both. Whilst local factors should not be ignored it may be important to situate them in a broader context. The final part of this chapter considers what general lessons may be learned from this highly specific study of a project's struggles with local circumstances.

## PART 1: THE HISTORY AND WORK OF T2 WARD

T2 was a long-stay ward at Bexley Hospital, a fairly typical large psychiatric hospital on the outskirts of London. The ward's patients came from Lewisham, some ten miles away. Most were middle-aged or older with a long history of hospitalization. They included some very difficult and disabled people. The ward had a successful resettlement record. Five group homes in Lewisham were established in conjunction with a housing association. Over 80 people in all were discharged in the ten years prior to the move from Bexley, all followed up and supported by the ward nursing staff. The ward succeeded in rehabilitating some of the hospital's most challenging patients. However, those with whom no progress was made were transferred to another ward for continuing care.

T2's origins can be traced back to the decision in 1972 for two female patients to be accompanied home for weekends to help prepare them for discharge. The success of this, and the sectorization of the hospital, led to the formation of a mixed ward where domestic activities were encouraged. A cooker and a fridge were purchased. A group of four women who were particularly close were prepared together and discharged to a group home. Eventually male patients were included in the resettlement programme and a selection procedure for admission introduced. The goal of rehabilitation to the community was incorporated into the ward aims and T2 became designated a 'rehabilitation ward'.

Developments were supported by the consultant psychiatrist, who represented the ward in disputes with the hospital administration and also pressed for additional resources. However, the new style of work was introduced step by step by the nursing staff, particularly the ward sister. After some years of argument she was allowed to work 9 to 5 rather than the usual nursing hourse to ensure uniformity of approach between the two shifts. A social worker and psychologist became involved. A team was formed and the ward became surer in its direction and philosophy.

The next phase began with the realization that the ward, then 30-bedded, was being more successful in managing the older long-stay patients than in dealing with the new, younger patients. There was difficulty in getting the latter group engaged in the ward's cooking, shopping and skills programmes; neither did they settle into the regular routines demanded of them by the hospital departments. It was also felt that dormitories offered inadequate personal space, and that the size of the ward mitigated against the development of a domestic atmosphere. Consequently, the ward was divided into two, T4 for the younger patients (for reasons that were never clear the hospital's administration objected to T4 either having a proper name or being called T3!), and T2 continuing to cater mostly for the older group.

In the converted ward were six cubicles where the patients slept, each cubicle with two beds. Cooking and washing facilities were on the ward and there was access to a transitional flat, also based in the hospital, called Lee House, to which patients moved for a period of six months to a year prior to leaving the hospital.

## T2 before the move – its work and culture

As had been hoped, the new, smaller T2 facilitated greater group cohesion and intimacy between staff and patients. The most immediately striking aspect of the ward as one walked onto it was its warmth and liveliness. The patients greeted you rather than ignoring you—you felt you existed in their minds, unlike many other long-stay wards. Curiosity as to the reasons for one's presence was expressed. There was an air of activity. The nurses were not in uniform, the patients were wearing respectable up-to-date clothing. People were in small groups, there were pictures and plants and cooking going on in the kitchen. Work was being done in good or bad heart—humour was encouraged and irritability tolerated.

T2's style of work was based not on an ideology or detailed set of principles, but on experience sustained by the belief in patients' potential for change. It was accepted that progress would be slow and that each person had to develop at his or her own pace. The style of work done with patients relied very heavily on staff doing things with them, showing them how to do things, instructing them, commenting on how they were doing. Often this occurred in a small group that shopped or cooked together. In addition a sense of belonging was cultivated, belonging to a ward culture that set clear norms of behaviour. The ward's expectations were repeatedly linked with those in the community. Thus although patients were not given deadlines for when they were expected to leave the ward they were constantly reminded that it was not a permanent home. Continuity was nevertheless emphasized, and it was made clear that links would be maintained.

The method of communication with patients was noticeably direct—staff said what they felt (if appropriate), e.g. saying they were angry with someone if they were, explaining to the patients why they were raising a particular issue at the morning meeting. The daily morning meetings, where staff and patients got together, were the pivotal point of the day. it was here that difficult issues, such as how to respond to a disturbed patient's behaviour, were aired. In trying to get patients to say how they feel about things a fine balance had to be kept between preventing evasion of the issue and not being over-intrusive or pressurizing. The tone of the meetings varied enormously: sometimes they dealt only with routine matters, at other times with very personal ones.

Patients had a 'key worker' who was responsible for implementing care plans and for discussing problems, progress and future plans with her or him. As well as the more formal ward reviews, the lunchtime handover meeting was used to go over programmes in detail.

An important feature of the ward culture was the lack of pretence—there was no pretence that staff were in the same position as patients, although the belief was expressed that patients had the potential to learn. Similarly, although everyone's views were listened to there it was clear that the sister was in charge of the ward—there being an acceptance of both her authority and the consultant psychiatrist's authority. Disagreement was tolerated and openly discussed, as were staff's and patients' good and bad qualities.

Compared to most wards T2 was a pressurizing environment. Pressure was of two kinds—personal pressure applied by someone working with the patient and the demands of the ward culture itself. For example, it was made clear on admission that all patients expected to take their turn in routine duties such as laying the tables. Unlike the details of individual programmes this was not negotiable.

A major question for the ward team was how much pressure it was legitimate to apply. Too much pressure on a patient could lead to a breakdown, but too little could lead to no progress at best, relapse at worst. A constant dilemma, therefore, mentioned often by the sister, was whether to allow people the freedom to act in a way that might result in a deterioration in their clinical state. A fine balance had to be maintained between clinical and ethical demands.

Related to the question of pressure was the problem of how to respond to people's 'illness'. The ward endeavoured to work with the 'healthy' part of the patient's personality but inevitably the patients' psychosis posed the largest obstacle to this. A problem for staff and patients was therefore how to respond to manifestations of 'illness' such as odd speech or behaviour. Were they to be ignored, tolerated, interpreted, modified, treated, or what? The staff's attitude contained a pragmatic mix of three elements. First, it was accepted that patients were ill in the traditional medical sense of suffering from a condition that legitimately interfered with their capacity to function normally. For example, occasional extremes of behaviour were excused on the grounds that the person was ill. Secondly, and in contrast, much everyday 'illness behaviour' was seen as a way of avoiding involvement. Thus questions were repeated if they received an unintelligible reply and efforts made to ensure that symptoms weren't used to opt out of ward activities. The third element was the attempt to understand someone's illness when a clear possible meaning presented itself. For example, a patient who left an empty bottle with its cap off overnight in the hope that the bottle will somehow be full in the morning might be asked whether she felt empty inside.

The consultant and sister were central influences on T2s development. Their roles contrasted somewhat with the democratic ethos of the multidisciplinary team approach so favoured nowadays, being stirkingly analogous to those of father and mother. The consultant was protector of the ward's interests, acquiring resources for it, defending it against attacks, maintaining order when things threatened to get out of hand. Although not physically present for much of the time he remained a very powerful figure for the patients. The sister was a constant presence on the ward, attending to the details of the patients' care, helping them towards independence. Put like this, it would be easy to criticize the ward for being old-fashioned—although this would risk begging the question of the importance of parental functions.

T2 slowly assumed its own identity and became more independent of its base institution. Not surprisingly it met with resistance from within the hospital—as exemplified by the battles over uniform and nursing hours. Patients attended hospital departments less and less, nearly all activities ultimately being conducted on the ward. Most recently, the issue of dependence was played out in terms of the catering arrangements. T2 wanted to do all its own catering. The hospital objected. The question was: could T2 cater for itself or did it need to be sustained by the institution? It was decided to postpone implementing the new arrangements. The issue would be decided with the move into the community.

## Leaving hospital

The most recent phase of the ward's development was signalled by the decision to leave the hospital. The idea owed more to practical than ideological considerations. With so many patients discharged and being followed up at great distances it seemed logical to base the service in the district of origin of the patients. This would also make it easier to admit people who needed a short period of intensive rehabilitation, would facilitate liaison with other local agencies, and allow for the possibility of 'day patients'. In short, it seemed sensible to move the district rehabilitation service to the district itself.

A building was identified in the form of a damaged ex-home for adolescents managed by the housing department. Number 215 Sydenham Road is a large Victorian house in a pleasant residential area. It is situated on a main road next door to a church, opposite a pub, and close to local shops. Preliminary enquiries suggested that the housing department was quite happy for the health authority to repair and use the building. That was the easy bit. Nearly three years later the ward has just left its institutional base.

Unlike many community care initiatives the Sydenham Road project thus emerged from institutional surroundings. Although all were keen to leave, the ward's institutional past was valued, again in contrast to projects whose inspiration is an outright rejection of what has gone before. For both T2's staff and patients the move from hospital to the community was intended to be a further step in a natural progression, an attempt to transfer and build upon a well established identity in a new setting.

## PART 2: PREPARING TO MOVE

For the project to proceed further a working relationship needed to be established with the health authority administration in Lewisham and North Southwark. By chance, at the same time as T2's staff began to think of moving out of hospital, the health authority had produced a document outlining its strategy for developing community-based services for its long-stay patients. T2's request to move out of hospital therefore seemed timely, and the project was adopted as a pilot for the district's new developments despite the fact that the management structure required to implement it was not in place. The events that followed highlighted the complex interactions between political, organizational and psychological levels of functioning in the project's development.

### The steering group

A steering group was established to sort out operational and management issues relating to the transfer of staff and patients from Bexley and the transfer of control of the building from the local authority to the health authority. The terms of reference of the steering group were ill-defined, however, and for some while it appeared that anyone with an interest in the project felt entitled to come to the meetings. The only people who seemed absent were those whose consent was essential for decisions to be binding. Most notable of these absentees were the housing department respresentative whose agreement was required for legal formalities regarding the building, and the consultant psychiatrist who was needed to endorse operational policies that impinged on clinical practice. Furthermore, the group's decision-making powers within the health authority's planning structure were unclear and no effective joint planning structure existed between health and local authorities. There was thus no obvious way of either making decisions or resolving conflicts. The steering group was such in name only.

Against this background problems began to emerge regarding the control and ownership of the project. The bone of contention was the building. Years of neglect had left it badly vandalized, and it required considerable repair and conversion work which the health authority had agreed to pay for. Although not an asset that had previously been in great demand the building soon became the focus of a major dispute. The housing department refused to transfer management of the building unless the health authority agreed to certain stipulations in the operational policy, most notably that admission and discharge be determined by a special needs housing group, rather than by the consultant. This unexpected insistence on changes in the service's modus operandi as a precondition of cooperation seemed quite at odds with the housing department's hitherto peripheral involvement. Not surprisingly, the consultant would not countenance it, whilst the administration, getting rather edgy about the large sum of money it had committed, wanted a compromise, or at least a form of words which looked like one.

The dispute is open to numerous interpretations. It could be seen as primarily a battle over control; as an ideological or political conflict; as a conscious or unconscious attempt at sabotage; or simply the inevitable product of poor management. The clash between the consultant and housing department representative possibly reflected deep ideological differences between local and health authorities regarding the appropriate model and management of mental illness. From the former's perspective the consultant's refusal to compromise was seen as typical medical intransigence. However, from his point of view he was defending the project against outside threat. More subtly, the consultant also represented an element of the health authority's true position, which the administration preferred to have stated by him rather than risk a direct confrontation with the local authority. Similarly, the housing department articulated another element of the health authority's position which it preferred to have stated by the housing department rather than risk direct confrontation with the consultant: namely that it did want more say over the project than T2's team were happy with. The playing out of the dispute as a battle between the housing department and the consultant therefore left the way open for the administration to get what it wanted by appearing to play a 'mediating' role.

Although precise motivations remain obscure the dispute is probably best seen as a political battle over control. T2's staff were made painfully aware that, at the very least, *they* were no longer in command of what they felt to be their project.

The issue generated great anxiety and emotion, evident in both the intensity of activity outside the steering group and the near-paralysis of activity within it. Sometimes it seemed as if the point of the project had been lost altogether. At one particularly fraught meeting an architect who had been invited along to report on plans for converting the building mentioned in passing that once the work was completed 'you will have a good building'. This remark transformed the atmosphere of the meeting, which suddenly became more relaxed and workmanlike. The group's being reminded of the value of the project, temporarily lost touch with, helped it regain its functioning and the threat of disaster seemed to subside. The building seemed to represent the project itself—at one moment in ruins, too costly to repair, at another worth working for. In fact, it was only once work on the building began that the 'building work' required of the group began in earnest and the project was able to 'get off the ground' at all.

### The staff

The transition from hospital to community-based services requires both the re-thinking of professional roles and re-definition of the relationship between clinical and administrative tasks. This is bound to generate much anxiety in those involved, particularly in pioneering projects such as Sydenham Road. It was clear early on from the way everyone went round saying 'we must sort out the staffing' but no-one actually did anything that it was not going to be easy. In fact, it took well over a year before anyone from the receiving district discussed staffing issues with anyone from Bexley. Two related issues dominated proceedings: the extent to which the professional composition of the staff team should remain the same and the extent to which a community-based T2 should retain the same model of work.

T2, as has already been noted, had a very traditional staffing structure. The ward team intended to keep the basic pattern and employ mostly nurses in the new unit, with the consultant as head of the team, the sister as head of home, and one occupational therapist, psychologist and social worker. It was argued that the system had worked reasonably well at Bexley, so why not retain it for the moment? This was objected to on two grounds: (1) that this would lead to Sydenham Road's being too nurse dominated and (2) that it would lead to its being too 'medical' (i.e. too consultant-dominated).

On the face of it there was some substance to the objections: community-based work probably is different from hospital-based work, and nurses may not be especially qualified for it (although who is?). In addition, the move to the community gave patients a different status since they were closer to being tenants of the local authority. This latter issue was further complicated by the fact that Sydenham Road was to be neither strictly a treatment facility in the traditional medical sense, nor an ordinary residential facility.

However plausible, the ward staff (correctly) perceived these objections to be motivated by the view that T2's style of work was too 'institutional', although criticisms were not spelt out. They resented the insinuation that they were doing something wrong and felt robbed of the opportunity to defend themselves by the refusal to make criticisms explicit. Their feelings were illustrated by the incident which gave this chapter its title: the sister heard on the grapevine of a plan to appoint Lewisham/North Southwark nurses in place of some of the existing staff who had planned to transfer with the ward. The sister was furious. Joining the morning group, where the occupational therapist was doing a crossword with the patients, she interrupted quite innocently 'can anyone think of the name of the bird that pushes birds out of their nest and takes over the nest for itself—I was trying to think of it all last night and I couldn't.' One of the patients soon piped up 'cuckoo', to the sister's evident relief.

Clearly, the sister felt that there was a plot afoot to push her and her staff out of the nest and to take it over. The problem thus arises of specifying the nature of the threat experienced. Most obvious was the threat to the T2 staff's job security and an implicitly low valuation of their professional abilities. More basic, perhaps, was the feeling that the identity the ward had built was under attack and going to be taken away.

Why should either the health or local authority attack T2's identity? Leaving aside whatever justified criticisms there might be of T2, and the differing demands of hospital- and community-based work, it is worth considering more closely the terms in which the discussion was couched. The view seemed to be that staff engage in one of two ways of being. The first is called 'institutional' and is characteristically linked with the hospital, with something authoritarian, old and outmoded, with lack of ack-nowledgment of the patients as individuals and a correspondingly exces-sive encouragement of dependence. Its attitude to mental illness is called 'medical' and involves a limited understanding of patients' needs and states of mind. The T2 staff felt identified as representatives of this way of being and naturally resented it. The alternative way is linked with 'the community' and is felt to be new and progressive, more respectful of individuals' rights and needs, encouraging of independence and democra-tic, non-institutional and non-medical in orientation. The health and local authorities saw themselves as supporters of this way of being, and wished to adopt a management structure and work practices that accorded more closely with it than they perceived T2 as doing.

Spelt out as above, the position of the health and local authority seems quite reasonable. It is possible to see how T2's reluctance to accept changes to its staffing structure could be seen as institutional rigidity. However, a rather different light is cast on the situation if one considers that it is the health and local authorities, not T2, which had the history of non-involvement with the chronically mentally ill—the health authority sending its patients to Bexley and the local authority refusing requests for supported housing for those well enough to be discharged. In contrast, whatever its failings, T2 had a long history of involvement in rehabilitation and resettlement. From this perspective it is not surprising that the ward saw themselves as moving into an unwelcoming environment. The determination to maintain continuity during the move was therefore felt to be important not just as a matter of principle but in order to contain staff and patients' anxiety. On many occasions the sister emphasized that things would 'carry on as usual' following the move. She felt this was important to prevent 'healthy anxiety' becoming 'panic'.

Although in the event all ward staff who wanted to transfer to Sydenham Road were appointed, the issue highlighted differing conceptions of the project: whilst the district was getting excited about something that represented a break from the past, the ward was primarily concerned with minimizing discontinuity. It is questionable whether the terms in which the arguments were couched correctly identified the issues at stake; and interesting that the language used put T2 on the defensive despite being both the initiators of the project and the group with the best record of previous involvement.

## The patients

'Community care' is supposed to be partly about moving patients from unhealthy institutional environments to healthier, more normal community settings. It is thus essential to consider the patients' experience of such a move. The literature on quality of life and care (as summarized by Lavender, 1985) pays particular attention to whether the client is treated in a more caring, respectful manner once out of hospital and to the provision or otherwise of material necessities. This emphasis can neglect the significance of people's experience of mental illness in their relationships with the hospital, its staff and residents. It might be expected that a change in setting would highlight these issues, which in the daily run of things may be hard to uncover because they provide the unarticulated background to life in hospital. Their importance is illustrated by a discussion that took place several months before the move.

The patients were shown a videotape about the Italian experience of closing mental hospitals as a lead in to discussing the move. Much disagreement was expressed at the idea of closing mental hospitals. One patient felt that they (the T2 patients) shouldn't be in hospital but in Sydenham because they weren't 'mental'. On the other hand hospitals were necessary for people who were, like S— downstairs, who was 'dirty', didn't wear 'nice clothes' and 'loses her mind'. Someone else agreed that they should be in a hostel like Sydenham Road, but felt they should have access to the hospital if they needed it. The same patient felt that he personally shouldn't be in hospital but in prison because all he did was take things that didn't belong to him. Another patient felt that there should be places like hospitals for people to come into when they couldn't cope, but that otherwise people should be allowed to go home (rather than go to Sydenham Road). She admitted (for the first time) that she had been having visions for years and said that she must therefore be mad, mustn't she? 'You've got a point there', someone replied. Someone else said 'we are perfectly insane. Of course we are, we can't argue about that.' Someone else said she felt trapped by the word 'mental'. Anger was expressed at attitudes to the mentally ill—'people with problems, we should be called', said one patient.

The prospect of moving from hospital raised the question of where 'madness' was to be located, both geographically and psychologically. Their basic concept of the hospital was as a place for people who are 'mad' and there was general agreement that such a place was needed. However, that raised the additional question whether they personally needed to be in such a place, i.e. were they mad or normal. One person disowned any awareness of her 'madness' and located it in the person downstairs, with the people who were moving being seen as sane; in contrast, the man who claimed they were perfectly insane disowned his sanity.

Given that the hospital was seen as somewhere for mad people, and the community as a place for normal people, it is not surprising that the patients found it hard to understand Sydenham Road. If they were being discharged from hospital did that mean that they were no longer ill? If they were still ill would that be tolerated at Sydenham Road? Why were they going to Sydenham Road? Sydenham Road was unlike hospital (which is for madness) or the community (which is for normality). Although obvious in a way this was quite difficult for the patients to grasp. Psychologically, the move was not a straightforward one into 'the community'. For all patients the meaning of the move depended in part on their relationship to their own 'madness'.

In another meeting at which the move was being discussed the problem of a place for, and tolerance of, 'madness' was raised explicitly for the whole group. A patient complained about another patient who was harassing and swearing at her offensively, and also screaming and upsetting other patients at night. The sister suggested that this might be because the patient was not well, was not being herself. It was agreed that this may be the case, but strong feelings were expressed to the effect that even so such behaviour was unacceptable and reprehensible. During this discussion the patient in question got up and sat at a table away from the group, saying nothing and seemingly not listening. The discussion moved from the gross intolerance of the patient who had raised the question—'I've got enough problems of my own without having to put up with anyone else's—to a slightly more sympathetic but nonetheless critical attitude. Then someone said that the thought the patient was quite a nice person really when you actually spoke to her. This seemed to change the atmosphere and the patient came back to the group. Almost simultaneously the patient who had initially complained got up and left. She said she wasn't going to go to Sydenham Road.

This incident vividly acted out the problem of what to do about madness. Initially it was not tolerated, and the 'mad' patient left the group. Then it was accepted but criticized. Finally, it was accepted and the sane 'nice person' part of the patient was also recognized. It is only then that she rejoined the group. Simultaneously, the complaining patient (the same one who thought hospitals were necessary for people like those downstairs), left the group saying she wouldn't go to Sydenham Road. It was hard for her to acknowledge that their 'madness' was to be transferred with them to the new setting. The group as a whole, however, was more accepting of this. The material suggests that 'Sydenham Road' came to represent somewhere where both madness and sanity could be housed. If this is so then it is possible to predict that the new setting would be subject to more intense conflicts than settings which are clearly either hospital or community, since part of its definition is that both sane and insane aspects of people have to be acknowledged simultaneously.


PART 3: DISCUSSION

The shift to community care necessitates complex organizational change as well as an innovative approach to service delivery. Any successful service development will inevitably involve both. As Sarason (1972) points out, the creation of new settings often proceeds on the belif that if the right combination of resources, motivation and shared purpose can be found then the mistakes of the past can be avoided. This both assumes that the problems of the past are easily avoided and diverts attention from characteristic processes and problems that arise in the creation of any new setting. These include establishing agreement on values, the formation of a leadership structure and the development of a working core group. In trying to draw some general lessons from Sydenham Road's attempt to negotiate these it may be helpful to distinguish three interrelated sets of difficulties: (1) problems related to the project's prehistory, (2) problems arising from the management of the planning process, and (3) problems relating to the task or goal of the project.

## The influence of history

It is important to adopt an historical stance towards planning, as failure to do this is likely to lead to repetition of precisely those patterns of behaviour it is hoped are being replaced. There are a number of ways in which 'history' plays its part. First, there are the constraints imposed by the previous experience of the individuals involved. This limits both the range of options likely to be considered and the possibilities of change from previous patterns. The steering group suffered from a lack of acknowledgment of its relative inexperience in planning community-based facilities and also of the significance of the project's origins in T2. A striking feature was the lack of 'reality orientation'—several members had never visited T2 and there was no attempt to visit other similar projects to learn from their experience.

More important perhaps than individuals' personal histories are their institutional histories. Although the large hospital tended to get landed with the negative connotations of the term, both local and health authorities are of course institutions with patterns of functioning often no less 'institutional', if under less public scrutiny. Thus, whatever their conscious intentions members of the steering group brought with them attitudes and styles of interaction that were all too familiar. For example, it was not long before problems between clinicians and managers or local and health authorities emerged, each party characteristically feeling that their point of view was not being registered by the others—evidently a phenomenon that is not easily going to be left behind in the move to the community!

At a deeper level the 'history' that is most relevant to be aware of is the history of involvement (or lack of it) with severe mental illness. There was no getting away from the project's origins in Bexley Hospital, nor the low priority that had traditionally been given to the long-stay patient group by the health and local authority. An odd process seemed to occur whereby T2 staff were implicitly held responsible for the poor state of affairs represented by large psychiatric hospitals when the truth was the reverse—the poor state of affairs (if that is what it was) was if anything a consequence of the health and local authorities history of non-involvement with the long-term mentally ill. It is arguable that in the name of 'progressive' operational policies (as against the allegedly 'institutional' practices advocated by T2's representatives) the health and local authorities were inadvertently repeating the same pattern of non-involvement except in a more modern guise.

## Managing the planning process

'Planning' is commonly thought to involve the design and implementation of a project, with all relevant parties getting together to draw up a blueprint and a timetable, resolving outstanding issues and safely guiding the project towards its practical realization. This rather cosy conception represents what one might call planning without the process. It assumes that planning can be divorced from its social and organizational context, and that a group exists with shared goals and values. Neither of these assumptions was justified in the case of 215 Sydenham Road: there was no pre-existing planning framework and the numerous agencies and professions involved had differing goals and loyalties.

A broader conception of planning is to view it as a process of accommodation between a number of complex structures. Proper management of this process of accommodation is essential and occurs most easily in the context of satsifactory inter- and intra-agency relationships. In the present case there was no history of good relationships between the main agencies involved. Exisitng relationships were therefore bound to be strained by a project which required considerable accommodation and cooperation as well as constituting a threat to established status quo.

In these circumstances the first objective should have been to establish a steering group whose relationship to the wider organizational context was sufficiently stable and well-defined to enable it to function effectively. However, this was never done, in part because the project did not fit easily into any coherent overall strategy and in part because the importance of this initial step did not seem to be fully recognized. It therefore became impossible to define satisfactorily the terms of reference or the composition of the group.

The lack of clear relationship to external structures impeded the internal workings of the group. Its areas of authority were poorly delineated. This made it hard to establish a method of making decisions or dealing with conflicts. Leadership was made difficult not for lack of 'leadership qualities'—there was if anything an excess of people who were leaders in other contexts—but because it was unclear what powers a leader would have.

The problems in the constitution of the steering group were probably a symptom as much as a cause of the antagonisms that surfaced. Ill-feeling manifested itself either in a lack of energy in the group's machinations, or in rows such as that over the building, an incident which illustrated how powerful the forces are which underlie the tortuous and seemingly emotionally flat workings of committees. One of the functions of the steering group should have been to provide a setting where destructive rivalries could be managed and contained. In the event, the group's structural weaknesses led to an increased vulnerability to dysfunction and disintegration. Because the group had such difficulty functioning as a working group much of the real bargaining went on outside it. This in turn had a demoralizing effect on those who were not party to such negotiations, and inhibited the development of a sense of shared achievement.

The steering group thus found it hard to function in a creative manner. Its functioning sometimes had as much to do with inter-professional and inter-agency power struggles as a desire to take responsibility for ensuring the project's success. There was great difficulty in synthesizing competing conceptions of the project. The dispute over the building and the operational policy is an example. Although it was recognized that a solution would have to incorporate elements of everyone's ideas ultimately, a deliberately ambiguous form of words was adopted to resolve the situation—not so much a solution as a cover-up and postponement of the difficulties. This suggested sadly that the best that could be hoped for at that time was the peaceful coexistence of different forces within the project rather than their successful integration. It survived—but only just.

## The task

Although it is tempting to blame the severity of the steering group's problems on poor organization and management it is arguable that these in turn reflect difficulties of the task itself. Disagreement regarding the nature of the task existed at several levels. Basic agreement was lacking on what was meant by 'community care', and this made it hard to resolve issues of control, membership, and ownership of the project. Open discussion of these was made harder by the confusion over whether the project was to be conceived of as an essentially new venture on the part of the health authority, local authority or both; or whether it was meant to be basically a re-location and development of an already existing service. Differences in emphasis were reflected in the problems those involved perceived themselves as having. The ward's main objective was to preserve its integrity of functioning in the new managerial and social environment. In contrast, the district's main aim was to set up a service whose management structure and operational policy were compatible with its financial, strategic and philosophical objectives.

A more fundamental question is how far the difficulties experienced by the project relate to one of the primary tasks of any psychiatric service, the management of psychological disturbance. Bott (1976) has argued that staff in the traditional mental hospital suffer from a basic contradiction in the task that they are expected to perform on behalf of society. On the one hand they are expected to manage severe disturbance because it is felt to be unmanageable elsewhere; on the other hand they are expected to pretend that this is all for the patient's own good. One of the functions of the institution is to deal with this conflict between 'caring' and 'controlling'. At ward level this can be experienced in terms of the conflict between freedom and restrictiveness. Although unavoidable, the conflict can be managed in better or worse ways. One method of dealing with it is to transport disturbance away from the immediate vicinity—the 'solution' represented by the large hospitals. However, it is only likely to be managed more constructively in the community if its existence is recognized. A particularly acute version of it is thus likely to arise if the movement out of hospitals is fuelled by anti-institutional attitudes because the demand is for staff to continue managing disturbance at the same time as eliminating the methods that hitherto enabled them to do so. This demand was felt most directly by the T2 staff, but in fact was one that was implicit in the whole group's task. However, there was little recognition of it. Instead, what seemed to happen is that each subgroup experienced the others as being uncaring and controlling. Thus the T2 staff felt that the health and local authorities weren't interested in them or the patients, but merely with getting things to accord with a certain ideal version of how things should be; whilst the T2 staff tended to get looked upon as not being concerned primarily with the individuals under their care but rather with the preservation of an allegedly 'institutional' way of being.

Bott's argument depends on the idea that the characteristic problems of institutional settings are partly a response to the institution's task. If this is so, then it would be expected that new settings created to fulfil similar tasks will encounter comparable difficulties, even if manifested in a different form. The view that moving out of hospital into the community means leaving institutions behind may have contributed to a lack of exploration of this point. This is a shame, because there is in fact a highly relevant literature, classic studies including Stanton and Schwarz's (1954) investigation of the mental hospital and Menzies' (1960) paper on social systems as a defence against anxiety. These authors, writing from a psychoanalytic perspective, interpret seemingly irrational aspects of the institution's organization, such as deindividualized care practices, as having a defensive function—shielding staff from the emotional impact of contact with severe psychological disturbance and distress. For example, the traditional division of nurses' jobs into discrete tasks helps protect them from contact with individual patients' suffering or death. The division of roles between members of a multidisciplinary team in a psychiatric hospital may sometimes have a similar function. This applies in the wider context of the institution or society, as well as at the level of clinical practice within a ward. Thus, one might say that mental hospitals perform the function of protecting society from contact with 'madness'—in which case it is not surprising that a project such as Sydenham Road caused so much organizational disruption. The most important implication of this perspective is that the problem of change cannot be bypassed by creating something new. If staff in institutions behave as they do in response to the institution's task then change will be resisted unless more constructive methods of dealing with the task evolve. Similarly, new settings are unlikely to be successful unless they build upon a recognition of the reasons for the faults of the old.

## CONCLUSION

The experience of Sydenham Road illustrates two major points, the first relating to the planning process and the second to the task of mental illness services. The literature on resettlement tends to conceive of planning in a technical, administrative sense, ignoring the dynamics of service development—despite the fashion for referring to 'change management'. Texts on community care focus on technical issues such as joint planning, management structures and funding (e.g. Audit Commission, 1986; NFHA, 1987). Although tempting to solve apparently organizational problems with organizational solutions—such as better information and planning mechanisms—analysis suggests that they may be manifestations at an organizational level of deeper problems in the nature of the services it is intended to provide. These problems have a history that is embodied in the experience and ideas the participants bring to the task *and* in the organizational structure within which planning is taking place. 'Planning' should not therefore be conceived of as a tedious administrative task, but as a process in which basic issues are negotiated, albeit often in a tortuous and barely recognizable way. An important management role, therefore, is to maintain some awareness of both the project's history and these basic issues, thereby providing a sense of reality by which discussion can be guided and goals assessed.

The second point relates to the manner in which institutions are conceived. Sydenham Road's experience illustrates how once an institution exists the problems that it was a response to often only become clearly visible again once the institutional structure is disturbed. This was evident, for example, both in the conflicts within the steering group and in the patients' response to the move. An institution may thus be conceived of as an invariant frame embodying problematic areas which only become evident when the frame is disrupted. This is similar to the concept discussed by Bleger (1966). He points out that the meaning of a behaviour can only be understood in relation to a frame, and that the frame, however silent, nevertheless has a meaning itself. It is possible that in creating community-based services the meaning of the frame has been forgotten and needs to be studied again in the process of change. We cannot assume that we know about it because we have never known what it is like to be without it.

It will also be important to study people's new frames and understand them before they too become invisible. This means extending the concept of rehabilitation to include an understanding of the dynamic processes involved. If this is not done there is the danger that (to paraphrase an ex-resident of T2) on arriving in the community 'we shan't know what to do there when we get there'.


ACKNOWLEDGMENTS

The material presented here is part of a larger study of the Sydenham Road Project funded by Lewisham and North Southwark Health Authority. Thanks to everyone involved on T2, especially Dorothy Gatula, for their help with this study. Thanks also to Jon Stokes of the Tavistock Clinic for discussions which helped clarify many of the ideas presented.


REFERENCES

Audit Commission (1986). *Making A Reality of Community Care*, HMSO, London.
Bleger, J. (1966). Psycho-analysis of the Psychoanalytic frame, *International Journal of Psychoanalysis*, **48**, 511.
Bott, E. (1976). Hospital and society, *British Journal of Medical Psychology*, **49**, 97–140.
Lavender, A. (1985). Quality of care and staff practices in long-term settings. In F. N. Watts (ed.) *New Developments in Clinical Psychology*, Wiley, Chichester.
Menzies, I. (1960). A case-study in the functioning of social systems as a defence against anxiety. *Human Relations*, **13**, 95–121.
National Federation of Housing Associations (1987). *Housing: the foundation of community care.* NFHA/MIND.
Sarason, S. (1972). *The Creation of Settings and the Future Societies*, Jossey Bass, New York.
Stanton, A., and Schwarz, M. (1954). *The Mental Hospital*, Basic Books, New York.

Community Care in Practice
Edited by A. Lavender and F. Holloway
© 1988 John Wiley & Sons Ltd

Chapter 14

# The Development of Residential Accommodation in the Community

JOHN HOWAT, PETER BATES, JOE PIDGEON and GILL SHEPPERSON

Housing for the chronically mentally ill cannot be considered in isolation from general housing policy and the operations of the benefit system any more than it can from the ability of health, social services and voluntary organizations to provide appropriate care and support. Unfortunately the current policies, preoccupations and endeavours of these agencies are disjointed, and this has prevented the emergence of an integrated view of how services should develop (Audit Commission, 1986; Social Services Committee, 1985).

Concerns about the policy of community care have been expressed from a number of viewpoints. Some perceive an underlying crisis of the welfare state in which government promotes community care in order to save money (Sedgewick, 1981; Scull, 1984). Others are concerned about the likely increased burden to be placed upon families (National Schizophrenia Fellowship, 1975). These views may be contrasted with earlier critiques of institutional care such as the liberal–individualist (Szasz, 1973), deviance theorist (Scheff, 1963), critic of professional entrepreneurialism (Scull, 1979) and existential analyst (Laing, 1967).

This is a report from the front line in an area where the closure of institutions is proceeding extremely rapidly. One of the major psychiatric hospitals will close in 1988 and the other is planned to go by the early 1990s. If this happens the large conurbation of Nottingham will be almost totally reliant on community-based residential care for the mentally ill. The only exceptions will be acute inpatient services and a small forensic unit.

Despatches sent under such circumstances inevitably lack the comprehensive vision and calm strategic insight that characterize the view from headquarters. No apology is offered for this bias and limitation, as the aim is to complement more abstract and generalized accounts. The aim is also to give a description of the current state of residential accommodation for the mentally ill in Nottingham in terms of its elements and their characteristics as a 'system'. The service will be placed within its local historical context. The chapter will describe objectives and future plans in order to highlight issues which are relevant to mental health care systems.

## MENTAL HEALTH SERVICES IN NOTTINGHAM

### The area

Nottingham health district contains a population of 610,000, and is the second largest in England. Three-quarters of this population live in the conurbation, which is relatively compact. In broad socio-demographic terms Nottingham shows no outstanding features which mark it out. The age structure of the population is typical of that of English cities of its size. More than 50 per cent of housing in the city is in public ownership. Nottingham has a significant black ethnic minority whose residence is concentrated in the remaining older housing stock in the inner residential zone.

The majority of the inner of ring nineteenth-century working-class housing around the central business district was replaced during the 1960s and 1970s. The new development at that time was mostly through expansion of more peripheral housing estates with only four large complexes of deck access and high-rise housing. As in many other industrial cities these latter have proved to be structurally and socially problematic. The City Council has already in the last decade demolished two, and have advanced plans to remove another.

The pattern of employment shows diversification between manufacturing and service sectors and there is no single, dominant industry. Major elements include garment manufacture, tobacco products, cycles and pharmaceuticals. Levels of unemployment and general economic prosperity have not fluctuated widely in the past, and lie in an intermediate position between the depressed North and West Midlands and the more affluent South-East. There has been a deterioration in employment prospects in the 1980s at close to the national average trend.

The surrounding area comprises a mixture of contiguous suburbs of the city, commuter villages, farm land and a few mining areas (most of the large Nottinghamshire coalfield lies to the north in the neighbouring health district).

## Mental health services

Acute psychiatric services have been fully sectorized since 1985. Each of the six sectors is served by a community mental health team, hospital acute ward and day hospital (in either hospital or community). The sector teams are also responsible for five long-stay wards containing 'elderly graduate' patients.

Services for the psychiatry of old age are well developed and provide comprehensive care for those over 65, except for graduates in care. There is a full range of specialist services including a recently developed forensic service which is now responsible for one long-stay ward. The rehabilitation and community care services manage all other long-term care in hospital and all such residential and day care in the community.

The area is served by two psychiatric hospitals. Mapperley Hospital is situated within the city and has served Nottingham since 1880. Mapperley is said to have been the first mental hospital in England to take the symbolic step of unlocking all its wards in 1952. Its then medical superintendent, Duncan MacMillan, was an energetic proselytizer of community care and between 1948 and 1963 the number of resident patients fell from 1300 to half that number (Howat, 1979). Mapperley now provides acute inpatient care to half of the district, specialist services, part of the psychogeriatric service and most of the long-stay beds. At the end of 1987 there were 350 beds.

Saxondale Hospital is the former county asylum. It opened in 1902 and lies 9 miles from the centre of the city, to the east. This places it away from its main catchment area. In addition to Nottingham it has, until recently, served the other two health districts within the county. Admissions ceased in 1986 and apart from over 100 long-stay patients from Central Notts Health Authority there remain only part of the psychogeriatric service and 40 long-stay graduate inpatients. The hospital will close in late 1988.

There is in addition a district general hospital (DGH) psychiatric unit within the major teaching hospital, Queens Medical Centre. It contains 80 acute beds and a psychogeriatric assessment unit. The psychiatric beds opened in stages between 1983 and 1986. They serve the remaining half of the district and are supported by an acute day hospital.

## Social services

Until recently the only specific provision for mental health within the district managed by social services was a psychiatric day centre on its fringe. This deals with a wide range of mental health problems and has both short- and long-term clients. There is also a hospital-based social work department which is well integrated with the NHS services.

Between 1984 and 1987 mental health social work teams were established in each of the acute sectors. These social workers form part of the community mental health team together with occupational therapists, nurses, psychologists and psychiatrists. Referrals are taken to the team which shares a common base. The actual style of practice, rate of development and degree of engagement with primary care and other community resources varies from sector to sector.

### The voluntary sector

The contributions made by voluntary organizations to direct care provision are described later in the text. There are local MIND and National Schizophrenia Fellowship groups which campaign actively, and voluntary organizations are becoming more actively involved in the planning of services.

A significant development since 1985 has been the setting up of a Patients' Councils Support Group based on the model established in the Netherlands. At present patients' councils are based mainly in hospital where they help residents to express their views on 'non-clinical' aspects of care (Barker and Peck, 1987). A further step in the movement towards greater service user participation and empowerment is the newly formed Nottingham Advocacy Group with plans for both patient and citizen advocacy schemes similar to those operating in the mental handicap field.

### Strategic planning

There is no strong local tradition of collaborative planning between agencies. There are few problems created by non-coterminosity of administrative boundaries, but the size of the district and reorganization have inhibited key officer relations (Glennerster, 1983).

The increasing non-viability of Saxondale and the decision to close it at an early date very much 'emerged' during the 1980s. This has been a mixed blessing. Much planning has been closure-driven rather than innovative, community-centred and needs-based. Nonetheless consultation over closure plans has raised the profile of forgotten services with the public and local authorities. The imminent availability of institutional funding has also helped to confirm alternative schemes, but not as much as might have been expected (Webb and Wistow, 1986).

The current strategic plan envisages the closure of Mapperley Hospital by 1994. Acute and specialist services will move to a second DGH unit with all other care provided in the community. Implementation should be improved by the use of a computer model to align staffing, funding and patient need through the stages of transition. Longer-term services will be replaced first as a policy desideratum. There will also be much greater emphasis on training, evaluation and user participation.

## DEVELOPING RESIDENTIAL CARE

Nottingham Rehabilitation and Community Care Services (RCCS) are in practice the long-term division of the NHS mental illness unit. RCCS does, however, include a closely integrated social work team and aspires to an interdisciplinary approach to practice and management. The service has a central role in planning and coordination all NHS long-term care. It also provides all long-term residential and day care in the community and almost all hospital-based services.

Although notable and well-documented instances stretch back over more than two decades (Clark, 1981; Bennett, 1978), widespread accept-ance of rehabilitation as a specialism in psychiatry is recent (Wing and Morris, 1981). In some areas the rehabilitation service is ancillary in the sense that it provides specific inputs such as occupational and industrial therapy to the general mental illness services. Elsewhere the service undertakes integrated care but is hospital-based only, sometimes with responsibility for all long-stay patients. A few rehabilitation services have sought to be more comprehensive and have encompassed residential care in hospital and community together with day care and community after-care. This last model is increasingly being accepted as the most appropriate for new patterns of care (Royal College of Psychiatrists, 1986).

The Nottingham service was established at the beginning of 1982 through a reorganization of staff and services at Mapperley Hospital. This was united with the service at Saxondale in 1984. Development has been through the re-utilization of capital and revenue as older institutional services have closed, with only one relatively small injection of funding through joint finance.

### The 1982 position

On initial establishment the service possessed a range of resources entirely based within the psychiatric hospital and an outline remit conceived in terms of a traditional view of rehabilitation. This concentrated upon assessment, training, resettlement and supportive aftercare. An initial evaluation of prospects by the new team led to the following general conclusions which have dictated strategy since then.

1. Residential and day care units should be dispersed and reduced in size. They should relate appropriately to each other, to generic services and to the broader community.
2. More day care was required and more people were capable of living in normal accommodation provided adequate training and support were provided.
3. The setting up of a community team was a priority. This would help to link dispersed units, support clients living more independently and provide a much-needed counterpoint to the institutional perspective.
4. There were no models from British practice of a comprehensive community service and a flexible response would be necessary. One consequence of this was an acceptance that services might move to accommodation which had a relatively short useful lifespan. Disposability would be a virtue in an era of rapid change.
5. Services for the chronically mentally ill could not be divorced from general psychiatry but nevertheless demanded an adequate overview of need, and in some crucial areas much greater integration for effective delivery.
6. Users of services suffered from lack of realistic choice and effective power. Support would be given to all attempts to redress this balance but occasions would arise at a time of rapid change when this priority could find little expression. To a lesser extent the same would be true for staff members.

## The climate of change

The first five years of the service might have been a period of steady planning, development and monitoring of the changes which seemed desirable. However, the inevitably early closure of Saxondale, following its destabilization by the removal of acute services, dictated events and imposed a timetable upon them. In the absence of adequate pump-priming funding, a great deal of expedient planning has been necessary. This has freed capital and revenue expenditure which has provided an infrastructure for community care.

At the same time NHS reorganization led to changes in district boundaries, management structures and key personnel. This considerably hindered development of a strategy and the establishment of cooperation at a critical level with other agencies. Staff of the service were committed to community care and did not retreat into a defensive position. Much of the change which has occurred has been of the 'do-it-yourself' type with an associated involvement of staff in service design and property procurement. Nevertheless, because of the instability there has been a concentration on bricks and mortar at the expense of the development of flexible and innovative schemes. In particular, little has been done to improve the marginalized status of users of the service.

## THE NEW RESIDENTIAL SERVICES

These are described below as they exist in late 1987, together with a brief indication of the management agency, current functions and, for recent developments, the hospital service which they have replaced (if any).

### MacMillan Close (RCCS)

This unit, which opened in May 1987, replaced two 20-bed hospital rehabilitation wards. It provides 28 residential places and 20 day places. Most referrals come from the acute psychiatric services either from admission wards or direct from the community. The principal functions are assessment and active rehabilitation with a usual maximum stay of nine months.

MacMillan Close consists of twelve modified modern townhouses on a main road next to Mapperley Hospital but more closely adjacent to similar private housing. Residents have inpatient status and the unit is staffed by nurses and occupational therapists. It can be regarded as a 'hospital–hostel' and in many ways the design is a compromise. Its main advantages are opportunistic—cheapness, speed of construction and adaptability together with a great improvement in physical living circumstances and some normalization. The main drawback is one of scale. Overall this mixed model of care has the advantage in a transitional period of being able to cope with referrals at an early stage where capability or risk are uncertain.

### Transitional hostel (RCCS)

The unit opened in May 1987 and has been much afflicted by developmental vicissitudes of funding, planning permission and property finding. The title is provisional and the unit is in temporary accommodation in a satellite building at Mapperley. It replaced services at Saxondale Hospital, but is not a resettlement project. It is a staffed NHS hostel with eight places and is aimed at younger otherwise potentially new long-stay patients whose needs were less well met by the previous alternatives of 'revolving door' readmission to acute wards and structured rehabilitation activities. It will move to ordinary housing early in 1988.

### Broomhill House (RCCS)

This is a twelve-place NHS hostel with less intensive staffing, which opened in May 1987. The initial use is for resettlement of long-stay inpatients from Saxondale. The twelve residents were the most handicapped in the Saxondale Unit and chose to go as a group. If, however, continued residence at Saxondale had been an option most would have chosen to stay there. Staff and residents worked together for two years in hospital in preparation. This period is probably too long and real benefits became evident only after the move.

The building is a large house in a suburban area. After six months of operation all residents are functioning more independently, using normal community services, and prefer their new living circumstances. Initial local resistance at the stage of pursuit of planning permission has changed to an unproblematic acceptance with an increasing degree of integration. Although this development is typical of those which have been criticized as 'mini-institutional' this staff group has been the most active in using principles of normalization and the residents positively welcoming (their choice) to short-term relief care 'guests'.

### Hughendon Lodge (Anchor Housing Association and RCCS)

A joint venture which provides twelve single-bedroom places in a newly built unit, it is registered as a residential home for the mentally disordered. The housing association is responsible for construction, management and staffing, which is by a manager and care assistants. Further support of appropriate type and intensity is provided by the community rehabilitation team. Assessment is a joint responsibility. RCCS have placement priority and guarantee to meet the costs due to vacant places. There are no other revenue costs to the NHS who provided the site with the costs of construction being met by a repayment mortgage.

Hughendon Lodge opened in May 1987. It primarily provides a service to older residents with moderate dependency needs. The initial group came both from hospital and less suitable community placements. An important long-term role is expected to be as part of a range of provision for those ageing in care.

Anchor are primarily a housing association providing for the elderly and this was their first development of its type. There has been a high degree of cooperation on policy, staff appointment and support. Satisfaction expressed by residents is high, the regime tolerant and the physical quality of the accommodation excellent. The single rooms offer privacy and relative independence for a residential home. For example, postal deliveries are direct to each resident's letterbox.

## Family placement scheme (RCCS)

This scheme began formally in 1984 but built upon three years' experience of similar informal arrangements. It is principally administered by the rehabilitation social work team with support from other psychiatric social workers and other members of the community rehabilitation team. The aim was to provide a framework which would link informal and substitute carers in the community with the recovering mentally ill, who might benefit from living as part of a family, sharing all household facilities.

All carers in the original informal scheme were staff of Mapperley Hospital. The scheme was created by staff in long-stay areas who felt that a number of patients were ready to move on, but unsuitable for the limited range of existing options in the community. The accommodation offered was in the form of supervised lodgings, often with supplementary day care. The philosophy was mixed, with its stress on family living and normalization as ideals contrasting with the exclusive use of professionally experienced carers.

Unquestionably many of those placed benefited from the move from the institutional setting to a more relaxed family atmosphere. However, there were no formal arrangements for assessment or monitoring of progress, nor criteria agreed for placement or displacement. There were no guidelines for standards of desirable or adequate care and the dual status of the carers as staff of the hospital and members of the foster family made the normalization of relationships problematic. In particular, the notion of rehabilitation as a continuing process was an alien one for these early placements as the stability of the scheme depended on residents' needs and activities remaining unchanged (to allow the carers to continue in their original jobs).

The formal scheme attempted to draw upon the strengths of what already existed using a model derived from children's fostering schemes. Monthly support meetings were established, in the course of which a strong core identity of the carers group emerged. At the same time changes in the levels of DHSS remuneration brought a steady stream of inquiries from potential carers wishing to offer accommodation to the recovered mentally ill. This increase in interest was certainly due in part to publicity given to local psychiatric hospital closures.

These prospective carers were encouraged to attend the support group, which almost all did. This was valuable as the strong group identity of the existing carers and their desire to maintain good practice had a direct counselling effect, unmediated by professional staff. For families proceeding beyond this point the next step is assessment by two staff of the scheme. There are now guidelines for good practice based upon *Home Life* (DHSS, 1983), references are taken up and arrangements for monitoring standards and progress established.

Even with these safeguards there remain a number of problems, especially with long-term placement. It is difficult for any family to make a commitment to the indefinitely prolonged care of any individual (not least one without blood ties). This implies a need for monitoring, support and the availability of alternative accommodation in the event of displacement. When complementary day care is also provided it diminishes the burden on the family and broadens the range of rehabilitative opportunity for the resident.

Despite public advertisement and considerable effort from the team, the current number of placements is only 21; not much greater than in the original informal scheme. The more rigorous procedures must have played a part in restricting its growth. If less regard had been paid to the risk of abuse of those placed and the families involved, and if the potentially available rate of benefit had been fully exploited, the number could have been very much larger. It is particularly noteworthy that any entrepreneurial manipulation which increases the payment to the family decreases the disposable income available to those placed.

Nevertheless the scheme has valuable qualities. Its existence discourages unmonitored alternative arrangements and provides a benchmark of good practice. The scheme is an addition to a hitherto limited range of options for sheltered accommodation. Increasingly it is being used for short-term placement either as a form of respite care or as a stepping stone towards more independent living.

**Group homes (voluntary organizations)**

In 1982 there were ten group homes in the district. These were managed by Guidepost Trust and MIND, and their establishment was largely due to the enthusiasm of individual staff members in the two psychiatric hospitals. The extent to which assessment and preparation was carried out varied considerably, and there was no systematic arrangement for professional support or liaison.

The residents resembled those described in studies of group homes (Pritlove, 1985), as most were middle-aged and had come from long-stay inpatient care. The homes provided permanent rather than transitional accommodation, and residents were full tenants. Volunteer support groups were responsible for rent collection, repairs, social support and seeking professional help in crisis.

One of the first tasks of the rehabilitation service was to review the functioning of the existing homes together with the sponsoring voluntary organizations. At the same time the potential for development of further group homes was evaluated. As a result, assessment and training were increased with particular emphasis on relationships within the group to supplement existing programmes which focused mainly on domestic competence. As a first step a pair of semi-detached houses was obtained on the perimeter of the Mapperley site, opening on to the main road. One was used as a domestic training area and the other as an unstaffed pre-discharge halfway house.

A CPN and social worker from the community rehabilitation team (CRT) were nominated for each group home to act as key workers for the residents. They also attend all meetings of the volunteer care group for that home. A group home forum was established, consisting of members of the CRT and representatives of the voluntary organizations for discussion of broader issues of policy, problems and development. Two further group homes were opened. The twelve homes house approximately 36 residents at any time. As the system evolved, and a clearer impression was gained, it emerged that many of the group homes were functioning poorly as social units in a number of ways. In some cases one resident was acting either as the dominant leader or linchpin carer for the group. In others a chronically disturbed member was a source of anxiety to co-residents, or the group had little or no social contact outside the home. Volunteers often found it difficult to confront such issues because of their close identification with the project, lack of knowledge of appropriate alternatives and, most frequently, lack of confidence that professional support would be available if a crisis ensued.

Some residents did move on to other accommodation and at times of crisis the new collective responsibility of the rehabilitation services seemed to be helpful, as community staff were able to arrange short-term intensive support, including residential care or day care, at short notice and on a flexible basis. The movement was both to higher and lower levels of independence.

Group homes have been an important and relatively common alternative to long-term psychiatric hospital care. They offered one model of a relatively normal set of circumstances for living compared with such hospitals and did so at low cost, with company and independence (Capstick, 1973). However, the service in Nottingham is now looking towards the provision of shared accommodation in a more flexible way. This demands good relationships with providers of housing and a willingness to offer a service which is orientated away from the identification of earmarked residential resources with fixed, attached inputs of care and support.

Existing group homes have changed functions as their residents' needs have emerged. One is now a fairly independent congregation of bedsits and two others, by way of contrast, are staffed part-time by a worker paid by the voluntary organization to bolster current residents' endeavours. Filling vacancies in group homes has proved to be a serious problem, but this can be reduced if there are well-developed arrangements for community placement and a lively network of communication among current and potential residents.

## St Stephen's Lodge (MIND)

A ten-place hostel for longer-term residents established as a replacement for a previous venture which had experienced difficulties in achieving its aim to be a halfway house.

## Hospital care

At the end of 1987 the residual complement of long-stay hospital beds consists of 65 at Mapperley occupied by 'younger' patients. Following a recent reorganization, 45 form part of RCCS with the remainder joining the forensic service as a longer-term 'disturbed' provision. There are, in addition, 90 further beds at Mapperley and 40 at Saxondale whose occupants are almost all over 70 years of age.

## Other voluntary sector

A number of projects which cater primarily for the homeless and probation services clientele make useful contributions which increase the quantity of provision and range of choice of hostels and sheltered housing.

## The Private Sector

The rapid decline in the inpatient population of Mapperley between 1948 and 1963 (Howat, 1979) was not accompanied by any systematic or even sporadic new provision in the community other than the 'hospital-supervised lodging scheme'. This scheme, which metamorphosed into the large current private residential homes sector, was responsible for the absorption of most long-stay patients discharged during the latter phase of this period (Howat and Kontny, 1982).

There has never been any direct local authority residential provision for the mentally ill in Nottingham and the contribution of the voluntary sector has rarely exceeded ten places. Furthermore there is little evidence that the psychiatrically disabled were gaining access, whether privileged or otherwise, into alternative sheltered accommodation except for the range of hostel and allied accommodation schemes primarily aimed at the needs of offenders and the homeless. Until recently the choice available to the chronically mentally ill has been restricted to various forms of institutional living, or 'independent' life at home, with or without families, with the latter bearing a considerable burden (Brown et al., 1966).

The most unusual feature of accommodation/care in the community in Nottingham is the large private sector. This presents an opportunity to examine the inherent problems in such residential care for the chronically mentally ill. Twelve such homes provide 150 places for the mentally ill. Most were originally established in the 1960s as 'hospital-supervised lodgings' under the sponsorship of Mapperley Hospital. Proprietors were initially guaranteed day care, holiday relief readmission of residents to hospital and a same-day crisis intervention service from social workers or CPNs. Most of these establishements were former lodging houses: they were concentrated near the city centre and were large, with over 20 residents in some cases. Almost all residents shared bedrooms (up to five per room) and there was little privacy.

In 1977 the DHSS resgulations set them apart from the usual board-and-lodgings providers and most applied for registration. In fact such homes were eligible for registration under the National Assistance Act, 1948, but until 1977 there were no advantages for proprietors in doing so and none in fact were so registered. By 1978 most of the homes were registered by the local authority, which also made loans to cover work necessary to meet fire regulations and paid a weekly care allowance for each resident. In return proprietors agreed to continue to offer accommodation to the mentally ill for a period of ten years.

One explanation for these arrangements might be the local authority's embarrassment over its own lack of residential provision, and pressure from the health authority which might have wished to divest itself of responsibility for its original creation. In addition, by 1978 many residents and proprietors were ageing and the prospect of closure and readmission on a large scale was looming ominously, especially since contemporary DHSS levels of payment did not make residential homes the attractive business proposition they were later to become. In 1982 there was an acceleration in the locally set levels of payment which continued until 1985 when central limits were imposed for each client group. During this period the weekly rate doubled to £130 per resident. In the meantime the 1984 Registered Homes Act consolidated previous legislation and was accompanied by a code of practice which was endorsed by the Secretary of State (DHSS, 1983).

The code of practice formed the basis for local guidelines and the Social Services Department went further by appointing a homes adviser specifically for homes for the mentally disordered. A liaison group was set up consisting of the adviser and members of the community rehabilitation team (CRT). The majority of residential homes residents are clients of the rehabilitation service, with 50 per cent receiving day care from this source and a further 15 per cent elsewhere. This is in effect a large subsidization of the private sector by statutory agencies.

A social worker and CPN from the CRT act as key workers for each home. The rehabilitation service is also a major provider of more intensive residential care for crisis readmission and reassessment. In return it has proved possible to negotiate criteria for placement and aftercare, and in some cases key workers have been able to influence management regimes in the homes. In addition the homes advisory service has agreed steady reductions in bed numbers towards an immediate target of a maximum of two per room and the ultimate objective of single rooms for all residents who wish them.

These homes are becoming an increasingly unattractive proposition to the newer long-term mentally ill who have experienced more active rehabilitation. This is in part because of their size, overcrowding and restrictive regimes. Another important consideration is that the DHSS personal allowance for residents is only £9 weekly and most prefer independent accommodation or the range of alternative provision which is slowly emerging. Also, those younger people with higher levels of long-term dependency need more intensive care than residential homes can provide.

A decline in new placements will leave an ageing and increasingly handicapped population of residents. Unlike their contemporaries in long-stay beds in psychiatric hospitals, whose needs have been placed on planning agendas by run-down and closure policies, they are largely forgotten. At present Supplementary Benefit payments contribute almost £1 million per annum to the costs of these residential homes in Nottingham. As the Audit Commission (1986) observe in their comments on the

'Perverse effects of social security policies', this leads to 'placing an undue emphasis on residential care, where other services may be more suitable for the client and cost less'.

## COMPLEMENTARY SERVICES

### Day care

In 1982 RCCS took over a 40-place day centre and a 100 place day unit for industrial therapy at Mapperley. These were the remaining elements of more than 300 hospital-based day care places created in the 1960s to support former long-stay patients discharged to 'hospital-supervised lodgings' and elsewhere. Their style was supportive and insular with little turnover and no links with the outside community.

In September 1987 a new day centre opened in the community. Early in 1988 the Mapperley day centre will follow and the industrial therapy unit will be converted into a dispersed skills and practical activities network (SPAN) with a new emphasis on the development of transfer skills and the use of satellite premises. Preparatory pilot exercises have included the successful development of a workers' cooperative jointly with social services' psychiatric day centre. In addition a consortium approach to day care has been agreed on principle with social services and there are plans to open another jointly managed day service before the Saxondale closure in late 1988. The network of day care has been further expanded since 1985 through four voluntary sector drop-in centres supported by joint finance and other more occasional and ad hoc enterprises. The emerging model is incerasingly one of resource centres and day services with two-way traffic in the use of buildings. Already the local MP holds constituency surgeries in the new day centre.

### Community rehabilitation team

At present this consists of twenty staff including CPNs, social workers, occupational therapists, clinical psychologists and psychiatrists. Seven new posts were funded through joint finance and the remainder relocated in the run-down of institutional care. The team provides the links between the elements of the dispersed service. Among the team's functions are:

1. The provision of specialist professional services to residential and day care units of the rehabilitation and community care services.

2. A major part in the assessment of new referrals.
3. Aftercare and support to those living independently.
4. Specialist support to non-statutory residential facilities, e.g. group homes and registered homes.
5. Liaison with general psychiatric teams, generic services and other relevant agencies such as those working with the homeless.
6. Service development.

Within the multidisciplinary team a keyworker is assigned to each client and takes responsibility for coordinating overall rehabilitation and care, seeking services from other professionals within and outside the team. Team members have been instrumental in the setting up of a homelessness and mental health group. They provide an advisory and liaison service to the facilities for the homeless and have conducted a survey of mental health problems among their clientele.

## FUTURE DEVELOPMENTS

### Ordinary housing

Recent developments in providing sheltered accommodation in the form of hostels and greater support by peripatetic staff to those living 'independently' have increased the range of appropriate provision. They have also highlighted the existence of a large number of people with long-term but changing disability whose needs are best serviced through the use of normal housing with flexible support.

Two dispersed intensively supported housing (DISH) schemes will be established by 1989. The first of these will provide support to 25 people currently living in the community with families, in group homes or alone. The second, which will be more intensive, will replace 25 of the remaining long-stay beds. New housing will be required, and this will be provided by a consortium of four housing associations in addition to, but dispersed among, their general provision. Support for each scheme will come from a community support team. The project will be managed by a group consisting of representatives from the NHS, housing associations, social services and, for the first time, users. Once again, most funding will come from direct savings made from closure. Subsequently the plan envisages 20 more long-stay beds being replaced by a community provision, the form of which is yet to be decided. The final 20 long-stay beds for those with behavioural disturbance will remain in hospital.

## The elderly

By the end of 1988 three schemes will be in place for the settlement of the remaining 40 elderly long-stay patients in Saxondale. These are a sheltered ordinary housing project, a second hostel similar to Hughendon Lodge and a local community hospital which will also provide long-stay psychogeriatric beds. During the period of run down and closure of Mapperley more such developments will take place to meet the needs of the remaining 90 elderly long-stay patients there.

## Special needs

A small (six-place) project using cluster flats and support has been agreed with the community mental handicap team and a housing association. It will cater for young people who become entrenched in one service or the other but who have difficulties (usually behavioural) requiring help from both.

Planning is at an early stage for a support network for those with multiple disabilities as a result of acquired brain damage. Discussions are taking place involving the many statutory agencies with responsibility and concerned voluntary organizations.

## CONCLUSIONS

1. Ordinary housing with flexible support should form the basis of sheltered accommodation for the chronically mentally ill in the community (Bayliss, 1987). Its development has been critically inhibited by the difficulties faced by all public housing agencies, the tendency for managers to prefer 'packaged' schemes and the continual changes and uncertainties in the operation of the benefit system.
2. The rapid closure of hospitals presents service planners with a dilemma. The developments that best meet the needs of existing institutional residents are frequently not those suited to the next generation. Properties should be regarded as disposable.
3. Much greater attention must be paid to staff training for community care.
4. More thought and effort should be given to the evaluation of new services and the development of information systems that prevent people 'falling through the net'.
5. The contribution of the voluntary sector in Nottingham has added to the

range and quality of provision. This has not been true of the private sector. These circumstances are unlikely to alter unless there is politically inspired major structural change. It is argued that the case for the latter is weak when there is much evidence of innovation, decentralization and empowerment of the user/consumer by existing statutory and voluntary agencies. For these services any market is, in any case, an internal one.

6. Real choice for the service user depends upon an adequate and available range of services, access to information and increased participation in decision-making within. Conflict with the providers of care is not inevitable in this process. Realizing this aim will be difficult, but if the move to community care is to be justified there is no alternative.

## REFERENCES

Audit Commission (1986). *Making a Reality of Community Care*, HMSO, London.

Barker, I. and Peck, E. (1987). *Power in Strange Places: user involvement in mental health services*, GPMH, London.

Bayliss, E. (1987). *Housing: the foundation of community care*, NFHA/MIND, London.

Bennett, D. (1978). Community psychiatry, *British Journal of Psychiatry*, **132**, 209–20.

Brown, G. W., Bone, M., Dalison, B., and Wing, J. K. (1966). *Schizophrenia and Social Care*, Oxford University Press, London.

Capstick, N. (1973). Group homes: rehabilitation of the long-stay patient in the community', *Proceedings of the Royal Society of Medicine*, **66**, 1229.

Clark, D. H. (1981). *Social Therapy in Psychiatry*, Churchill Livingstone, Edinburgh.

COHSE (1983). *The Future of Psychiatric Services*, Centurion Press, London.

DHSS (1983). *Home Life—A Code of Practice for Residentail Care*, Centre for Policy on Ageing, London.

Glennerster, H. (1983). *Planning for Priority Groups*, Martin Robertson, Oxford.

Howat, J. G. M. (1979). 'Nottingham and the hospital plan: a follow-up study of long-stay in-patients', *British Journal of Psychiatry*, **135**, 42–51.

Howat, J. G. M., and Kontny, E. L. (1982). The outcome for discharged Nottingham long-stay in-patients, *British Journal of Psychiatry*, **141**, 590–4.

Jones, K. (1982). Scull's dilemma, *British Journal of Psychiatry*, **141**, 221–6.

Laing, R. D. (1967). *The Politics of Experience*, Penguin, Harmondsworth.

National Schizophrenia Fellowship (1975). *Schizophrenia—The Family Burden*, NSF, Surbiton.

Pritlove, J. (1985). *Group Homes—an Inside Story*, Joint Unit for Social Services Research, Sheffield.

Royal College of Psychiatrists (1986). *Psychiatric Rehabilitation Updated*, Royal College of Psychiatrists, London.

Scheff, T. (1963). The role of the mentally ill and the dynamics of mental disorder: a research framework, *Sociometry*, **26**, 436–53.

Scull, A. T. (1979). *Museums of Madness*, Allen Lane, London.

Scull, A. T. (1984). *Decarceration*, 2nd edition, Polity Press, Oxford.

Sedgewick, P. (1982). *Psychopolitics*, Pluto Press, London.

Social Services Committee (1985). *Second Report (Session 1984–5): on community care with special respect to adult mentally ill and mentally handicapped people*, HMSO, London.
Szasz, T. (1973). *The Manufacture of Madness*, Paladin, London.
Webb, A., and Wistow, G. (1986). *Planning, Need and Scarcity*, Allen & Unwin, London.
Wing, J. K., and Morris, B. (1982). *Handbook of Psychiatric Rehabilitation Practice*, Oxford University Press, Oxford.

*Section E*

# *Conclusion*

Community Care in Practice
Edited by A. Lavender and F. Holloway
© 1988 John Wiley & Sons Ltd

Chapter 15

# Conclusion

## FRANK HOLLOWAY and ANTHONY LAVENDER

This book has reviewed the development of community-based alternatives to the mental hospital from a number of perspectives. It has attempted to provide a range of informed opinion on the key issues in the field. No single viewpoint has been identified as reflecting the whole truth of a complex area of policy and practice. Often the debate on community care is reduced to a series of ideological statements that confuse opinion with evidence. This is a familiar phenomenon: trends in social policy tend to be dictated by opinion-makers, particularly those who can convey their ideas in clear and colourful language (Jones and Fowles, 1984). Empirical evidence takes longer to have its impact.

The recent accelerated development of community care in Britain has coincided with a period of severe constraint on the finances of both the National Health Service and local government. The latter has historically been seen as the appropriate lead agency in the provision of community care through social service and housing departments. However, the record of cooperation between the health service and local authorities is poor (Audit Commission, 1986). The mentally ill have not been seen as a priority by local authorities, and the health service remains the key provider to this group. The prospects for a major shift in responsibility away from the NHS remain remote, without a concerted effort from central government.

Both in Britain and the United States the development of community care has involved an increasing use of social security benefits as a source of funding. Benefits tend to offer a perverse incentive towards the provision of residential care, rather than the development of a flexible package of help that involves a range of community support and ordinary housing (Audit Commission, 1986). In America, which is farther down the deinstitutionalization road than Britain, major industries have developed that provide nursing homes for the elderly and 'board and care homes' for younger people (Jones et al., 1983). Facilities serve very mixed groups of

297

people who cannot cope in society, for a profit. Nursing homes can undoubtedly provide a cheap alternative to the mental hospital, but at the cost of poorer quality of care and worse clinical outcome (Linn *et al.*, 1985).

The growth of the private residential sector in Britain, which has until recently tended to serve elderly people with predominantly physical disabilities, is a matter of major concern. Private care is notoriously difficult to regulate, and although the entrepreneurial spirit fosters innovation and a degree of flexibility, private providers must inevitably be concerned to maximize their profit. Residents who present difficulties that cost money or disturb the running of the institution will understandably be moved on to the residual public sector, which will retain a responsibility to take all patients referred to it. Conversely, by its very nature, the private sector is unlikely to engage in rehabilitation and resettlement of people who do not require long-term care. The lack of adequate assessment before placement in private residential care (over and above ability to pay) is also striking (Royal College of Psychiatrists, 1987).

Community care may also be linked to another form of privatization: the shift in the burden of caring from the state to the family and the local community. Historically institutional care for the mentally ill developed as a response to perceived failures in both the private madhouses and informal care by the community. The cycle may repeat itself unless the evolving services that replace the traditional psychiatric hospital pay adequate attention to the role of the family and the immediate social environment in the support of the continuing care client.

Although there are no blueprints available for the ideal alternative to the mental hospital, some other principles governing service development can be stated with confidence. It is particularly important in a climate of stable or diminishing real resources that activities are prioritized. One priority must be those people suffering from chronic and severe disabilities. Failure to meet their needs, so spectacularly apparent on the streets of American cities, will not only produce enormous unnecessary suffering, but may call into question the entire community care movement.

Good quality community-oriented services do exist. They are pro-active: that is, they actively seek out those known to be in need, rather than awaiting the recurrent crisis of hospital admission. They offer a broad therapeutic approach to the problems of clients and their families, with much effort devoted to helping those in contact with the service integrate into the community. Compared with the traditional mental hospital, care is much less medically based (which is not to deny the role of, for example, drug treatment in the management of the symptoms of mental illness). This broad therapeutic approach requires a range of skilled and well-trained staff working in a coordinated way that enables them to support each other and provide the user with a high-quality service. In this context the treatment and care provided should be in the form of an individualized programme that is the result of a careful assessment carried out in close consultation with the user/client/patient.

One area that has not been adequately explored is the role of the general medical practitioner and the primary health care team in the care of the chronically mentally ill (Jones *et al.*, 1983). Certainly the GP will now be faced with providing physical and possibly psychiatric care to patients formerly managed within the mental hospital. The manner in which the care provided by GPs is to be integrated into the new community-based services needs careful thought. The solutions are likely to be specific to each locality, but close liaison between primary care and the continuing care services is clearly essential. Although principles of geographical responsibility for service provision, continuity of care and specialist teams focused on the needs of those experiencing chronic disability are rightly emphasized, there is an equal and possible contradictory need to ensure that service users can exercise a degree of choice. Traditionally GPs have been the jealous guardians of choice in referral to specialist services, and this facility should somehow be retained in the brave new world of catchment area psychiatry.

Community-based care presents numerous challenges to service planners and providers. The ability of non-hospital alternatives to the psychiatric hospital to provide acceptable care for people who are persistently dangerous to themselves or to others, or whose behaviour is highly socially unacceptable, is unclear. Experience from hospital hostels in Britain and community-oriented psychiatric services in America suggests that a small minority of patients will require long-term care in well-staffed units on a hospital site (Goldberg *et al.*, 1985; Gudeman and Shore, 1984). The alternative to adequate provision for this client group is likely to be prolonged stay on an acute psychiatric ward, or discharge from the mental health system to homelessness or prison.

Working in a new style of service will require staff to adopt new roles and develop new skills. It is vital that adequate attention is paid to the training needs of staff who will work in the community-orientated service. Without adequate, and continuous, trianing there is no reason to believe that the quality of care outside the traditional institution will be any better than that within it. Training must be a priority within services undergoing transition.

Appropriate training, adequate and sensitive supervision and attention to the design of the jobs that staff are asked to carry out will all have a preventative effect against the development of 'burn-out' amongst staff (Lamb, 1982; Currie, 1986). Staff within the large institutions frequently show signs of burn-out, lacking enthusiasm, feeling bored, frustrated and resentful of their patients or clients and no longer enjoying their working lives. Such feelings may develop rapidly amongst staff who are pitched ill-prepared into the new community services.

There are important lessons to be learnt about the management of the new services, and the management of the painful transition from the old to the new (Towell and MacAusland, 1984), if the bad practices of the past are to be understood and avoided (Menzies, 1960). Analysis of the situations where the care in mental illness and mental handicap hospitals broke down into scandal has revealed a number of factors that make the occurrence of unacceptable practice more likely (Martin, 1984). These include not only lack of resources but isolation of the staff group, failure of professional supervision and an indifferent management concerned only with the smooth running of the institution. Dispersed community services will prove more difficult, and more costly, to manage than the centralized psychiatric hospital. It is vital that these services, particularly the residential and day care components, remain open to external influence and scrutiny. Closed systems are much more likely to develop poor-quality care. Elderly and dependent people without interested relatives are particularly vulnerable to abuse.

The abuses of the past have provided a powerful moral incentive for change. One major manifestation of change has been a growing interest in ensuring that the rights of patients are respected. Professionals have long seen their role as being an advocate for their patients' needs. However, radical critics of the mental health system would argue that such advocacy is inevitably self-seeking. Alternatives include the statutory oversight of patients' welfare (as partially embodied in the Mental Health Act Commission), advocacy from alternative professional or quasi-professional groups (such as lawyers or workers for voluntary agencies), the facilitation of non-professional befriending relationships and the empowering of patients to speak for themselves about their needs (Sang and O'Brien, 1984; Brown, 1981). No one approach is entirely satisfactory, but the realization that services must be more clearly responsive to the needs and desires of the users is entirely healthy and deserves reinforcement.

Given the constraints that currently attend the development of community care, and the well-articulated doubts about the wisdom of this policy, are there any grounds for optimism? There is good evidence that community-based alternatives for the mental hospital can provide very satisfactory care (Braun et al., 1981; Tessler and Goldman, 1982). Moreover, the decline of many large psychiatric hospitals now appears to be terminal. These hospitals continue to consume a very significant proportion of the resources available to the mentally ill, whilst appearing increasingly irrelevant to the needs of the populations they once served. The old pattern of care, wherein an isolated institution received the marginal in society and retained many in poverty and near degradation, has broken down.

The failure to collect adequate data on the process of deinstitutionalization in the United States was a major lost opportunity (Braun *et al.*, 1981). It is important that those attempting to develop high-quality community-based services for the continuing care client document their activities and remain open to external evaluation and review. In the absence of evidence about the success of new services we are in danger of 'romanticizing' the old institutions, or uncritically accepting that successor services are better. We must learn what kind of facilities work well for particular client groups, and be prepared to publicize the mistakes that will undoubtedly be made.

The task of improving the quality of care to a historically deprived and marginalized group is a daunting one. The contributors to this book, who come from a variety of professional backgrounds and hold a variety of ideological positions, are united in the belief that better services can be provided. The inevitable decline of an outmoded system of care offers an opportunity that must not be lost.

# REFERENCES

Audit Commission (1986). *Making a Reality of Community Care*, HMSO, London.

Braun, P., Kochansky, G., Shapiro, R., Greenberg, S., Gudeman, J. E., Johnson, S., and Shore, M. F. (1981). Overview: deinstitutionalization of psychiatric patients, a critical review of outcome studies, *American Journal of Psychiatry*, **138**, 756–59.

Brown, P. (1981). The mental patients' rights movement and mental health institutional change, *International Journal of Health Services*, **11**, 523–540.

Goldberg, D. B., Bridges, K., Cooper, W., Hyde, C., Sterling, C., and Wyatt, R. (1985). Douglas House: a new type of hostel ward for chronic psychiatric patients, *British Journal of Psychiatry*, **147**, 385–8.

Gudeman, J. E., and Shore, M. F. (1984). Beyond deinstitutionalization: a new class of facilities for the mentally ill, *New England Journal of Medicine*, **311**, 832–6.

Jones, K., and Fowles, A. J. (1984). *Ideas on Institutions*, Routledge & Kegan Paul, London.

Jones, L. R., Badger, L. W., Knopke, H. J., and Coggins, D. R. (1983). The emerging role of the primary care physician in the care of the chronically mentally ill, *Journal of Public Health Policy*, **4**, 467–83.

Linn, M. W., Gurrel, L., Williford, W. O., Overall, J., Gurland, B., Laughlin, P., and Barchiesi, A. (1985). Nursing home care as an alternative to psychiatric hospitalization, *Archives of General Psychiatry*, **42**, 544–51.

Martin, J. P. (1984). *Hospitals in Trouble*, Blackwell, Oxford.

Menzies, I. (1960. A case study in the functioning of social systems as a defence against anxiety, *Human Relations*, **13**, 95–121.

Royal College of Psychiatrists (1987). Private care for the elderly mentally ill, *Bulletin of the Royal College of Psychiatrists*, **11**, 278–82.

Sang, R., and O'Brien, J. (1984). *Advocacy; the U.K. and American Experience*, King's Fund Project Paper, 51, King's Fund Centre, London.

Tessler, R. C., and Goldman, H. H. (eds) (1982). *The Chronically Mentally Ill. Assessing Community Support Programmes*, Ballinger, Cambridge, MA.

Towell, D., and McAusland, T. (1984). Managing psychiatric services in transition, *Health and Social Services Journal*, 25. October.

# Appendix

THE GRIFFITHS REVIEW

The Secretary of State at the DHSS requested Sir Roy Griffiths 'to review the way funds are used to support community care policy and to advise on the options that would improve the use of these funds as a contribution to more effective community care' (DHSS, 1988). The Report's analysis of the failure to implement community care policies closely follows that of the Audit Commission (1986). Sweeping recommendations are made, including the creation of a ministerial post within the DHSS with responsibility for community care, the designation of social service departments as the priority agency for implementing community care and the consequent constriction of health authorities role to the provision of 'medically required' services.

Griffiths proposes that local authorities should be responsible for assessing local needs for community care, and as far as possible act entrepreneurially as care managers rather than providers of direct services to ensure these needs are met. (The private sector is seen as playing a key role.) A significant transfer of resources is envisaged from health authority and social security budgets to social services departments. Local authorities would take over the joint finance programme. Provision would be subject to means testing, with a long term emphasis on encouraging individuals to meet their own needs so that 'public resources are concentrated on those in greater need.'

These proposals are highly controversial. They require, for their successful implementation, a mass of legislation and a managerial revolution within social services departments, which would have to develop skills in epidemiology, service planning and management budgeting which they currently lack. The muted initial response from Government suggests that the implications of Griffiths are being very carefully weighed. It is likely to be some years before its impact (or lack of impact) is fully apparent. Chapter 5 assumes that the existing (1988) structure of services remains.

# Appendix

# Index

This book is to be ret    ied on or before
the last date s    d below.